NEUROBIOLOGY OF AMINO ACIDS, PEPTIDES AND TROPHIC FACTORS

TOPICS IN THE NEUROSCIENCES
Neuronal Control of Bodily Function: Basic and Clinical Aspects

Other books in the series, Neuronal Control of Bodily Function: Basic and Clinical Aspects

Ferrendelli, James A., Collins, Robert C., Johnson, Eugene M., Neurobiology of Amino Acids, Peptides and Trophic Factors.

NEUROBIOLOGY OF AMINO ACIDS, PEPTIDES, AND TROPHIC FACTORS

Edited by

JAMES A. FERRENDELLI
Washington University School of Medicine

ROBERT C. COLLINS
Washington University School of Medicine

EUGENE M. JOHNSON
Washington University School of Medicine

KLUWER ACADEMIC PUBLISHERS
BOSTON/DORDRECHT/LONDON

Distributors

for the United States and Canada: Kluwer Academic Publishers, 101 Philip Drive, Assinippi Park, Norwell, MA, 02061, USA

for the UK and Ireland: Kluwer Academic Publishers, Falcon House, Queen Square, Lancaster LA1 1RN, UK

for all other countries: Kluwer Academic Publishers, Distribution Centre, P.O. Box 322, 3300 AH Dordrecht, The Netherlands

Library of Congress Cataloging in Publication Data

Library of Congress Cataloging-in-Publication Data

Neurobiology of amino acids, peptides, and trophic factors / edited by
James A. Ferrendelli, Robert C. Collins, Eugene M. Johnson.
— (Topics in neurosciences)
"Proceedings of the third in a series of annual international
symposia" — Pref.
Meeting held Nov. 4–7, 1986 in St. Louis, Mo., co-sponsored by the
Research and Development Division of G.D. Searle & Co. and
Washington University; dedicated to Thomas Leo O'Donohue.
Includes index.
ISBN 0-89838-360-9
1. Neuroendocrinology — Congresses. 2. Amino acids — Physiological
effect — Congresses. 3. Neuropeptides — Physiological effect —
Congresses. 4. Neural transmission — Congresses. I. Ferrendelli,
James A., 1936– . II. Collins, Robert C. III. Johnson, Eugene
M., Ph. D. IV. O'Donohue, Thomas Leo, 1954–1987. V. G.D. Searle &
Co. Research and Development Division. VI. Washington University
(Saint Louis, Mo.) VII. Series.
[DNLM: 1. Amino Acids — physiology — congresses. 2. Neural
Pathways — congresses. 3. Neural Transmission — congresses.
4. Neuropeptides — physiology — congresses. 5. Neurophysiology —
congresses. WL 102 N49452 1986]
QP356.4.N475 1988
612'.814 — dc19
DNLM/DLC
for Library of Congress 87-34796
CIP

Copyright

Kluwer Academic Publishers, 101 Philip Drive, Assinippi Park, Norwell, MA 02061, USA

PRINTED IN THE UNITED STATES

CONTENTS

II. TROPHIC FACTORS

III. NEUROPEPTIDES

IV. SHORT COMMUNICATIONS

AUTHOR LISTING

LOCAL ORGANIZING COMMITTEE

J.A. Ferrendelli, Chairman
Seay Professor of Clinical Neuropharmacology
Washington University School of Medicine

R.C. Collins
Professor of Neurology
Washington University School of Medicine

E.M. Johnson
Professor of Pharmacology
Washington University School of Medicine

EXTERNAL ADVISORY COMMITTEE

M.H. Aprison
Indiana University School of Medicine
Indianapolis, Indiana

D.L. Felton
University of Rochester School of Medicine
Rochester, New York

R.C. Frederickson
G.D. Searle & Co.
Skokie, Illinois

D.H. Hellhammer
University of Munster and Max Planck Institute
Munster, Federal Republic of Germany

H.C. Hendrie
Indiana University School of Medicine
Indianapolis, Indiana

J.N. Hingtgen
Indiana University School of Medicine
Indianapolis, Indiana

R.C. Murison
University of Bergen
Bergen, Norway

H. Weiner
UCLA School of Medicine
Los Angeles, California

LIST OF PARTICIPANTS

Lloyd R. Allard
Department of Pharmacology
St. Louis University School of Medicine
St. Louis, Missouri 63110

Morris H. Aprison
Distinguished Professor of Neurobiology and Biochemistry
Indiana University School of Medicine
Indianapolis, Indiana 46223

M.D. Ard
Department of Anatomy and Neurobiology
Washington University School of Medicine
St. Louis, Missouri 63110

M. Flint Beal
Department of Neurology
Massachusetts General Hospital and Harvard Medical School
Boston, Massachusetts 02114

Margery C. Beinfeld
Department of Pharmacology
St. Louis University School of Medicine
St. Louis, Missouri 63110

C. Becker-Carus
Psychologisches Institut II
Universitaet Muenster
Muenster, Federal Republic of Germany

Floyd E. Bloom
Division of Preclinical Neurology and Endocrinology
Scripps Clinic and Research Foundation
La Jolla, California 92037

Richard Bunge
Department of Anatomy and Neurobiology
Washington University School of Medicine
St. Louis, Missouri 63110

Kenneth M. Carnes
Department of Anatomy and Neurobiology
Washington University School of Medicine
St. Louis, Missouri 63110

Robert C. Collins
Professor of Neurology
Washington University School of Medicine
St. Louis, Missouri 63110

R.P. Compton
Searle Research and Development
Division of G.D. Searle & Co.
St. Louis, Missouri 63198

Patricia C. Contreras
Searle Research and Development
Division of G.D. Searle & Co.
St. Louis, Missouri 63198

Erminio Costa
Fidia-Georgetown Institute for the Neurosciences
Georgetown University
Washington, D.C. 20007

Carl W. Cotman
Department of Psychobiology
University of California, Irvine
Irvine, California 92717

Debora A. DiMaggio
Department of Pharmacology
St. Louis University
St. Louis, Missouri 63104

J.A. DiMicco
Department of Pharmacology
Indiana University School of Medicine
Indianapolis, Indiana 46223

C.F. Eldridge
Department of Anatomy and Neurobiology
Washington University School of Medicine
St. Louis, Missouri 63110

Wayne Engleman
Searle Research and Development
Division of G.D. Searle & Co.
St. Louis, Missouri 63198

E. Fadda
Fidia-Georgetown Institute for the Neurosciences
Georgetown University
Washington, D.C. 20007

James A. Ferrendelli
Seay Professorr of Clinical Neuropharmacology
Washington University School of Medicine
St. Louis, Missouri 63110

Ian D. Forsythe
Laboratory of Developmental Neurobiology
National Institutes of Health
Bethesda, Maryland 20892

R.C. Frederickson
Searle Research and Development
Division of G.D. Searle & Co.
Skokie, Illinois 60077

Terry A. Fuller
Department of Psychiatry
Washington University School of Medicine
St. Louis, Missouri 63110

Nancy M. Gray
Searle Research and Development
Division of G.D. Searle & Co.
St. Louis, Missouri 63198

I. Gutberlet
University of Munster and Max Planck Institute
Munster, Federal Republic of Germany

Song Ping Han
Department of Pharmacology
St. Louis University School of Medicine
St. Louis, Missouri 63104

Gail Handelmann
Searle Research and Development
Division of G.D. Searle & Co.
St. Louis, Missouri 63198

R.D. Harken
Searle Research and Development
Division of G.D. Searle & Co.
St. Louis, Missouri 63198

Franz Hefti
Department of Neurology
University of Miami School of Medicine
Miami, Florida 33101

Dirk H. Hellhammer
Klin. Psychologie, Universitaet Trier
Trier, Federal Republic of Germany

H.C. Hendrie
Chairman and A.E. Sterne Professor of Psychiatry
Indiana University School of Medicine
Indianapolis, Indiana 46223

Joseph N. Hingtgen
Professor of Psychology and Neurobiology
Indiana University School of Medicine
Indianapolis, Indiana 46223

W.F. Hood
Searle Research and Development
Division of G.D. Searle & Co.
Chesterfield, Missouri 63198

Eugene M. Johnson
Professor of Pharmacology
Washington University School of Medicine
St. Louis, Missouri 63110

C. Kirschbaum
Psychologisches Institut II
Universitaet Muenster
Muenster, Federal Republic of Germany

N. Kleitman
Department of Anatomy and Neurobiology
Washington University School of Medicine
St. Louis, Missouri, 63110

A.P. Kozikowski
Fidia-Georgetown Institute for the Neurosciences
Georgetown University
Washington, D.C. 20007

P.A. Kreiter
Searle Research and Development
Division of G.D. Searle & Co.
St. Louis, Missouri 63198

Thomas H. Lanthorn
Searle Research and Development
Division of G.D. Searle & Co.
St. Louis, Missouri 63198

Pamela T. Manning
Department of Pharmacology
Washington University School of Medicine
St. Louis, Missouri 63110

Joseph B. Martin
Chief of Neurology
Massachusetts General Hospital
Harvard Medical School
Boston, Massachusetts 02114

Mark L. Mayer
Laboratory of Developmental Neurobiology
National Institutes of Health
Bethesda, Maryland 20892

Brian S. Meldrum
Institute of Psychiatry
DeCrespigny Park
London, England

J. Michel
Searle Research and Development
Division of G.D. Searle & Co.
St. Louis, Missouri 63198

Joseph B. Monahan
Searle Research and Development
Division of G.D. Searle & Co.
St. Louis Missouri 63198

F. Nicoletti
Fidia-Georgetown Institute for the Neurosciences
Georgetown University
Washington, D.C. 20007

Thomas L. O'Donohue (Deceased)
Searle Research and Development
Division of G.D. Searle & Co.
St. Louis, Missouri 63198

John W. Olney
Department of Psychiatry
Washington University School of Medicine
St. Louis, Missouri 63110

Ronald W. Oppenheim
Department of Anatomy
Bowman Gray School of Medicine
Winston-Salem, North Carolina 27103

Joseph L. Price
Department of Anatomy and Neurobiology
Washington University School of Medicine
St. Louis, Missouri 63110

Linda M. Pullan
Searle Research and Development
Division of G.D. Searle & Co.
St. Louis, Missouri 63198

Randy K. Rader
Searle Research and Development
Division of G.D. Searle & Co.
St. Louis, Missouri 63198

Steve Rapp
Searle Research and Development
Division of G.D. Searle & Co.
St. Louis, Missouri 63198

J.P. Ray
Department of Anatomy and Neurobiology
Washington University School of Medicine
St. Louis, Missouri 63110

Dikla Roufa
Searle Research and Development
Division of G.D. Searle & Co.
St. Louis, Missouri 63198

F.T. Russchen
Department of Anatomy and Neurobiology
Washington University School of Medicine
St. Louis, Missouri 63110

Clifford B. Saper
Department of Pharmacology
University of Chicago
Chicago, Illinois 60637

Anantha Shekhar
Department of Pharmacology and Toxicology
Indiana University School of Medicine
Indianapolis, Indiana 46223

R.G. Smith
Searle Research and Development
Division of G.D. Searle & Co.
St. Louis, Missouri 63198

David G. Standaert
Department of Pharmacology
Washington University School of Medicine
St. Louis, Missouri 63110

Judith M. Stone
Department of Pharmacology
St. Louis University School of Medicine
St. Louis, Missouri 63110

C. J. Strasburger
Klinik f. Innere Medizin
Med. Universitaet
Luebeck, Federal Republic of Germany

Frank C. Tortella
Neuropharmacology Branch
Walter Reed Army Institute of Research
Washington, D.C. 20307

Herbert Weiner
Department of Psychiatry
UCLA School of Medicine
Los Angeles, California 90024

Gary L. Westbrook
Laboratory of Developmental Neurobiology
National Institutes of Health
Bethesda, Maryland 20892

Christine Wilcox
Department of Pharmacology
Washington University School of Medicine
St. Louis, Missouri 63110

W.G. Wood
Klinik f. Innere Medizin
Med. Universitaet
Luebeck, Federal Republic of Germany

J.T. Wroblewski
Fidia-Georgetown Institute for the Neurosciences
Georgetown University
Washington, D.C. 20007

Qiao Yan
Department of Pharmacology
Washington University School of Medicine
St. Louis, Missouri 63110

PREFACE

This volume represents the proceedings of the third in a series of annual international symposia. The first, The Neuroregulation of Autonomic, Endocrine, and Immune Systems, was held in Indianapolis in the fall of 1985. The second, Psychological and Biological Approaches to the Understanding of Human Disease, was held in Bielefeld, Germany in the fall of 1986. The theme of this series concerns the communication between the central nervous system and the other major systems of the body, and the purpose is to monitor the frontiers of research into these neuronal/hormonal regulatory interactions and their application to medicine. The present volume deals with the role of peptides and amino acids in these information transfer processes. Great strides have been made in exploring the important role of amino acids and peptides in neuroregulation, and the ongoing biotechnology revolution promises significant scientific and medical advances throughout the next decade and beyond. The work described in this volume captures the great excitement and promise of this biomedical renaissance. This meeting was cosponsored by Searle/Monsanto and Washington University and held in St. Louis in the early fall of 1986.

A major contributor to these proceedings was Dr. Thomas O'Donohue whose chapter deals with his work in characterizing the endogenous ligands for the PCP and sigma opioid receptors. Tom's personality and career personified the dedication of this series to the principle of a broad multidisciplinary approach to scientific problems. Tom died accidentally on the evening of April 14, 1987. This volume is dedicated to his memory.

Tom O'Donohue had scientific maturity and leadership qualities remarkable for one his age and was building an outstanding career with a very bright future. He gained the respect and love of all he met and was establishing a growing network of friends and collaborators throughout the world. Tom left NIH and joined Searle/Monsanto as Director of CNS Research in the spring in 1986. His contributions to this new and exciting program were inspiring and growing daily. A tragic accident, however, denied Tom the chance of reaching his full potential. On April 22, 1987 those who knew and loved Tom gathered in Bethesda, Maryland, for a memorial service for this very special man. A number of close friends and coworkers shared their memories of Tom, and their words are reproduced on the following pages.

Robert C.A. Frederickson
Summer, 1987

ACKNOWLEDGMENTS

The editors and organizers wish to thank Searle Research and Development, G.D. Searle & Co. for their generosity in sponsoring this meeting. We wish also to thank the authors for the high quality of their contributions, which, above all else, made this a successful and important event.

It is also a pleasure to acknowledge with gratitude the invaluable assistance with organizational details provided by Drs. H. Hendrie and J. Hingten and Mrs. Shirley Newhouse.

Finally, we must express our gratitude to Mrs. Teddy Norris for her excellent job of preparing this material for submission to the publisher.

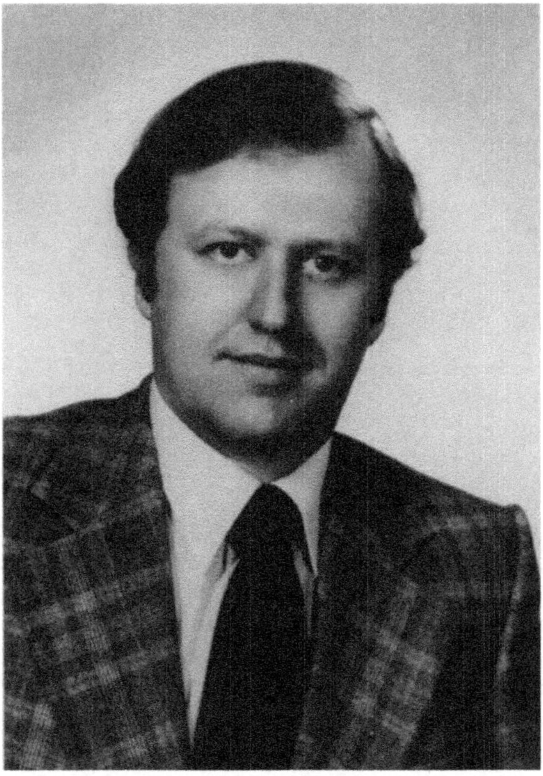

Thomas Leo O'Donohue
January 10, 1954–April 14, 1987

Dedication
THOMAS LEO O'DONOHUE
January 10, 1954–April 14, 1987

Memorial Services
Cedar Lane Unitarian Church
Bethesda, Maryland

Kenneth Torquil MacLean, Minister:

Let us be honest with death
Let us not pretend that it is less than it is:
It is separation;
It is sorrow;
It is grief.
But let us neither pretend that death is more than it is.
It is not annihilation;
As long as memory endures, his influence will be felt.
It is not an end to love;
The love we have known remains part of our lives.
It is not an end to joy and laughter;
Nothing would less honor a brave soul than to make our lives drab in counterfeit respect.
Let us be honest with death.

We gather this April day to affirm the gift of life, to give thanks for the life of Thomas Leo O'Donohue, to share memories of him and to express grief at his tragic and untimely death. We know we are all mortal; this death comes very hard.

Tom was born in Jersey City and grew up in New Jersey, the oldest of three sons of Thomas and Francis O'Donohue. He was the big brother to Kevin and

Terrance. He worked all his days. He had five paper routes. His parents think of him with pride and joy. They remember his laughter.

Tom played basketball in high school and loved it. He also liked to go fishing. After high school he hitchhiked to California. He might have played basketball in college in Bucknell, but by then he had discovered science, and his energy was focused on study and work. He met Gail Handelmann while he was at Bucknell and she was at Penn State, and they were inseparable almost from the beinning. They shared so much: their interest in science, their deep respect for each other's work and abilities, their determination to succeed, their great love. Tom and Gail were married in 1978.

After Bucknell, Tom came to Bethesda to work in the National Institutes of Health laboratory of Dr. David Jacobowitz. He is with us today to speak of his memories of Tom.

Remarks by Dr. Jacobowitz:

Tom came to my lab about 11 years ago and volunteered to work without pay, which I was not able to provide. He started with a small amount of savings. He made some money by giving blood at the NIH blood bank. He also worked in the evenings at a tavern as a bouncer. I just couldn't help admiring him for this. It soon became clear that Tom was no ordinary student. He was an extraordinarily hard worker and couldn't learn enough fast enough. He soon became a graduate student at Howard University Medical School, and I had the privilege to be his research adviser. Tom was very friendly with everyone in the laboratory. He collaborated in research with almost everyone and learned everything we had to offer. He believed that the way to study the brain was by a multidisciplinary approach — by looking at the brain through the microscope, by studying behavior of animals, and through biochemistry.

We began his thesis work by first studying the localization, or mapping, of a nerve chemical in the brain. We had one microscope to look through together — he looking with one eye and me looking with the other eye. We were cheek-to-cheek and how we loved it. This time period was the beginning of what we now called the neuroscience revolution, and Tom played a big part in it. Our first work at the microscope was a time of great excitement. Every slide yielded a new discovery. It was a time of magic. Tom and I were soon very close. He was no longer a student but a very close friend, in fact, my best friend. I confided in him all my problems and frustrations with the politics at NIH.

After completing his course work at Howard, Tom went on to be very productive in his thesis work on α-MSH and laid the foundation for much work that is going on today.

As a postdoctoral fellow in my lab, he identified three other peptides in the brain. He also identified an enzyme in the brain that processes endorphin **and**

much more. Five years ago he established his own unit in the Neurological Institute.

It was enjoyable for me to watch him progress in leaps and bounds. I enjoyed telling him about the new work in my lab and delighted in his enthusiasm for what was going on.

I feel very privileged to have known Tom. He was wonderful to work with and always so cheerful and pleasant.

Tom O'Donohue's accomplishments can only serve as an inspiration to all who knew and loved him. He was a natural leader who led by example and hard work and had the capacity to motivate and encourage others. His energy and enthusiasm were contagious.

In his laboratories at Monsanto and at NIH, he was the captain of his ship, and all who sailed with him knew it was nice to be aboard.

He always showed a willingness to share his talents, his enthusiasm, and his personal warmth.

He had boundless energy, coupled with a fierce sense of duty. His immense enthusiasm was easily transmitted to younger coworkers for whom he had an open heart. He found time to guide, stimulate, and encourage each member in his lab.

He left us a treasury of published works, a legacy of investigative courage, and an example of pure honesty in research.

We pray that time may ease the anguish of our bereavement and leave us only cherished memories.

Mr. MacLean:

Tom entered the graduate school of Howard University to continue his studies. Dr. Russell Miller is the Dean of the Medical School at Howard.

Remarks by Dr. Miller:

I wish to express my gratitude for the honor and privilege to have this opportunity to share my thoughts with you in this celebration of Tom O'Donohue's life and the many gifts he gave to all of us.

Tom O'Donohue was a student, a teacher, a scientist, a colleague, but most of all a friend. We first met at NIH when both of us were working in Dave Jacobowitz's laboratory. It was much later that I learned that Tom had been one of the normal volunteers at NIH, and on one occasion he had to be resuscitated after experiencing an untoward reaction to one of the experimental agents he was taking. Tom later informed me that this experience was one of the factors that convinced him it was time to go back to graduate school.

Tom enrolled in the Ph.D. program in Pharmacology in 1977 and was graduated in 1980. During these three years at Howard, I have delightful memories of our scientific and personal interactions. Also, during his graduate studies, he married a beautiful young scientist, Gail Handelmann.

During the relatively brief time that I have been involved in education, I have found that the most difficult task for students is not learning science or scientific principles or understanding them but very often students have difficulty in putting science in perspective, and the education they are receiving in the context of their life. I know that Tom did not have these difficulties, and I believe that is why he could become extremely productive very rapidly.

Tom's commitment was to more than science, however, it was to people. I recall an instance when he stayed up all night at a meeting trying to help a fellow student who was ill. He finally took his friend to a local hospital where he was diagnosed as having sickle cell crises, which had been precipitated by the high altitude in Colorado Springs. Tom went on to give his paper and present his colleague's work. "It was just something that needed to be done," he later told me.

During one of our conversations about science, Tom explained to me how he believed science was a tool to help people and that his efforts in the laboratory usually had as an end-point a better understanding into ways to improve human life. Our key phrase in examining a project or idea would be, "What's the pitch?" and in this way we tried to relate each project to some potential benefit to our society. By studying and learning the life sciences, he was enhancing his skills and ability to help others; also, as he learned about science and life, he learned about God. Scientific inquiry was an affirmation of his faith.

Sometime near the last year of graduate study, there was a process of role reversal when Tom began to teach me far more than I was teaching him, and then he began to teach other students, which continued to increase until his death. Tom held volunteer faculty appointments since 1981 in the Departments of Medicine, Pharmacology, and Genetics. He was patient and a kind man, who looked for the best qualities in everyone. He loved to teach; he derived great joy in helping and watching others develop educationally and scientifically.

Tom very much loved Howard University and especially the College of Medicine; during our last meeting he informed me that he was going to do as much as he possibly could for the medical school and the Department of Pharmacology. He would not accept the fact that his success and scientific contributions had already significantly benefited the university. My wife captured the essence of the relationship I had with Tom when she told me, "You see in Tom the best of yourself, and you want those qualities to be passed on to another generation of scientists."

Like Tom, I spent years studying medicine to better understand life. But there is no way to understand the mystery of life, to explain the unexpected, why some things happen, or words to convey one's feelings at the loss of life of a dear friend.

Although I have not gained special insights into life, I have learned to take solace in the knowledge that God is good and he takes care of his own. Tom is one of God's own.

Mr. MacLean:

To earn a Ph.D. in neuroscience in three years was a great achievement; it demonstrated exceptional abilities. Tom would deny that he was exceptional; he always said "I just worked hard." His colleagues knew that the statement was true and also that there was more to it than that. One of Tom's colleagues when he worked at the National Institutes of Health was Thomas Chase:

Remarks by Dr. Chase:

I had the privilege of knowing Tom O'Donohue as his supervisor during the period of his emerging scientific independence. Actually, at the time of our first meeting in late 1981, I hadn't properly reckoned on how far along that road to scientific maturity he figured he was: I thought I was interviewing someone to work as a staff fellow in my lab; but he started to negotiate an independent, section-sized resource in which to conduct his own research. And, of course, he got exactly that! But Tom was far more than just a good talker. He became an effective and accomplished scientist. When he left NIH in 1986, his bibliography listed more than 100 papers, 19 published during his last year here. His papers are among those most highly cited. In my view, Tom's most important contributions were to the group efforts which led to the discovery of new, central peptidergic pathways to the identification of the first mammalian cotransmitter neuron and to the isolation of a phencyclidine-like peptide from the brain and the development of an effective antagonist for this endogenous psychotomimetic.

What can we say about the ultimate impact of this research? Only time will tell. But among those placed in a position to formally evaluate his work, there was a remarkable convergence of opinion. Tom was held in exceptionally high regard. Our BSC called him "a major force, remarkably productive," and — rather aptly — "a big spark plug." In a particularly prophetic statement, the board also said that "it would be a major loss to lose such a major force."

And so it is. Tom earned the admiration and respect of his colleagues. He served on the editorial board of several journals; he was invited to organize and speak at numerous conferences; he became one of the prestigious Grass Travelling Fellows; he was selected to be a member of various NIH study sections, and — what I saw as a special source of pride — he received the Outstanding Young Scientist Award from the Maryland Academy of Sciences.

This was not all of TO'D. He was also a devoted husband, proud father, avid sportsman, and much more, as we have heard and will continue to hear. So, how did Tom manage to accomplish so much by the age of 33?

He was a clear thinker, inventive, logical, broad-based in relation to his span of information, yet well organized and clearly focused in relation to his own personal research. He was energetic, nearly irrepressible, but blessed by an inner calm and gentleness of spirit. He was a natural leader, friendly and open and direct, who attracted scientific collaborators and an ever widening circle of friends. He had an infectious zest for life, and for living it right, an unfailing sense of balance and fitness of things, but he was one who never attempted to foist his values on others.

Tom's passing came as a shock: the wrench of sudden, unexpected loss; the tragedy of early, premature death, with life in its ascendency, with extraordinary promise left unfulfilled. I'm reminded of the words of playwright Tom Stoppard who once said, "Life is a gamble, at terrible odds. If it were a bet, you wouldn't take it."

But Tom O'Donohue was not a man who shrank from the odds. Although we are now deprived of his physical presence, we will never lose sight of his spiritual legacy.

Mr. MacLean:

There were achievements and recognition as Tom's career developed — a growing list of published papers and, in 1985, the award as the Distinguished Young Scientist of Maryland for his discovery of multiple neurotransmitters in neurons in the brain. His scientific work was characterized by the same vibrant enthusiasm and generosity of spirit that one saw in the rest of his life.

Dr. Bibie Chronwall was another who knew him in the laboratory as both colleague and friend:

Remarks by Dr. Chronwall:

Tom started the unit of neuroendocrinology in the summer of 1982, and I had the great fortune to be recruited as the histologist within the first months. The pace in the lab was a combination of frenzy and euphoria. If Tom was wearing a flannel shirt and jeans with paint stains on them, then we knew it must be the weekend, or one of those funny federal holidays. You see, we worked most every day during the early years of Tom's independent endeavor. It was exciting and fun under his caring and inspiring leadership. We were encouraged to work independently in our specialities, but we never felt abandoned.

We were exploring a field of neuroscience that was soon to boom. For a while, we did "the neuropeptide of the week" and had the results, if not yesterday, at least by today. When Debbie DiMaggio's NPY antibody all of a sudden started to give immunohistochemical staining, his enthusiasm made what seemed at first an impossible task, just possibly doable, and in three days and two nights the distribution of NPY in the rat brain was mapped and another *Neuroscience* abstract was ready on the deadline.

Tom was never sick, didn't seem to need any sleep, and was very, very patient when dealing with our shortcomings. He was always there for us, be it to take down a bottle from the six-foot shelves, discuss an intricate experiment, the latest movie, or the appetizers at Le Marmiton. We grew into a close knit scientific family, working very hard, but also sampling Bethesda's many restaurants, or, on a rainy afternoon when everybody else was working, we could enjoy *Amadeus* from the best seats in the movie theater. On a lovely day like today, we would have phoned Gail to join us for lunch at Angler's Inn and a walk along the towpath to enjoy the redbuds.

Tom generously created opportunities for us to go to conferences and to make interesting contacts and to grow and succeed in our own fields, and his legacy is an enthusiastic, still functioning group. I wish to express my joy and gratitude to have been part of this first group, to have been his student, colleague, and friend all at once, and to have found such a multifaceted role model.

His laughter still rolls in our corridor, the POMC research continues in his spirit, and I often find myself asking "Hmmm, how would Tom have gone about this?"

Mr. MacLean:

It might be true to say that the most exciting events in Tom O'Donohue's life were the birth of his daughter Aiden in October 1985 and the birth of his son Ross in February of this year. He was so thrilled to be a father, and he loved those children so much — Tom was a joyous person. There were so many sources a joy in his life: his work, his dogs, his basketball, his children, his friends, and his beloved Gail.

She thought he might be the happiest person in the world, with his jokes and his warm laughter, his enjoyment of good food — the more exotic the better — his searching curiosity, and his creative imagination. He and Gail came to Cedar Lane in a searching mood and joined this congregation in 1985. They were just beginning to become involved here when they left to move to Chesterfield, Missouri, where Tom accepted a post with the Searle Pharmaceutical Company. Dr. Robert Frederickson, Senior Director of CNS Diseases Research at the Searle Company, has travelled from St. Louis to be with us today.

Remarks from Dr. Frederickson

There aren't words adequate to capture who Tom was and what he meant to those he touched. Nevertheless, all his colleagues in St. Louis and Chicago certainly experienced and felt everything that has been expressed so far this morning.

Tom presented a seminar at the Monsanto headquarters in St. Louis about two years ago. Afterward, several members of our group pulled me aside and asked how soon he would be aboard, they were anxious to work with this man. Tom did join us, not as an employee at that time, but as a consultant. We had a close collaboration on his endopsychosin project, and everyone soon recognized that Tom was a very special person. Excited by the challenge of helping to build the fledging CNS group, Tom eventually decided to join us as Director of Research in St. Louis.

I remember one day in the Spring of '86 I walked out the door of my condominium only to be unexpectedly met by Tom, Gail, Aiden, and Gail's parents. They were sightseeing and househunting, and the car had broken down. Tom and I set out to get help, but it was a weekend and everything was closed. However, we managed to find an auto store closed but with someone inside. Tom got this person's attention and convinced him to open the store. Tom went in and loaded up on cables and battery chargers — the best in the house. When we left, the storekeeper was behaving like a long lost friend and the problem had been solved.

This was typical of everything Tom did. There wasn't a problem or a barrier that Tom couldn't overcome with his creative intellect and immense charm.

In this industry, we are frequently faced with headcount restrictions and budgetary restrictions. These never hindered Tom. He would use his own network, within or outside of the company — or create a new one if necessary — and devise "convoluted schemes," as one of his students put it, to solve the problems. Therefore, almost every time I visited the St. Louis site, I would run into a new face.

Tom had very high standards. He worked very hard himself and expected a lot from his people, but he had a kind, understanding heart and was very sensitive and responsive to the needs of those around him. He was a warm person who could relate to anyone and everyone at all levels and in all situations.

A few days ago, his secretary found a young man in Tom's office perusing the books on his bookshelf. When she questioned him, he said there was no problem, he and Tom had been very close friends. A few days later we learned he was a new post doc who had joined the Monsanto group only two weeks earlier.

We all know Tom moved with ease in the highest scientific circles. A few weeks ago, he was asked to make a presentation to the Searle board, the highest of business circles. He wrote something up and gave it to me to review and comment on. But before I could, he got back to me and said to forget it, he had to rewrite it. With a broad grin and twinkle in his eye, he said someone up there had seen it and told him that it was too technical. He had to remove all those complicated words like agonist and receptor. Well, he gave that presentation, and it was a resounding success. He excited the board and they engaged him in a heated scientific discussion afterward, making suggestions that Tom accepted with good humor.

Tom'd door was always open, and he was always available regardless of his busy schedule — in fact, Tom and Gail's combined professional and family duties often meant that little Ross Hunter joined us for seminars and lab tours. Tom had a combination of gifts and qualities rarely, if ever, found in one man. His warmth and self-confidence bubbled over and rubbed off on those around him. He accomplished more in his short year with us than many do in a lifetime.

But, what I will probably remember most, is the specter of this giant of an irrepressible force coming toward me with a cheerful Irish grin on his face, and his hand outstretched, bursting forth with a buoyant, "Hi Bob, how's it going?" that dissoved all immediate stresses and worries. I believe that this simple expression of his warmth and intelligence is a personal remembrance we will all share.

When I mentioned today's service to Debbie DiMaggio, one of the students he brought to St. Louis, she got all excited and exclaimed, "Tom will be so sorry he has to miss it!" His very special force is still with us.

Mr. MacLean:

This was a man of many parts, one who crammed a great deal of living into 33 short years. Among his gifts was a superior talent for friendship. Joel Helke did not work with Tom. He knew him simply as a friend.

Unfortunately, Mr. Helke's words were not put to paper.

Mr. MacLean:

Each of us is left with images of Tom O'Donohue, the bright smile, the booming voice, the sharp mind, the dedication to science, the infectious enthusiasm, the natural way of the man. We think of him in the laboratory, bent over a microscope, or packing up the family and dogs for a walk along the towpath. These images may finally become clearer and sharper than the hurt.

Happy the man, and happy he alone,
He, who can call today his own:
He who, secure within, can say,
Tomorrow do thy worst, for I have liv'd today.
Be fair or foul, or rain or shine,
The joys I have possess'd, in spite of fate, are mine.
Not Heaven itself upon the past has power,
But what has been, has been, and I have had my hour.

I. EXCITATORY AMINO ACIDS

1. EXCITATORY AMINO ACID SYNAPSES: STUDIES OF NORMAL AND REORGANIZED PATHWAYS

CARL W. COTMAN

The acidic amino acids, L-glutamate and L-aspartate, appear to be the major excitatory transmitters in the central nervous system. Glutamate, for example, is enriched in select neurons, synthesized in nerve terminals primarily via the enzyme glutaminase, and accumulated by high-affinity uptake. Both endogenous and exogenously loaded L-glutamate exhibit Ca^{2+}-dependent release upon depolarization. Ablation of various neuronal pathways is associated with a modest decrease in glutamate levels and a greater loss of the high-affinity uptake system (for review see [1]).

The action of excitatory amino acids is mediated by at least four distinct receptors — the N-methyl-D-aspartate (NMDA), kainate (KA), quisqualate (QA), and 2-amino-4-phosphonobutyrate (AP4) receptors. NMDA receptors are involved in synaptic transmission as well as in phenomena such as long-term potentiation and learning. Kainate and/or quisqualate receptors appear to mediate most of the fast-excitatory synaptic responses at glutamate-using synapses. AP4 sites are found in the hippocampus, lateral olfactory tract, spinal cord, and retina. Hippocampal AP4 sites are most likely presynaptic.

In this contribution, the characteristics of binding sites in various brain regions are described along with their anatomical organization. In vitro autoradiography provides a new way to understand the anatomical organization of these receptor sites and to analyze their biochemical properties in discrete synaptic fields. Analyses in discrete fields allow direct comparisons between binding sites and the receptor characteristics determined by electrophysiological methods. In vitro autoradiography is also suitable for use in postmortem brain tissues obtained from patients with various neurological diseases. Re-

Ferrendelli, J.A., Collins, R.C. and Johnson, E.M. (eds), Neurobiology of Amino Acids, Peptides, and Trophic Factors.

cent data on excitatory amino acid receptors in Alzheimer's disease will be described.

1. IN VITRO AUTORADIOGRAPHIC ANALYSIS OF EXCITATORY AMINO ACID RECEPTORS

Excitatory amino acid receptors mediate synaptic transmission along many central nervous system pathways, participate in synaptic plasticity, and are involved in the genesis of various pathological conditions. The anatomical organization of the three well-described excitatory amino acid receptor classes, N-methyl-D-aspartate (NMDA), kainate, and quisqualate, has been described using quantitative autoradiographic techniques. Under the appropriate conditions, each of these receptors can be labelled by L-^{3}H-glutamate. In confirmation of these results, we have also used the selective radioligands D-^{3}H-amino-5-phosphonopentanoate, ^{3}H-kainate, and ^{3}H-AMPA and find anatomical distributions and pharmacological profiles identical to those found for L-^{3}H-glutamate binding to NMDA, kainate, and quisqualate receptors, respectively. AP4 sites have not yet been described in autoradiographic preparations.

In general, NMDA and quisqualate receptor systems are largely, but not completely, codistributed. NMDA and quisqualate receptors are found in high concentrations in the hippocampal CA1 region, cortical layers I-III, striatum, and lateral septum. Kainate binding sites are found to have a distribution complimentary to NMDA and quisqualate sites in the cerebral cortex, hippocampus, and thalamus. Kainate sites (^{3}H-kainate binding sites) predominate in the deeper cortical layers (V-VI), striatum, hippocampal stratum lucidum, anterior olfactory nuclei, and hypothalamus. The distribution of the glutamate uptake system corresponds to the distribution of the sum of the glutamate receptors [1].

2. ORGANIZATION OF NMDA BINDING SITES

NMDA-displaceable L-^{3}H-glutamate binding sites are found throughout the brain, with a predominance in the telencephalon (Figure 1-1) [2]. In cerebral cortex, NMDA sites are found in higher densities in frontal, anterior cingulate, and pyriform cortices. Lower concentrations are found in the parietal, posterior cingulate, and entorhinal cortices. There is a dense band of binding sites corresponding to layers I-III and an additional band in layer Va. Layer IV binding appears to be lowest in regions receiving specific thalamic innervation.

The hippocampus is particularly high in NMDA sites. The highest levels of binding in the entire brain are found over the stratum oriens and stratum radiatum of the CA1 field of the hippocampus. In CA3 these layers display moderately high levels, while the stratum lucidum and stratum pyramidale have distinctly low levels of binding. In the dentate gyrus, the outer molecular layer shows slightly lower levels of binding than does the inner molecular layer, while the infragranule and granule cell layers have quite low levels of binding.

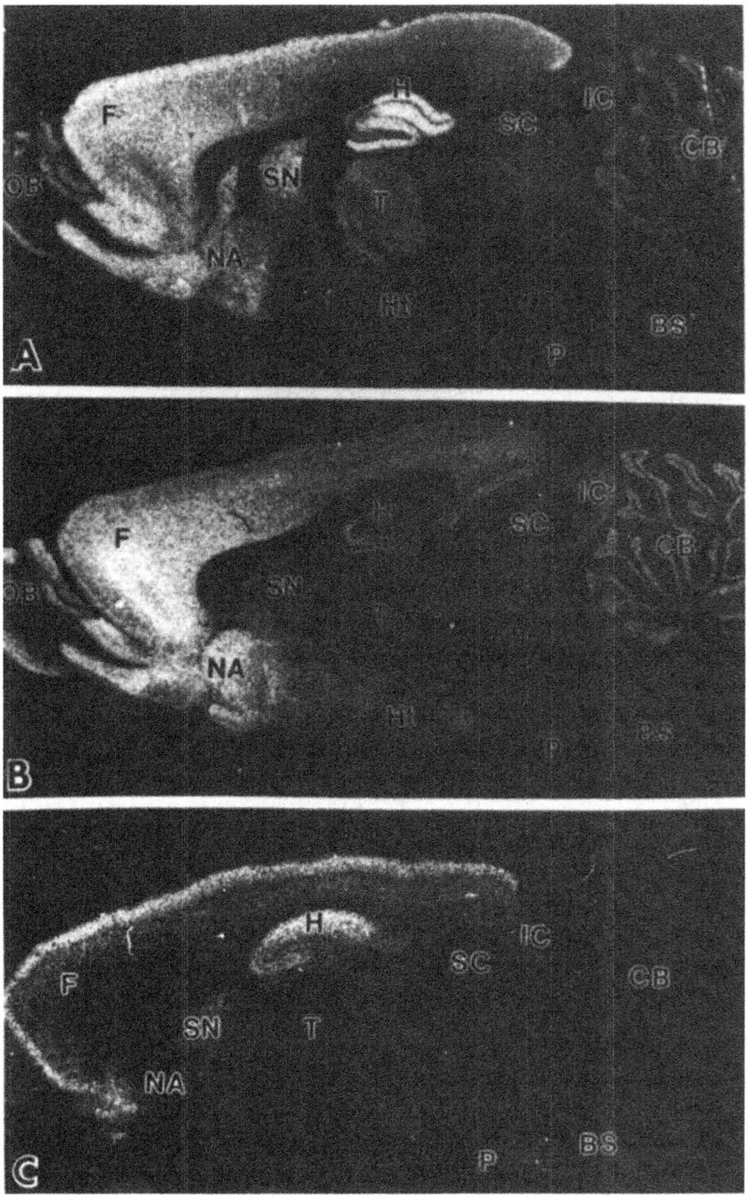

Figure 1-1. Receptor autoradiography. Sagittal sections of rodent brain displaying the distribution of various excitatory amino acid receptors. A. NMDA receptors labeled with ^{3}H-L-glutamate in the presence of KA and AMPA to displace binding to the QA and KA receptors respectively. B. Kainate receptors labeled with ^{3}H-KA. C. Quisqualate receptors labeled with ^{3}H-AMPA. OB = olfactory bulb; F = frontal cortex; NA = nucleus accumbens; SN = septal nucleus; H = hippocampus; T = thalamus; HT = hypothalamus; SC = superior colliculus; IC = inferior colliculus; CB = cerebellum; P = pontine nuclei; BS = brain stem.

Within the amygdala, there is a distinct pattern, that is also observed in the AMPA sites. Basolateral, lateral, posterior cortical, and the hippocampal-amygdaloid transitional area all exhibit higher receptor densities than do the central, medial, and anterior cortical regions. Septum shows higher levels in the lateral nucleus than in the medial component. Ventrally, the bed nucleus of the strai terminalis displays intermediate levels of binding, which were higher than the adjacent globus pallidus, ventral pallidum, and preoptic area. In the olfactory bulb, the external plexiform layer and the accessory bulb have higher concentrations than the other adjacent regions. More posteriorly, the anterior olfactory nuclei, olfactory tubercles, and the nucleus of the lateral olfactory tract show high levels of binding.

Thalamic regions, in general, have higher levels of NMDA sites than do the hypothalamic regions. Relatively low levels are found in the reticular nucleus and the zona incerta. Using D-^{3}H-AP5 as a ligand for NMDA receptors, the ventroposterior nucleus was distinctly labeled [3]. In both the lateral and medial geniculate, the dorsal subdivisions have higher levels of NMDA sites than the ventral subdivisions. Midbrain and brainstem regions display an overall low density of NMDA sites, with certain nuclei showing relatively higher levels of binding sites. These include the superficial and intermediate gray layers of the superior colliculus, dorsal medial interior colliculus, medial vestibular nucleus, cuniform nucleus, granule cell layer of the cochlear nucleus, parabrachial nucleus, nucleus of the solitary tract, central gray, the inferior olive, and the substantia gelatinosa of the spinal cord. In general, all along the floor of the fourth ventricle, medially located structures displayed moderate levels of NMDA sites, whereas ventrally located motor structures displayed no selective enrichment of binding sites. The cerebellum displayed overall low levels, with greater levels of binding in the granule cell layer than in the molecular layer. There was only a slight or no enrichment of NMDA sites found over the substantia nigra, the pontine nuclei, the red nucleus, the trigeminal nucleus, and the cerebellar molecular layer.

3. ORGANIZATION OF TCP BINDING SITES

Phencyclidine (PCP) receptors (sigma opiate-PCP sensitive) appear to be functionally coupled to NMDA receptors. NMDA-sensitive L-^{3}H-glutamate binding sites have a distribution remarkably similar to that of binding sites for the selective PCP ligand ^{3}H-TCP. However, relatively lower levels of TCP (^{3}H-1(1-(2-thienyl)-cyclohexyl)piperidine) sites are found in the cerebellar granule cell layer, while slightly higher levels are found in the ventral nuclear complex of the thalamus. Thus, it is possible that NMDA sites are not uniformly coupled to PCP receptors.

4. ORGANIZATION OF QUISQUALATE BINDING SITES

Quisqualate receptors appear to be labeled by ^{3}H-AMPA. In isolated membrane preparations [4] and autoradiographic preparations [5, 6], ^{3}H-AMPA binds to a distinct class of binding sites, which displays the same ligand specificity for quisqualate agonists as does the quisqualate receptor. As with the other two receptors, this binding site may also be labeled by L-^{3}H-glutamate [7, 8]. In general, quisqualate sites as labeled by ^{3}H-AMPA display a pattern similar to that of NMDA sites (Figure 1-1) [5].

5. ORGANIZATION OF KAINATE BINDING SITES

Kainate receptors can be selectively labeled in both autoradiographic and isolated membrane preparations by ^{3}H-KA [9–13]. In addition, L-^{3}H glutamate can also be shown to label KA sites in autoradiographic preparations [7]. As found for NMDA and AMPA binding sites, ^{3}H-KA binding sites are found predominately in the telencephalon (Figure 1-1) [11, 13]. However, within various regions, KA sites display a largely complimentary distribution to that found for the other binding sites. In neocortex, KA sites are located predominately in the superficial-most layer and in layers V and IV, with layer VI having a slightly higher density than layer V.

The hippocampus displays a very distinct pattern of KA binding sites. The highest density of KA binding sites in the rat brain corresponds to the stratum lucidum, and moderate concentrations are found in the inner portion of the dentate gyrus molecular layer. With the exception of the hilus and a portion of the stratum lacunosum-moleculare, the remainder of the hippocampus displays low levels of KA binding. Thalamic midline nuclei, reticular nucleus, zona incerta, and hypothalamus have moderate levels of binding, while the remainder of thalamus has low levels.

6. ALTERATIONS IN PLASTICITY OF EXCITATORY AMINO ACID RECEPTORS IN ALZHEIMER'S DISEASE

Are there changes in excitatory amino acid receptors in Alzheimer's disease? At one level, it is obvious that as neurons degenerate receptors will decline. It is less obvious, however, whether or not receptors are lost in the early stages of pathology or perhaps even increase in compensation for loss of nearby neurons. For example, with partial deafferentiation, receptors often are upregulated as a partial compensatory mechanism, and in some cases afferents sprout and reinnervate denervated areas. Our studies have focused on the hippocampus, where it is possible to carry out detailed studies in both rodents and man.

In Alzheimer's disease, one of the hallmark changes is the loss of neuronal populations that occurs throughout the course of the disease. In addition to a profound loss of cholinergic neurons, it has been shown recently that there is a loss of particular cortical associational neurons. Studies on brain tissues obtained postmortem from patients with Alzheimer's have demonstrated severe loss in select areas of the limbic system. Van Hoesen and colleagues reported that Alzheimer's disease is accompanied by a select loss of layer II and III stellate cells of the entorhinal cortex and pyramidal neurons of the subiculum [14]. These entorhinal neurons are the primary source of cortical input to the hippocampus. The loss of the entorhinal cortex plus the subiculum functionally isolates the hippocampus and may account for the loss of cognitive functions that are dependent on the hippocampus. Thus, any particular compensatory mechanisms that can occur to preserve and/or rebuild this vital entorhinal pathway would be extremely critical in the early course of the disease.

Research carried out over the past several years in animal models has shown that in response to the loss of entorhinal cells, the remaining undamaged neurons are capable of sprouting new connections and forming new functional synapses to replace those lost [15, 16]. This, temporarily at least, may offset the precipitous loss of neurons and could, in principle, stabilize circuitries.

Several inputs contribute to the restored circuitries (Figure 1-2). In animals in which the contralateral entorhinal cortex is spared, the small crossed entorhinal pathway sprouts and increases the innervation of this zone. This increased input is physiologically potent enough to now excite the partially-denervated granule cells [17]. Thus, the system is capable of restoring bilateral cortical input. It has been postulated that sprouting of this input is a major factor in the recovery of function that is seen following unilateral entorhinal ablation [18, 19].

Commissural/associational (C/A) afferents from CA4 neurons that innervate the inner one-third of the molecular layer also sprout in response to an entorhinal lesion. These fibers expand their terminal fields and sprout partway into the denervated zone. This expansion which can be observed by silver staining, auto-radiographic, or HRP methods occurs rapidly and completely repopulates the area of expansion [20–22]. Recently, it has been shown that the commissural/associational axons appear to use an excitatory amino acid as their neurotransmitter, and receptors for kainic acid, a glutamate analog, appear to be selectively concentrated in the inner zone [23, 24]. Corresponding to the expansion of the fiber plexus, the kainic acid binding sites also appear to increase in number in the zone where the fibers have sprouted [25]. This suggests that the appropriate receptors are available, then, to subserve synaptic transmission. These new synapses appear capable of enhancing the drive of the dentate granule cells [26]. Since these fibers form a recurrent excitatory loop, such sprouting may serve to amplify signals passing through this relay.

Based on the information described above in rodent models, it would be predicted that sprouting might occur in the brain of patients with Alzheimer's disease. However, there are several reasons why sprouting might not occur in the brain of Alzheimer's patients. It may be that the degenerative state of the brain is incapable or incompatible with regenerative growth responses. In other words, the system is in a pure state of catabolism such that anabolic reactions are unsuccessful. The system degrades more rapidly than it can possibly be rebuilt. The other major unknown is whether or not the gradual and partial loss of cells from a population is in itself capable of triggering regrowth.

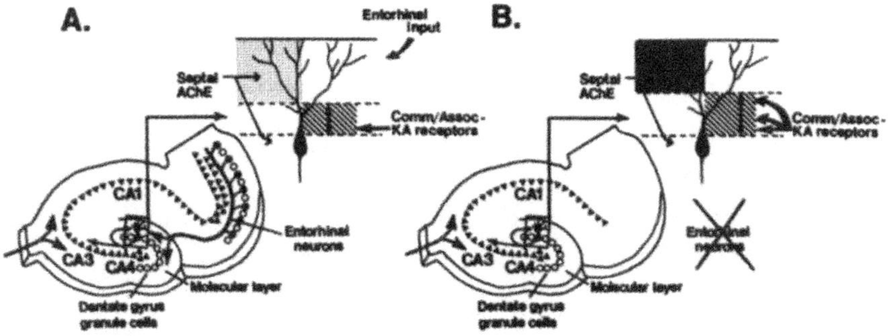

Figure 1-2. Changes in the dentate gyrus molecular layer following a unilateral entorhinal lesion. A. Normal distribution of entorhinal input to the outer two-thirds of the molecular layer, commissural/associational inputs (Comm/Assoc), and kainic acid (KA) receptors in the inner one-third of the molecular layer. Septal inputs occupy the outer molecular layer as well as a thin band of fibers in the supragranular zone. B. Following an entorhinal ablation the septal afferents, as well as commissural and associational afferents, sprout.

Specifically, in animal models, lesions which cause a rapid loss of input are used to trigger growth. In contrast, in Alzheimer's disease (AD), there is a slow, gradual loss of cells, which may or may not be a sufficient stimulus to incite regrowth.

Does the loss of entorhinal cells in Alzheimer's disease trigger sprouting and reactive synaptogenesis as in animal models with traumatic lesions? Do the commissural/associational fibers sprout in Alzhemier's disease brains? The kainic acid binding pattern in the hippocampus of control patients is similar to that observed in the rodent brain. A region of high density of kainic acid sites exists in the inner third of the molecular layer, the innervation zone of the C/A fibers.

In rodents with entorhinal lesions, these kainate binding sites become redistributed so that they occupy approximately one-half or more of the molecular layer (Figure 1-3). In the brains of Alzheimer's patients, the kainic acid binding sites also expand into the outer molecular layer so that they are now present in over half of the zone. This expansion is quite similar to that which occurs in rodents with entorhinal lesions. These results suggest that C/A fibers in the human brain sprout in response to pathologically-induced neuronal loss. As described elsewhere, cholinergic inputs also sprout in AD.

In the dentate gyrus, NMDA receptors are also present and appear to mediate long-term potentiation, a synaptic analog of memory. These receptors seem to be well-preserved in Alzheimer's disease, showing at best only small losses [27], in contrast to previous reports indicating a major neuronal loss of these receptor types [28]. Thus, many of the systems necessary to maintain function through a dentate gyrus integration center are preserved or are rebuilt in the course of neuronal loss.

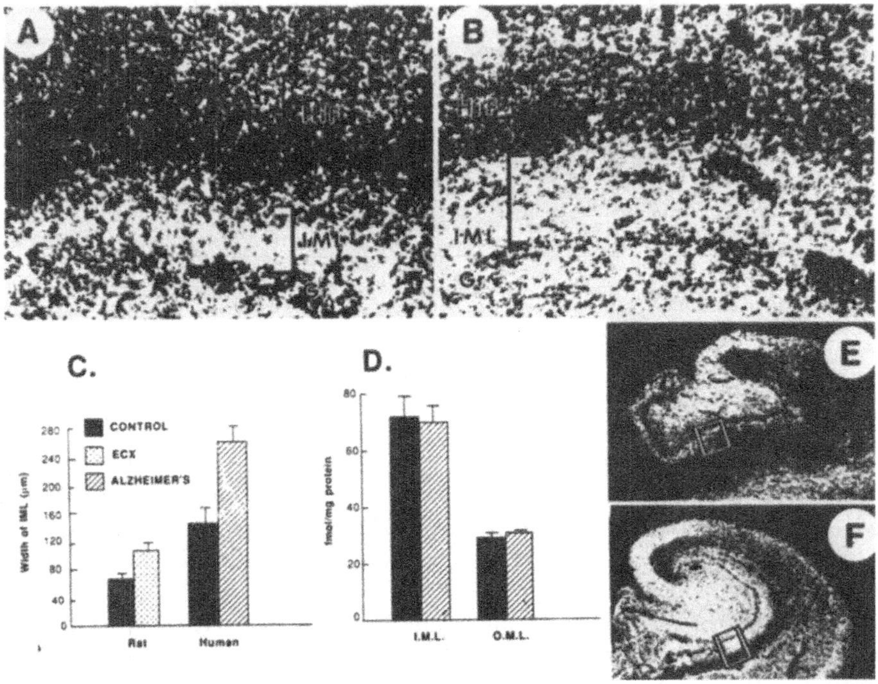

Figure 1-3. ^{3}H-kainic acid (KA) binding in the human hippocampal dentate gyrus. A. Autoradiographic distribution of ^{3}H-KA binding from a control subject. Receptors are concentrated in the inner molecular layer (IML) immediately subjacent to the granule cell layer (Gr). The outer boundary of the dentate gyrus is the hippocampal fissure (HiF). B. ^{3}H-KA binding in the Alzheimer's brain. Note that the receptor distribution has expanded to occupy over half of the molecular layer. C. Averaged widths of the ^{3}H-KA binding in the inner molecular layer compard between rats that have received an entorhinal cortical lesion (ECX) and controls, and Alzheimer's brains and controls. D. Total ^{3}H-KA binding in Alzheimer's brains and controls in the inner (I.M.L.) and outer (O.M.L.) molecular layers. No significant difference in total binding is seen between groups. E. Low power autoradiograph of ^{3}H-KA binding in the entire hippocampal formation from a control brain (E) and Alzheimer's brain (F). Boxes indicate similar areas to the higher magnifications shown in A and B.

7. NMDA AND TCP SITES IN AREA CA1 OF THE HIPPOCAMPUS

CA1 is vulnerable to AD neuropathology. A high density of NMDA and QA receptors is associated with stratum radiatum and stratum pyramidale of this region. In fact, stratum radiatum in the rodent contains the highest density of

NMDA binding sites in the brain. In contrast, KA receptor density is low. In AD, NMDA receptor densities in this region vary, with some cases showing little loss of receptors and other cases showing a pronounced loss. Further analysis of our cases revealed that loss of receptor density accompanied extremely severe cell loss in CA1. In AD cases with intermediate cell loss, receptor density is maintained, perhaps through compensatory mechanisms such as dendritic branching or receptor supersensitivity. In cases of severe neuronal loss, however, the compensation may no longer be adequate, and a loss of receptor density is observed.

No clinical parameter could be correlated with the greater neuronal loss or receptor density loss in CA1 of some patients. Parameters examined included age, postmortem delay, duration of illness, extent of atherosclerosis, and prolonged agonal state.

Phencyclidine can act as a noncompetitive NMDA antagonist, which appears to act by blocking the ion channel that is regulated by NMDA. To further evaluate the status of the NMDA receptor system in Alzheimer's disease, we examined the distribution and density of the associated phencyclidine binding sites labeled by ^{3}H-1(1-(2-thienyl)-cyclohexyl)piperidine, (^{3}H-TCP) [29]. In the normal hippocampus, the TCP binding site distribution was virtually identical to that found for NMDA receptors. Highest levels of binding were found in the CA1 strata pyramidale and radiatum and slightly lower levels in the dentate gyrus molecular layer. Moderate binding densities were observed in the CA3 region and low levels in the stratum lacunosum-moleculare and hilus of the dentate gyrus.

The hippocampus of some Alzheimer's patients showed significant loss of TCP binding sites in area CA1, whereas others had little loss. These results are similar to the findings for NMDA receptors. For each of the patients that were analyzed in the two studies (7 control and 7 Alzheimer's), the densities of the TCP sites were compared to those of NDMA sites in the hippocampal CA1 region. The densities of NMDA sites closely correlated to the TCP sites (correlation coefficient = 0.92). Thus, the densities of NMDA and TCP sites are very similar in individuals; those that show low levels of TCP sites also show low levels of NMDA receptors.

8. CONCLUSION

There are several fundamental conclusions that can be derived from autoradiographic studies on excitatory amino acid receptors. It is clear that autoradiography appears to reveal the major three subtypes of the glutamate receptor (NMDA, KA, and QA) and their anatomical organization. These correspond to the majority of sites to which glutamate binds. The sites can be labeled either by glutamate, with appropriate displacers, or by the direct ligand (e.g., ^{3}H-KA, ^{3}H-AMPA, ^{3}H-AP5). The pharmacological properties of the sites parallel those for the receptors studied electrophysiologically. The receptor sites are organized in a defined and precise manner in the CNS, and the overall pattern corresponds to the pathways proposed to use excitatory amino acids. All three sites are found primarily in telencephalic areas of the brain. NMDA, TCP, and QA sites are highest in hippocampal CA fields and in outer layers of the cerebral cortex. NMDA and TCP sites are very similar in their overall distribution, except for cerebellum and thalamus. KA sites in the cortex appear to be concentrated in the deeper layers. Autoradiography can be used on human postmortem tissues; these sites appear stable in postmortem tissues. In brains obtained from patients who have died of Alzheimer's disease, excitatory amino acid receptors in the dentate gyrus of the hippocampal formation appear to be preserved or actually increase. The increase appears associated with axon sprouting triggered by the loss of entorhinal neurons. It is our hypothesis that sprouting reactions serve to preserve and rebuild residual circuitry and act to preserve function in the early phases of the disease (see [16, 30–31] for discussion).

REFERENCES

1. Cotman, C.W. and Monaghan, D.T. Chemistry and anatomy of excitatory amino acid systems. In *Psychopharmacology: Next Generation of Progress*, Meltzer, H.Y. et al., ed., Raven Press, New York, 197–210.
2. Monaghan, D.T. and Cotman, C.W. (1985). Distribution of N-methyl-D-aspartate-sensitive L-^{3}H-glutamate binding sites in rat brain. J. Neurosci. 5, 2909–2919.
3. Monaghan, D.T., Yao, D., Olverman, H.J., Watkins, J.C. and Cotman, C.W. (1984). Autoradiography of ^{3}H-D-2-amino-5-phosphonopentanoate binding sites in rat brain. Neurosci. Lett. 52, 253–258.
4. Honore, T., Lauridsen, J. and Krogsgaard-Larsen, P. (1982). The binding of ^{3}H-AMPA, a structural analogue of glutamic acid, to rat brain membranes. J. Neurochem. 38, 173–178.
5. Monaghan, D.T., Yao, D. and Cotman, C.W. (1984). Distribution of ^{3}H-AMPA binding sites in rat brain as determined by quantitative autoradiography. Brain Res. 324, 160–164.
6. Rainbow, T.C., Wieczorek, C.M. and Halpain, S. (1984). Quantitative autoradiography of binding sites for ^{3}H-AMPA, a structural analogue of glutamic acid. Brain Res. 309, 173–177.
7. Monaghan, D.T., Holets, V.T., Toy, D.W. and Cotman, C.W. (1983). Anatomical distributions of four pharmacologically distinct ^{3}H-L-glutamate binding sites. Nature 306, 176–179.
8. Monaghan, D.T., Yao, D. and Cotman, C.W. (1985). ^{3}H-L-glutamate binds to kainate, NMDA and AMPA-sensitive binding sites: An autoradiographic analysis. Brain Res. 340, 378–383.
9. Foster, A.C., Mena, E.E., Monaghan, D.T. and Cotman, C.W. (1981). Synaptic localization of kainic acid binding sites. Nature 289, 73–75.
10. London, E.D. and Coyle, J.T. (1979). Specific binding of ^{3}H-kainic acid to receptor sites in rat brain, Mol. Pharmacol. 15, 492–505.
11. Monaghan, D.T. and Cotman, C.W. (1982). Distribution of ^{3}H-kainic acid binding sites in the rat CNS as determined by autoradiography. Brain Res. 252, 91–100.
12. Simon, J.R., Contrera, J.F. and Kuhar, M.J. (1976). Binding of ^{3}H-kainic acid, an analogue of L-glutamate, to brain membranes, J. Neurochem. 26, 141–147.
13. Unnerstall, J.R. and Wamsley, J.K. (1983). Autoradiographic localization of high-affinity ^{3}H-kainic acid binding sites in the rat forebrain, Eur. J. Pharmacol. 86, 361–371.
14. Hyman, B.T., Van Hoesen, G.W., Damasio, A.R. and Barnes, C.L. (1984). Alzheimer's disease: Cell-specific pathology isolates the hippocampal formation. Science 225, 1168–1170.
15. Cotman, C.W. and Nieto-Sampedro, M. (1984). Cell biology of synaptic plasticity. Science 225, 1287–1294.
16. Cotman, C.W. and Anderson, K.J. (1988). Synaptic plasticity and functional stabilization in the hippocampal formation: Possible role in Alzheimer's disease. In *Physiologic Basis for Functional Recovery in Neurological Disease*, S. Waxman, ed., Raven Press, New York, 313–336.
17. Steward, O., Cotman, C.W. and Lynch, G.S. (1973). Re-establishment of electrophysiologically functional entorhinal lesions: Innervation by the contralateral entorhinal cortex. Exp.

Brain Res. 18, 396–414.
18. Scheff, S.W. and Cotman, C.W. (1977). Recovery of spontaneous alternation following lesions of the entorhinal cortex in adult rats: Possible correlation to axon sprouting. Behav. Biol. 21, 286–293.
19. Loesche, J. and Steward, O. (1977). Behavioral correlates of denervation and reinnervation of the hippocampal formation of the rat: Recovery of alternation performance following unilateral entorhinal cortex lesions. Brain Res. Bull. 2, 31–39.
20. Lynch, G., Gall, C. and Cotman, C.W. (1977). Temporal parameters of axon "sprouting" in the brain of adult rat. Exper. Neurol. 54, 179–183.
21. Zimmer, J. (1973). Extended commissural and ipsilateral projections in postnatally deentorhinated hippocampus and fascia dentata demonstrated in rats by silver impregnation. Brain Res. 64, 293–311.
22. Scheff, S.W., Benardo, L.S. and Cotman, C.W. (1980). Decline in reactive fiber growth in the dentate gyrus of aged rats compared to young adult rats following entorhinal cortex removal. Brain Res. 199, 21–38.
23. Monaghan, D.T. and Cotman, C.W. (1982). Distribution of ^{3}H-kainic acid binding sites in the rat CNS as determined by autoradiography. Brain Res. 252, 91–100.
24. Monaghan, D.T., Holets, V., Toy, D. and Cotman, C.W. (1983). Anatomical distributions of four pharmacologically distinct ^{3}H-L-glutamate binding sites. Nature 306, 176–179.
25. Geddes, J.W., Monaghan, D.T., Cotman, C.W., Lott, I.T., Kim, R.C. and Chui, H.C. (1985). Plasticity of hippocampal circuitry in Alzheimer's disease. Science 230, 1179–1181.
26. West, J., Deadwyler, S., Cotman, C.W. and Lynch, G. (1975). Time-dependent changes in commissural field potential in the dentate gyrus following lesions of the entorhinal cortex in adult rats. Brain Res. 97, 215–233.
27. Geddes, J.W. and Cotman, C.W. (1986). Plasticity in hippocampal excitatory amino acid receptors in Alzheimer's disease. Neurosci. Res. 3, 672–678.
28. Greenamyre, J.T., Penney, J.B., Young, A.B., D'Amato, C.J., Hicks, S.P. and Shoulson, I. (1985). Alterations in L-glutamate binding in Alzheimer's and Huntington's diseases. Science 227, 1496–1499.
29. Monaghan, D.T., Geddes, J.W., Yao, D., Chung, C. and Cotman, C.W. (1986). ^{3}H-TCP binding sites in Alzheimer's disease. Neurosci. Lett. 73, 197–200.
30. Geddes, J.W., Monaghan, D.T., Cotman, C.W., Lott, I.T., Kim, R.C. and Chui, H.C. (1985). Plasticity of hippocampal circuitry in Alzheimer's disease. Science 230, 1179–1181.
31. Cotman, C.W., Geddes, J.W., Monaghan, D.T. and Anderson, K.J. (1987). Excitatory amino acid receptors in Alzheimer's disease. In *The Neurochemistry of Aging*, P. Davies, ed., Cold Spring Harbor Laboratory, Cold Spring Harbor, 27, 66–84.

2. CONDUCTANCE MECHANISMS ACTIVATED BY L-GLUTAMATE

GARY L. WESTBROOK, MARK L. MAYER, AND IAN D. FORSYTHE

There is little doubt that L-glutamate, and perhaps other similar endogenous compounds, are major excitatory neurotransmitters in the mammalian CNS. Thus the role of excitatory amino acids both in the mediation of fast excitatory postsynaptic potentials (epsps) in numerous pathways, as well as their role in pathophysiological situations, is receiving increasing attention. The surge in scientific interest in this area can be traced to two important developments. First, the receptor classification scheme based on studies by Watkins and colleagues in the spinal cord which defined three receptor subtypes, activated selectively by N-methyl-D-aspartic (NMDA), kainic (KA), and quisqualic (QA) acids [1]. This classification has been particularly useful for studies of the NMDA receptor subtype for which a potent and selective antagonist, 2-amino-5-phosphonovaleric acid (AP5), has been available for several years [2]. An important corollary of this classification has been the recognition that L-glutamate acts at more than one receptor type, but with a particularly high affinity for the NMDA receptor [3]. The use of selective agonists and antagonists has also allowed rapid progress in the understanding of the regional and cellular localization of excitatory amino acid receptors on CNS neurons, as discussed by Drs. Cotman and Fagg in this volume. The second important development has been the use of in vitro preparations, especially dissociated cell cultures for studies of the ion channels linked to these receptor subtypes. Dissociated neuron cultures allow the use of the voltage clamp and patch clamp methods necessary for detailed studies of ion channels, and, in addi-

Ferrendelli, J.A., Collins, R.C. and Johnson, E.M. (eds), Neurobiology of Amino Acids, Peptides, and Trophic Factors.

tion, essentially eliminate the problems of drug delivery and tissue reuptake associated with such studies in more intact preparations [4].

We review here our studies of conductances activated by excitatory amino acids on cultured spinal and hippocampal neurons as well as how these conductances contribute to stimulus evoked epsps between cultured neurons. Our results suggest that NMDA receptors are associated with a voltage-dependent conductance permeable to calcium and monovalent cations, whereas kainate/quisqualate receptors are linked to a voltage-insensitive cation conductance with essentially no calcium permeability. Monosynaptic epsps between neurons in both spinal cord and hippocampal cultures show two components — a fast epsp with properties similar to kainate/quisqualate responses and a slow component, lasting up to 500 msec due to activation of NMDA receptors. The unique features of this slow epsp, i.e., voltage-dependence and calcium permeability, may have important consequences both for the short-term modulation of neuronal excitability as well as for more long-lasting changes in synaptic efficacy. Such results suggest that an endogenous excitatory transmitter for these monosynatpic epsps could act simultaneously as a classical fast transmitter and as a neuromodulator.

1. METHODS

Cell cultures of spinal cord were prepared from embryonic mice by previously described methods [5]. Hippocampal cultures were prepared from 17-day mouse embryos by similar procedures, except that neurons were grown on confluent astrocyte feeder layers at low density ($0.5-1.5 \times 10^5$ cells per 35 mm dish). This resulted in isolated groups of 2–5 neurons used for studies of synaptic interactions between adjacent neurons. Electrophysiological recordings were made with patch electrodes in the whole-cell configuration [6] in either current clamp or voltage clamp mode. Experiments were conducted at room temperature (25–28 °C.) and drugs applied by local perfusion (see, e.g., Ref. 7 for details). For synaptic experiments, epsps were evoked either by extracellular stimulation using an agar-plugged glass micropipette or, more commonly, by intracellular stimulation of the presynaptic neuron.

2. TWO DISTINCT CONDUCTANCE MECHANISMS

The first clue that the depolarizing action of L-glutamate resulted from activation of more than one specific ion channel came from current clamp studies in cat motoneurons in vivo by Engberg and colleagues. They demonstrated that depolarizations evoked by NMDA or DL-homocysteic acid were associated with increases in membrane resistance, whereas depolarizations evoked by kainate were associated with decreases in membrane resistance [8, 9]. An example of this behavior in cultured spinal cord neurons is illustrated in Figure 2-1; the voltage deflection resulting from repetitive hyperpolarizing current pulses was used to measure membrane resistance. Of note, the L-glutamate-evoked depolarization shows little change in membrane resistance, consis-

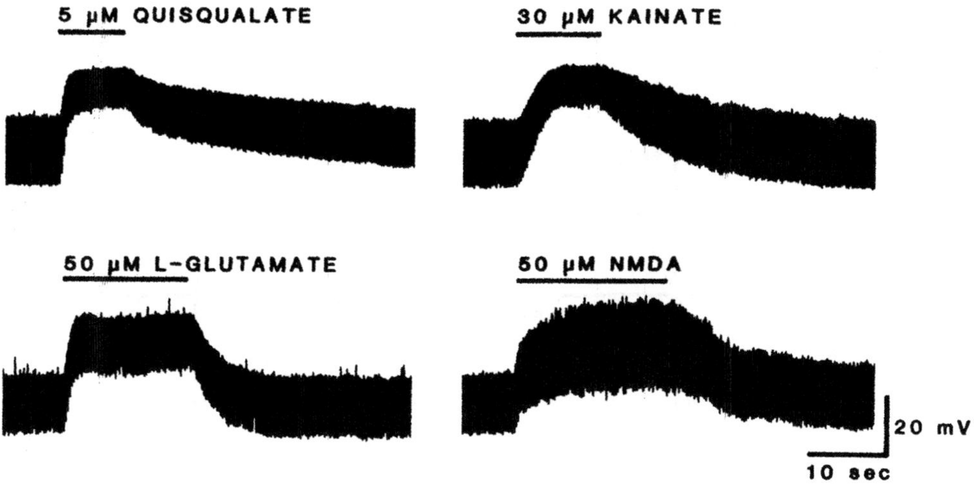

Figure 2-1. Depolarizations evoked by brief pressure applications of excitatory amino acids to cultured spinal cord neurons. Responses of equal amplitude evoked by quisqualate and kainate are accompanied by a decrease in the amplitude of the hyperpolarizing electrotonic potentials, i.e., an increase in membrane conductance, whereas the response to NMDA results in an apparent increase in membrane resistance and the response to L-glutamate shows no apparent change in membrane conductance. Whole-cell current clamp recording using a KCl-based intracellular solution; the extracellular solution was HEPES-buffered saline with 2 mM Ca^{2+} and 1 mM Mg^{2+}. (Taken from Mayer & Westbrook [24] with permission).

tent with its mixed agonist action [5, 10]. The basis of these agonist-specific changes in membrane resistance are now clear from current clamp and voltage clamp studies of neurons in cell culture, which demonstrated that there are two distinct conductance mechanisms activated by excitatory amino acids, a voltage-dependent conductance linked to NMDA receptors and a voltage-insensitive conductance linked to kainate/quisqualate receptors [5, 11, 12]. L-glutamate activates both conductances in a dose-dependent manner, with lower concentrations acting primarily on the conductance linked to NMDA receptors [5].

As shown in the left panel of Figure 2-2A, under voltage clamp the inward current activated by NMDA has a region of negative slope conductance at membrane potentials hyperpolarized to −35 mV. This means that depolarization of the neuron, e.g., by incoming synaptic traffic, will increase the availability of NMDA-receptor channels. This "regenerative" characteristic is at least part of the explanation for the increased tendency for neurons to fire action potentials in bursts during applications of NMDA, as shown in the left panel of Figure 2-2B (see also discussion of Figure 2-3 below.)

2.1. Mg^{2+} — blocks NMDA-receptor channels

Our studies initially focused on the mechanism responsible for voltage-dependence of the NMDA-activated conductance. For other ion channels,

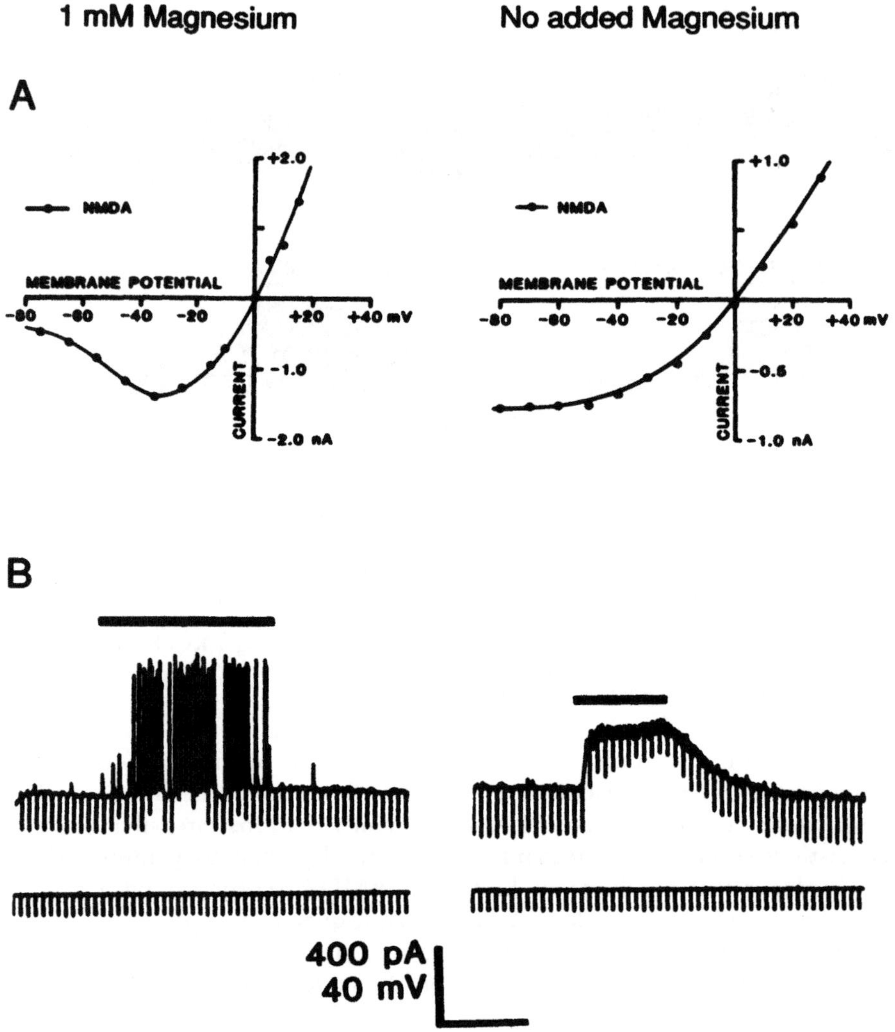

Figure 2-2. A. Current-voltage plot of peak amplitude of responses evoked by brief pressure applications of NMDA from one neuron in a bath containing 1 mM Mg^{2+} (left panel) and another neuron in a "Mg^{2+}-free" bath (right panel). Note that on removal of extracellular Mg^{2+}, the I-V plot loses the negative slop region characteristic of responses evoked by NMDA. Results using two microelectrode voltage clamp; the bathing medium also contained 5 mM Ca^{2+} (see text). B. The burst firing associated with application of NMDA reflects the voltage-dependent action of Mg^{2+}. At left, application of 100 μM NMDA evokes a burst of action potentials; on removal of Mg^{2+}, NMDA evokes a larger depolarization, shunting the membrane resistance, and no action potentials occur. (Modified with permission from Mayer & Westbrook [20].

such as the tetrodotoxin-sensitive sodium channel or voltage-dependent calcium channels, the voltage sensitivity of the channel results from a voltage-induced conformational change in the channel protein, leading to "gating" of the channel between the closed and open stages. However, the voltage-dependence of the NMDA-activated conductance has a quite different mechanism — Mg^{2+} ions enter and block the open channel [13, 14]. The channel-blocking action is voltage-sensitive and increases with membrane hyperpolarization, since the charged blocking ion senses the transmembrane voltage within the channel in its open state. As a result, removal of Mg^{2+} from the extracellular fluid removes the negative slope from the current-voltage (I-V) relationship of the NMDA-activated conductance (Figure 2-2A, right panel). As is seen in the right panel of Figure 2-2B, removal of Mg^{2+} also changes the nature of the depolarizing response to applications of NMDA; in Mg^{2+}-free medium, the same concentration of NMDA induces a much larger depolarization, which shunts the membrane resistance without inducing a burst of action potentials.

The blocking effect of Mg^{2+} is quite potent. Nowak et al. [14] demonstrated that with low concentrations (1–10 μM) of Mg^{2+}, NMDA-receptor channels show the flickering block characteristic of the fast open channel block seen with the action of a variety of charged molecules on acetylcholine receptor channels [15–17]. A simple sequential kinetic model for channel block includes three states,

closed — open — blocked,

with the blocking rate being a function of voltage and $[Mg^{2+}]$. This is a useful model for describing the interactions of Mg^{2+} with the NMDA receptor channel at low Mg^{2+} concentrations; however, several features of NMDA-receptor channels already demonstrate that a more complex model will be necessary to describe the action of Mg^{2+} at physiological concentrations, i.e., 0.8–1.0 mM. For example, an important prediction of the sequential model is that the total charge transfer during opening of a single channel should remain constant in the presence of blocker, i.e., the total time the channel spends in the open state after initially opening is invariant. At the single channel level, this means that the burst duration should increase as the blocker concentration increases, but in the presence 100 μM Mg^{2+} , the burst duration actually decreases [14]. At the level of the macroscopic current, the sequential model also fails to predict the observed negative slope conductance of the macroscopic current. The explanations for this are yet to be clarified, but may included either "closed" channel block [16, 18] or enhanced desensitization [19].

2.2. Implications of channel block for neuronal excitability

Since channel block by Mg^{2+} underlies the voltage dependence of the NMDA-activated conductance, this means that factors that alter the degree of channel block will also alter the voltage-dependence of the conductance. As predicted by the sequential channel blocking model, these will include the extracellular

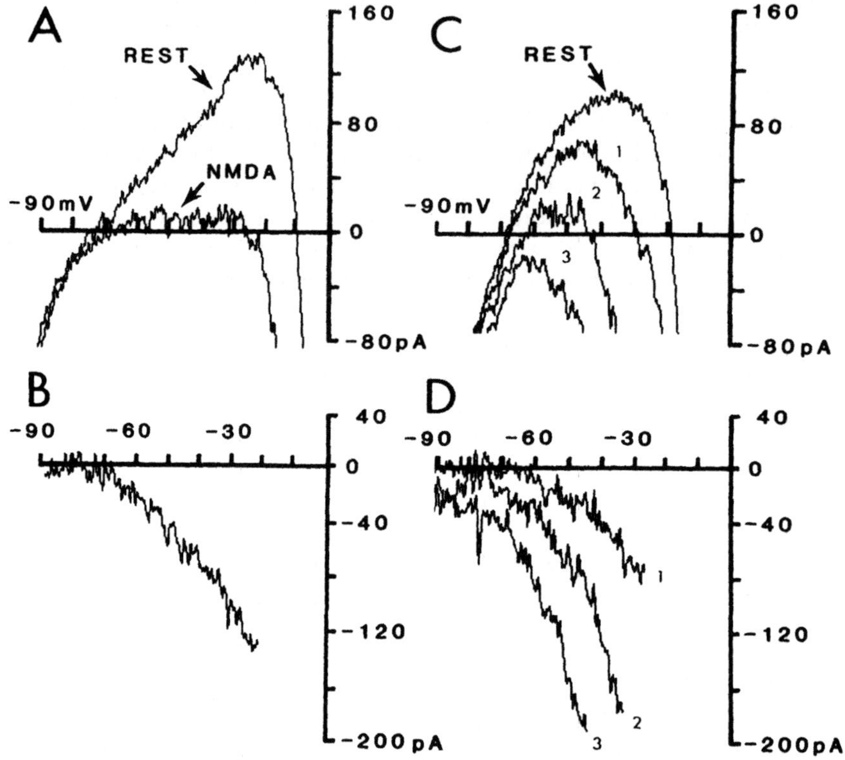

Figure 2-3. Interaction of the NMDA-activated conductance with voltage-dependent calcium currents in cultured spinal cord neurons under voltage clamp. A, C. Whole-cell current-voltage plots recording at rest and during application of 50 μM NMDA in response to a ramp voltage clamp from -100 to 0 at 0.42 mV/ms. Whole-cell patch recording; intracellular solution contained C_s^+ to block outward K^+ currents and 5 mM Mg-ATP to reduce rundown of Ca^{2+} currents. B, D. Difference I-V relationship obtained from A and C reflects I-V behavior of the NMDA-activated conductance. Note that the threshold for inward current of the whole-cell I-V relationship is shifted to increasingly negative potentials with increases in the dose of NMDA. Holding current at -70 mV was taken as 0 pA. (Taken from Mayer and Westbrook [24] with permission.)

$[Mg^{2+}]$, and since the block by Mg^{2+} is noncompetitive [14, 20], a higher effective agonist concentration will lead to a greater percentage reduction of agonist-induced current. In addition, the voltage-dependent NMDA conductance will interact with other voltage-dependent membrane conductances in determining the overall current-voltage relationship of the cell. An example to illustrate this is shown in Figure 2-3. In Figure 2-3A the I-V relationship of a spinal cord neuron in response to a ramp voltage stimulus is shown as "rest" (the neuron is loaded with Cs^+ to reduce outward current). The downward current deflection positive to -20 mV reflects activation of conventional voltage-dependent calcium channels. On application of NMDA in 1 mM $[Mg^{2+}]_o$ (Figure 2-3A, "NMDA"), the slope conductance of the neuronal

I-V relationship decreases markedly and shifts the threshold for net inward current to a more hyperpolarized voltage (−30 mV in this example). The threshold for inward current through NMDA channels (Figure 2-3B) is much more hyperpolarized than for the voltage-dependent calcium current (i.e., the L-type channel [21]), thus the NMDA conductance would serve to increase neuronal excitability by augmenting "Ca^{2+}" spikes and enhancing burst firing. As can be seen in Figure 2-3C, increasing the dose of NMDA leads to even further shifts in the threshold for inward current of the membrane I-V relationship. This effect is entirely a result of the Mg^{2+}-induced voltage dependence of the NMDA-activated conductance and not a result of any direct calcium permeability of the NMDA-receptor channel (see below).

2.3. Action of other divalent cations on NMDA channels

Several other divalent cations, including Co^{2+}, Mn^{2+}, and Ni^{2+}, also cause a voltage-dependent block of NMDA-receptor channels similar to Mg^{2+} [20, 22]. However, Cd^{2+}, a potent blocker of voltage-sensitive calcium channels, has essentially no blocking action on NMDA responses at micromolar concentrations [13]. This can be a useful tool in differentiating responses to NMDA-receptor channels from those due to conventional voltage-sensitive calcium channels. The rank order of potency of divalent cations as NMDA channel blockers correlates with the rate constant for exchange of water molecules in the inner hydration shell [23], suggesting that the slow rate of substitution of water molecules could be a limiting factor in the permeation (or block) by these ions in the pore of the NMDA channel (see Ref. 24 for further discussion of this point).

Recently the effects of the Group IIB transition metal cations, Zn^{2+}, Hg^{2+}, and Cd^{2+}, on responses to NMDA on cultured hippocampal neurons have also been examined [25]. Zn^{2+} is of particular physiological interest since it is present in high concentrations in the hippocampus and is released from mossy fiber terminals with activity [26, 27]. These results demonstrate that Zn^{2+} at low micromolar concentrations is a potent antagonist of responses evoked by NMDA but not by kainic acid. The antagonism by Zn^{2+} is not competitive, but, in contrast to the action of Mg^{2+}, the effects of Zn^{2+} are not sensitive to the membrane voltage. This suggests that the site of action of zinc is not within the open channel but, rather, is near the external surface of the membrane. Millimolar concentrations of Cd^{2+} had a similar action, but Hg^{2+} did not antagonize NMDA responses, thus the effects of zinc are unlikely to be the result of reduction of -S-S- bonds.

3. IONIC PERMEABILITY OF NMDA CHANNELS

3.1. Reversal potential measurements

Voltage dependence of responses to NMDA, coupled with the blocking action of some divalent cations, led to the suggestion that NMDA activated a voltage-sensitive calcium conductance [28]. Studies using Ca^{2+}-sensitive electrodes either intracellularly or extracellularly have also suggested that calcium influx accompanies responses to L-glutamate or NMDA [29, 30]. However, in physiological saline, the reversal potential of responses to excitatory amino acids is similar and close to 0 mV [5, 14], more consistent with ion channels that have a nonselective permeability to monovalent cations similar to the acetylcholine receptor channel. For responses to KA and QA, as expected for a channel permeable to sodium and potassium, a decrease in extracellular sodium did shift the reversal potential to a more hyperpolarized potential; however, little or no reversal potential shift occurred for responses to NMDA, suggesting that ions other than Na^+ and K^+ contributed to the response [20]. As reviewed below, several different experimental approaches using cultured neurons have now demonstrated that the NMDA-receptor channel has a significant permeability to Ca^{2+}; calcium's action in the channel is complex in that it both permeates the channel and shows competition with permeant cations (Na^+ and K^+) as well as with blocking ions such as Mg^{2+}. To investigate the relative permeability of the NMDA channel to calcium as well as monovalent cations, the reversal potential under voltage clamp of responses to NMDA was measured as a function of the extracellular sodium and calcium concentration. At a constant sodium concentration of 105 mM, increasing $[Ca]_o$ from 0.1 to 50 mM resulted in a progressive shift of the reversal potential from −7 mV to +30 mV [31, 32]. Recently, Ascher and Nowak [33] have reported similar results for single channel currents activated by NMDA. Using the extended constant field equation, our results are reasonably well fit by a $P_{Ca}:P_{Na}$ of 10.6, assuming $P_{Na} = P_K = P_{Cs}$. Similar calculations on the reversal potential of responses evoked by kainic acid showed essentially no measurable calcium permeability with a $P_{Ca}:P_{Na} = 0.15$ [32]. The $P_{Ca}:P_{Na}$ ratio of 10.6 for the NMDA channel compares to 0.22 for the acetylcholine receptor channel ($[Ca]_o = 20$ mM [34]), while conventional voltage-sensitive calcium channels show much greater selectivity for calcium over sodium and potassium, e.g., $P_{Ca}:P_{Cs} > 1000$ for calcium channels in guinea pig heart ventricular cells [35].

3.2. Ion interactions

Although the extended constant field equation provides a useful method, in this case, to compare relative calcium permeabilities, it is only a valid description of channel permeation if movement of ions through the channel obeys the so-called independence principle, i.e., there is no interaction between ions or binding of ions within the channel. However, at $[Na^+]_o < 50$ mM and in the presence of 10 mM $[Ca]_o$, the reversal potential for responses evoked by NMDA deviates from the values predicted by the extended constant field equation, i.e., there is an apparent increase in $P_{Ca}:P_{Na}$ at low sodium concentrations, indicative of competition between the permeating ions [32].

There is also interaction between divalent cations that primarily act as blockers of the NMDA channel (e.g., Mg^{2+}) and those divalent cations that can permeate the channel (e.g., Ca^{2+}). As seen in the left panel of Figure 2-2, there is usually some residual nonlinearity at hyperpolarized potentials in the current-voltage relationship of the NMDA-activated conductance, even in the apparent absence of Mg^{2+}. It was initially assumed this was due to small amounts of Mg^{2+} (measured at 3–5 μM in our experiments [20]); but we also considered whether $[Ca^{2+}]_o$ at millimolar concentrations could also have a voltage-dependent blocking action. However, when $[Ca^{2+}]_o$ was reduced from 5 mM to 0.1 mM, the voltage-dependent block of the NMDA-activated conductance actually increased, suggesting instead that the residual micromolar $[Mg^{2+}]_o$ was a more effective blocker at low $[Ca^{2+}]_o$. This effect was confirmed by comparing the NMDA-activated conductance at low and high $[Ca^{2+}]_o$ (Figure 2-4). At 5 mM, $[Ca^{2+}]_o$ partially relieved the block due to residual Mg^{2+}, and thus the NMDA-conductance was increased at potentials negative to −80 mV [32]. On the other hand, at depolarized voltages, high $[Ca^{2+}]_o$ decreased the NMDA-activated conductance, consistent with a competition of Ca^{2+} with permeant monovalent cations. Of note, the single channel conductance of NMDA-receptor channels is lower in high calcium solutions between 0 and −60 mV [22]. These studies underscore the idea that for the NMDA channel, rather than two categories of cations — permeant and blocking ions — there is a continuum of behavior from essentially pure blocking ions such as Mg^{2+} to highly permeant cations.

3.3. Optical measurements of calcium influx

These reversal potential measurements demonstrate that the NMDA channel is permeable to calcium but do not indicate whether this results in a significant transient change in free cytoplasmic calcium. Since Na^+ is clearly the major charge carrier through NMDA channels near the resting potential, and considering the ionic interactions described above, it could be argued that there is little calcium influx associated with the operation of these channels under physiological conditions. In view of the postulated interlocking functional roles of calcium and NMDA receptors, we attempted to directly measure intracellular calcium transients in response to activation of excitatory amino acid receptors using the calcium indicator dye arsenazo III (see Ref. 7 for details of method). Single spinal cord neurons were loaded with approximately 1 mM arsenazo using patch electrodes in the whole-cell mode. Since depolarization alone results in calcium influx due to activation of conventional voltage-sensitive calcium channels, we performed our experiments under voltage clamp. Thus we could separate calcium influx via agonist-gated ion channels from that due to voltage-activated calcium channels. As shown in Figure 2-5, responses to NMDA were associated with increases in $[Ca]_i$. Traces a and b show optical absorbance signals recorded simultaneously at wavelengths of 1) 660 nm (the wavelength at which changes in $[Ca]_i$ evoke maximal increases in absorbance) and 2) 570 nm (the isobestic wavelength used to control for movement related artifacts). The differential signal (570–660), labeled Δ T, detects

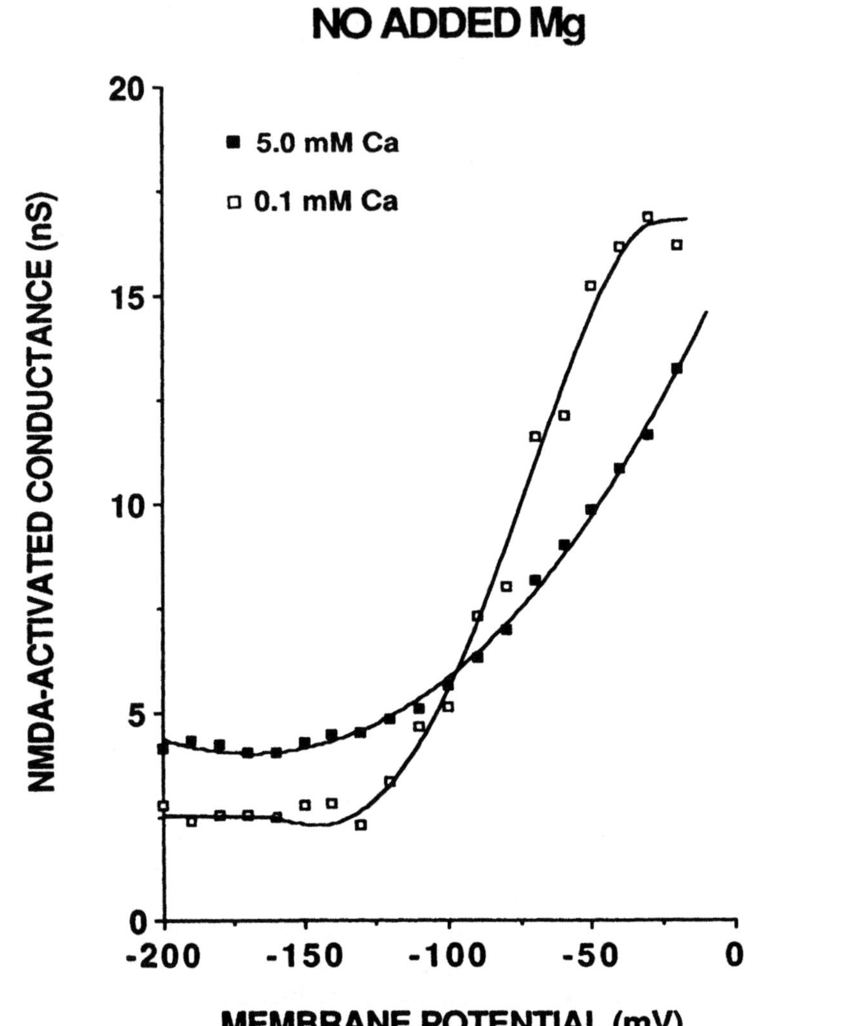

Figure 2-4. Conductance-voltage plots illustrate ion interactions within the NMDA-receptor channel. Chord conductance calculated from inward currents evoked by NMDA during a series of 30 msec voltage jumps from a holding potential of −50 mV. Bath contained no added Mg^{2+} and either 5 mM Ca^{2+} or 0.1 mM Ca^{2+}. Note that at membrane potentials negative to −90 mV, the conductance is larger in 5 mM Ca^{2+}, reflecting relief of Mg^{2+} block by calcium ions; however, positive to the "crossover" voltage of −90 mV the conductance is less in 5 mM Ca^{2+}, reflecting an interaction of Ca^{2+} with permeant monovalent cations. Lines drawn by eye. Whole-cell patch recording from two spinal cord neurons using a discontinuous single-electrode voltage clamp. (Taken from Mayer and Westbrook [32].)

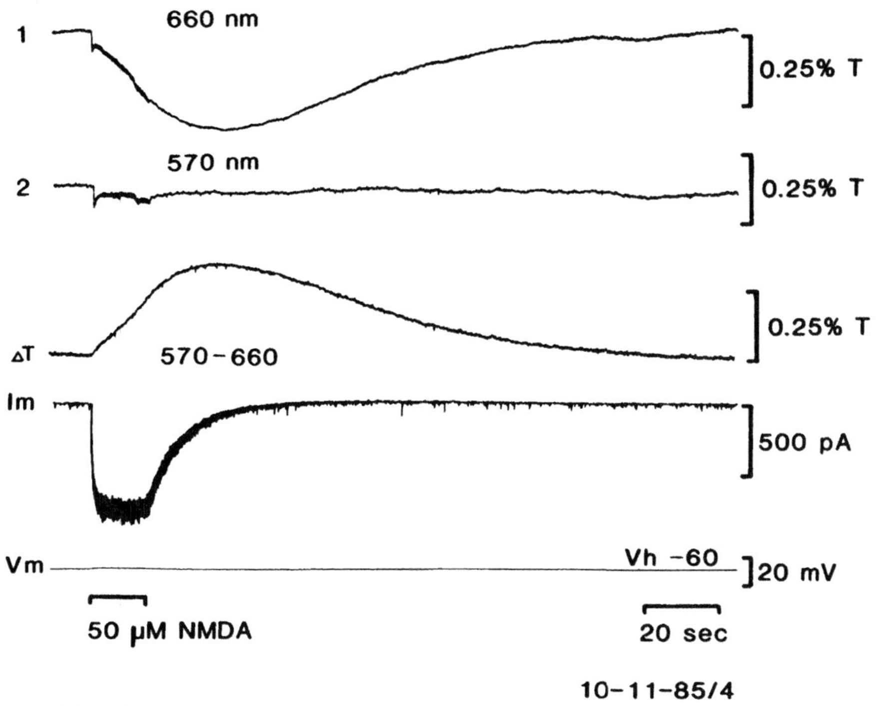

Figure 2-5. NMDA increases $[Ca]_i$ in spinal cord neurons under voltage clamp measured with the calcium indicator dye arsenazo III. Traces a and b show transmittance changes at 660 and 570 μm in response to application of 50 μM NMDA; small deflections at the beginning of traces are due to movement-related artifacts. The ΔT trace is the differential transmittance (570–660) that detects optical absorbance changes when arsenazo III binds Ca^{2+}; an upward deflection reflects an increase in $[Ca]_i$. A large inward current evoked by NMDA (Im) at a holding potential (Vm) of −60 mV accompanies the agonist-evoked calcium transient. Whole-cell recording with patch electrode containing 0.7 mM arsenazo III. (For further details see Ref. 7 from which this figure was taken with permission.)

the change in absorbance due to binding of Ca^{2+} by arsenazo III, an upward deflection, indicating an increase in $[Ca]_i$. In contrast to NMDA, responses evoked by KA or QA under voltage clamp were associated with minimal calcium transients. Responses evoked by L-glutamate did have associated calcium transients that could be blocked by Mg^{2+}, consistent with an action on NMDA receptors [36].

Calcium transients in response to NMDA were dose-dependent and varied with the driving force for inward current through NMDA channels. It was conceivable that the calcium transient was not due to transmembrane calcium flux but rather resulted from release of calcium from intracellular stores, especially since some excitatory amino acids have been reported to stimulate turnover of phosphatidylinositol [37, 38]. However, NMDA-evoked calcium transients were blocked by high concentrations of Mg^{2+} in parallel with the block of inward currents, demonstrating that ion flux through NMDA channels was responsible for the calcium transient [7]. In solutions with no added Mg^{2+}, the peak inward current and peak calcium transient occurred at a membrane potential near −60 mV. We could also record NMDA-evoked calcium transients in physiological levels of Mg^{2+} [36]. Since Mg^{2+} shifts the point of maximal inward current of the NMDA-evoked current-voltage relationship to more depolarized potentials (−35 mV in 1 mM Mg^{2+} [20]), it is likely that under physiological conditions depolarization from −60 to −30 mV would result not only in a larger NMDA-evoked current, but also a larger calcium influx. Thus it seems likely that calcium influx through NMDA channels occurs at membrane potentials hyperpolarized to that required to activate conventional voltage-gated calcium channels (see, e.g., Figures 2-3A and 2-3B). It is conceivable that calcium influx through NMDA channels could be especially significant at membrane potentials subthreshold of conventional calcium channels. For example, this may explain why conjunctive depolarization of the postsynaptic neuron can trigger long-term potentiation (LTP) in the CA1 region of the hippocampus [39–41].

Although more detailed investigations, especially at the single channel level, will be necessary to develop a complete biophysical description of ion permeation and block of NMDA channels, a qualitative summary of the interaction of Ca^{2+} and Mg^{2+} is now possible (Figure 2-6). Mg^{2+} ions enter the channel and bind to a site deep within the channel, thus blocking the flow of permeant ions; this block is increased with membrane hyperpolarization. Ca^{2+} can enter the channel and compete with Mg^{2+} (not necessarily at the same binding site, but perhaps by electrostatic repulsion) and displace Mg^{2+} from its binding site, leading to permeation of both Ca^{2+} and monovalent cations through the channel.

4. SYNAPTIC ACTIVATION OF NMDA RECEPTORS

Several antagonists, including kynurenic acid, cis-2,3-piperidine dicarboxylic acid (PDA), and γ-D-glutamylglycine, block responses to KA, QA, and NMDA, and these have been used to investigate the receptors activated by synaptic stimulation both in vivo and in vitro (see Ref. 24 for review). These studies were remarkably similar in demonstrating that fast epsps, at pathways thought to use an excitatory amino acid as the transmitter, were mediated by a KA/QA receptor type. Although the NMDA-receptor antagonist AP5 could be shown to have an effect on "polysynaptic" activity (e.g., see Ref. 42), the mechanism by which this occurred was unclear. In addition, studies of the synaptic currents underlying fast epsps between single Ia afferents and motoneurons in vivo [43] and between cultured spinal cord neurons [44] have indicated a relatively voltage-insensitive conductance mechanism compatible with that seen with the responses evoked by KA or QA.

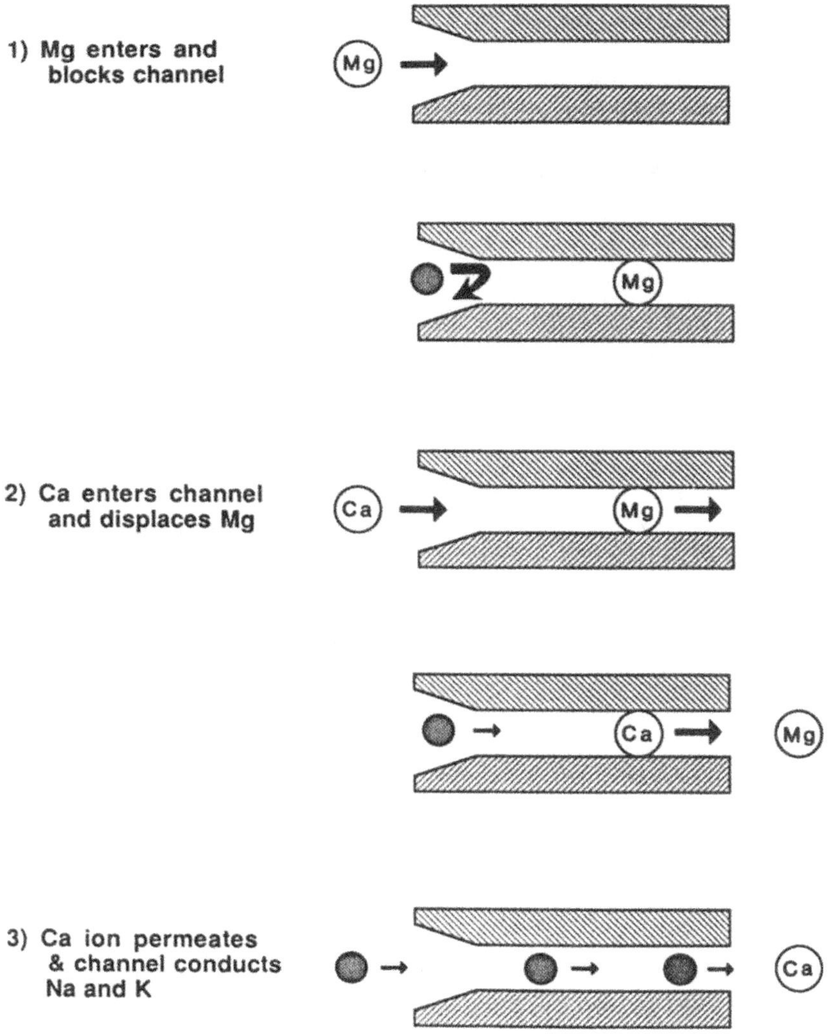

Figure 2-6. Schematic representation of permeation of divalent cations through NMDA-receptor channels. See text for details.

Based on this evidence, it was possible that NMDA receptors were either extrasynaptic or that there was a subset of primarily local circuit neurons that operated via a NMDA-receptor mediated synaptic mechanism. However, several recent studies in vitro have indicated that NMDA receptors can be directly activated at synapses in neocortex, hippocampus, and spinal cord [45–49]. In most cases, these evoked epsps were monosynaptic and contained both an early component due to activation of KA/QA receptors and a slower component that was blocked by the specific NMDA-receptor antagonist, AP5.

To investigate the synaptic activation of NMDA receptors in greater detail, we have examined the behavior of monosynaptic epsps evoked by stimulation of an adjacent neuron in either spinal cord or hippocampal cultures (SC-SC or HPC-HPC epsps). To facilitate study of activation of NMDA receptors, experiments were usually performed in a Mg^{2+}-free solution containing 50–100 μM picrotoxin to block ipsps. Both SC-SC and HPC-HPC epsps had two pharmacologically distinct components: a fast component blocked by PDA or kynurenate [44, 50, 51] as well as a slow component that was blocked by AP5 or Mg^{2+}, consistent with a NMDA-receptor mechanism [49]. Ketamine, which blocks responses evoked by NMDA in a voltage-dependent manner [52, 53], also blocked the slow epsp. An example of such a dual receptor epsp between two spinal cord neurons is shown in Figure 2-7. Perfusion of the synaptic pair with 100 μM Mg^{2+} blocked a slow component of the epsp, which is shown after digital subtraction in the lower trace. The NMDA-receptor mediated component has the same latency as the fast component but has a much slower time to peak as well as a duration of up to 500 msec. The duration of the slow epsp always exceeded the membrane time constant of the postsynaptic neuron, indicating that the duration was a function of persistent activation of NMDA receptors. Since NMDA receptors are activated by lower concentrations of L-glutamate than are non-NMDA receptors, it is conceivable that activation of NMDA receptors would outlast the brief transient of high concentration of transmitter necessary to activate non-NMDA receptors, and, in this sense, L-glutamate seems the ideal transmitter candidate to explain these results.

In Figure 2-7, the peak of the epsp was reduced by Mg^{2+}, which could be due to a presynaptic inhibitory effect of Mg^{2+} on transmitter release or to a particularly early developing NMDA-receptor mediated component for this epsp.

In the presence of Mg^{2+}, the synaptic current (epsc) underlying SC-SC or HPC-HPC epsps, measured under voltage clamp, also shows a fast and a slow component. Previous studies have demonstrated that the fast epsc between cultured spinal cord neurons is voltage-insensitive, with a decay time constant less than 1 msec [44], consistent with activation of KA/QA receptors. However, a much slower component of the synaptic current is voltage-dependent and Mg^{2+}-sensitive, as expected for the activation of NMDA-receptor channels. Figure 2-8 shows an HPC-HPC epsc at holding potentials between −60 mV and +40 mV. An I-V relationship of the fast current component (triangles) is nearly linear, while the NMDA-receptor mediated component (circles) is voltage-dependent in the presence of 100 μM Mg^{2+}. In this example, the ratio of the fast:slow conductance at +40 mV was approximately

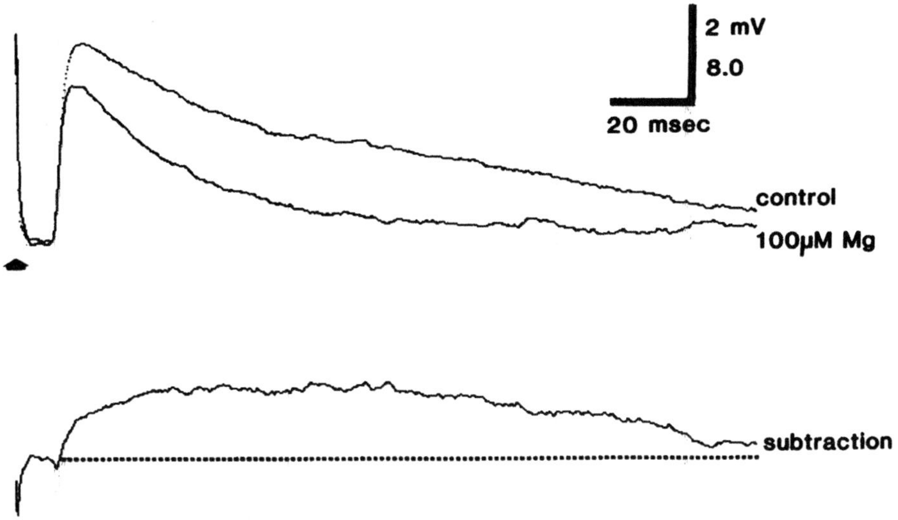

Figure 2-7. Monosynaptic epsps between spinal cord neurons have both fast and slow components. A monosynaptic epsp ("control") was evoked by extracellular stimulation of a nearby presynaptic neuron in a bath containing no added Mg^{2+}, 1 mM Ca^{2+}, and 100 μM picrotoxin. During perfusion with 100 μM Mg^{2+}, the decay of the epsp was much more rapid. The slow Mg^{2+}–sensitive component of the epsp is shown in the digitally subtracted record at bottom. Similar results were obtained with AP-5 and ketamine, demonstrating that the slow component of the epsps is due to activation of NMDA receptors. Whole-cell current clamp recording; intracellular solution contained $KMeSO_4$. Large arrow at beginning of traces indicates time of presynaptic stimulation. (Taken from Forsythe and Westbrook [49].)

5:1. For other epsps, this ratio varied from about 1:1 to 20:1; in a few cases no slow component could be detected [49].

5. FUNCTIONAL IMPLICATIONS

Recent studies from different preparations and brain regions clearly indicate that both non-NMDA (KA/QA) and NMDA receptors are activated at many, if not all, pathways that use an excitatory amino acid, probably L-glutamate, as a transmitter. This is particularly intriguing in view of the unique features of the NMDA-receptor mediated conductance: voltage-dependence and calcium permeability. The voltage-dependence of the NMDA-receptor channel can, in the short term, serve to increase neuronal excitability by augmenting burst firing; calcium influx through NMDA channels may further increase the tendency to rhythmic bursting through activation of calcium-dependent K^+ channels [54, 55]. In addition, calcium permeability of the NMDA-receptor channel may serve to link a number of phenomena, such as LTP in the CA1 region of the hippocampus, which are both calcium-dependent [56–58] and blocked by NMDA receptor antagonists [59–61]. Excitotoxic neuronal

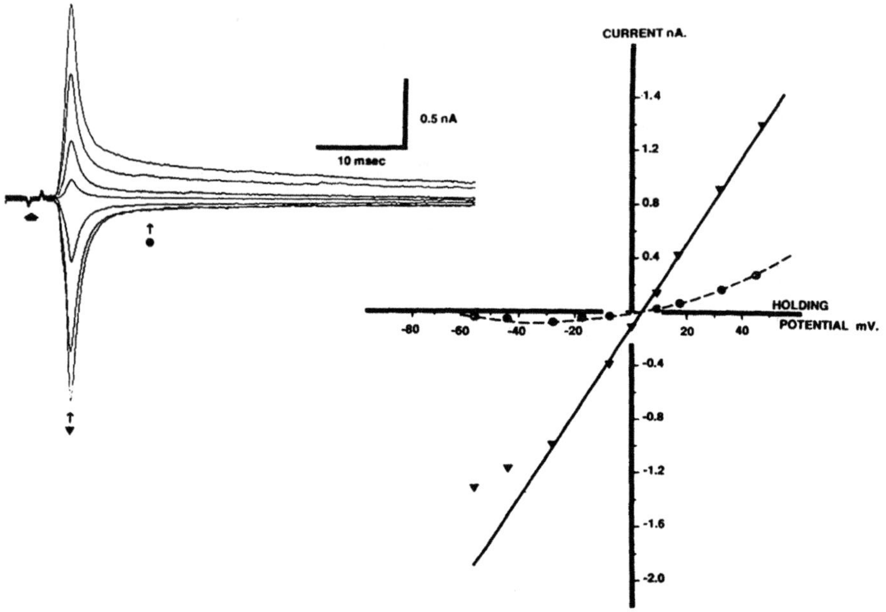

Figure 2-8. The slow epsp shows voltage-dependent behavior characteristic of NMDA-receptor channels. Voltage clamp of monosynaptic excitatory postsynaptic current (epsc) between two hippocampal neurons. Synaptic currents at left were evoked at a series of holding potentials from −60 mV to +40 mV in a bath containing 1 mM Ca^{2+} and 100 μM Mg^{2+}. Arrow indicates coupling artifact from stimulation of presynaptic neuron. I-V plot of the synaptic current at two different times are plotted at right. Note that the late component is voltage sensitive and shows a negative slope conductance at membrane potentials negative to −35 mV similar to the NMDA-activated current-voltage relationship (see Figure 2-2A). Plotted values of the early component shown at voltages hyperpolarized to −40 mV underestimate the peak epsc amplitude due to voltage escape of the voltage clamp and were ignored in estimating slope conductance. (Taken from Forsythe and Westbrook [49].)

damage may also fit these criteria [62]. The details of this relationship could be of fundamental importance not only to an understanding of excitatory neurotransmission in the CNS, but could also help to define the border between synaptic plasticity and abnormal hyperexcitability if, indeed, similar mechanisms control both phenomena.

REFERENCES

1. Watkins, J.C. and Evans, R.H. (1981). Excitatory amino acid transmitters. Ann. Rev. Pharmacol. Toxicol. 21, 165–204.
2. Davies, J.D. and Watkins, J.C. (1982). Actions of D and L forms of 2-amino-5-phosphonovalerate and 2-amino-4-phosphonobutyrate in the cat spinal cord. Brain Res. 235, 378–386.
3. Olverman, H.J., Jones, A.W. and Watkins, J.C. (1984). L-glutamate has higher affinity than other amino acids for [^{3}H]-D-AP5 binding sites in rat brain membranes. Nature 307, 460–462.

4. Garthwaite, J. (1985). Cellular uptake disguises action of L-glutamate on N-methyl-D-aspartate receptors. Br. J. Pharmacol. 85, 297–307.
5. Mayer, M.L. and Westbrook, G.L. (1984). Mixed-agonist action of excitatory amino acids on mouse spinal cord neurons under voltage clamp. J. Physiol. (Lond.) 354, 29–53.
6. Hamill, O.P., Marty, A., Neher, A., Sakmann, B. and Sigworth, F.J. (1981). Improved patch-clamp technique for high-resolution current recording from cells and cell-free membrane patches. Pflügers Archiv. 391, 85–100.
7. MacDermott, A.B., Mayer, M.L., Westbrook, G.L. Smith, S.J. and Barker, J.L. (1986). NMDA-receptor activation increases cytoplasmic calcium concentration in cultured spinal cord neurones. Nature 321, 519–522.
8. Engberg, I., Flatman, J.A. and Lambert, J.D.C. (1979). The actions of excitatory amino acids on motoneurones in the feline spinal cord. J. Physiol. (Lond.) 288, 227–261.
9. Lambert, J.D., Flatman, J.A. and Engberg, I. (1981). Actions of excitatory amino acids on membrane conductance and potential in motoneurones. In *Glutamate as a Neurotransmitter*, DiChiari, G. and Gessa, G.L., eds., Raven Press, New York, pp. 205–216.
10. Westbrook, G.L. and Mayer, M.L. (1984). Glutamate currents in mammalian spinal neurons: Resolution of a paradox. Brain Res. 301, 375–379.
11. MacDonald, J.F. and Porietis, A.V. (1982). DL-Quisqualic and L-aspartic acids activate separate excitatory conductances in cultured spinal cord neurons. Brain Res. 245, 175–178.
12. MacDonald, J.F., Porietis, A.V. and Wojtowicz, J.M. (1982). L-aspartic acid induces a region of negative slope conductance in the current voltage relationship of cultured spinal cord neurons. Brain Res. 237, 248–253.
13. Mayer, M.L., Westbrook, G.L. and Guthrie, P.B. (1984). Voltage-dependent block by Mg^{2+} of NMDA responses in spinal cord neurones. Nature 309, 261–263.
14. Nowak, L., Bregestovski, P., Ascher, P., Herbet, A. and Prochiantz, A. (1984). Magnesium gates glutamate-activated channels in mouse central neurones. Nature 307, 462–465.
15. Adams, P.R. (1976). Drug blockade of open end-plate channels. J. Physiol. (Lond.) 260, 531–552.
16. Adams, P.R. (1976). Voltage jump analysis of procaine action at frog end-plate. J. Physiol. (Lond.) 268, 291–318.
17. Neher, E. and Steinbach, J.H. (1978). Local anaesthetics transiently block currents through single acetylcholine-receptor channels. J. Physiol. (Lond.) 277, 153–176.
18. Lingle, C. (1983). Blockade of cholinergic channels by chlorisondamine on a crustacean muscle. J. Physiol. (Lond.) 339, 395–417.
19. Clapham, D.E. and Neher, E. (1984). Substance P reduces acetylcholine-induced currents in isolated bovine chromaffin cells. J. Physiol. (Lond.) 347, 255–277.
20. Mayer, M.L. and Westbrook, G.L. (1985). The action of N-methyl-D-aspartic acid on mouse spinal neurons in culture. J. Physiol. (Lond.) 361, 65–90.
21. Nowycky, M.C., Fox, A.P. and Tsien, R.W. (1985). Three types of neuronal calcium channel with different calcium agonist sensitivity. Nature 316, 440–443.
22. Nowak, L. and Ascher, P. (1985). Divalent cation effects on NMDA-activated channels can be described as Mg-like or Ca-like. Soc. Neurosci. Abs. 11, 953.
23. Diebler, H., Eigen, M., Ilgenfritz, G., Maas, G. and Winkler, R. (1969). Kinetics and mechanism of reactions of main group metal ions with biological carriers. Pure Appl. Chem. 20, 93–115.
24. Mayer, M.L. and Westbrook, G.L. (1987). The physiology of excitatory amino acids in the vertebrate central nervous system. Prog. Neurobiol, 28, 197–276.
25. Westbrook, G.L. and Mayer, M.L. (1987). Micromolar concentrations of Zn^{2+} antagonize NMDA and GABA responses of hippocampal neurons. Nature 328, 640–643.
26. Assaf, S.Y. and Chung, S.H. (1984). Release of endogenous Zn^{2+} from brain tissue during activity. Nature 308, 734–736.
27. Howell, G.A., Welch, M.G. and Frederickson, C.J. (1984). Stimulation-induced uptake and release of zinc in hippocampal slices. Nature 308, 736–738.
28. Dingledine, R. (1983). N-methylaspartate activates voltage-dependent calcium conductances in rat hippocampal pyramidal cells. J. Physiol. (Lond.) 343, 385–405.
29. Bürhle, C.P. and Sonnhof, U, (1983). The ionic mechanism of the excitatory action of L-glutamate upon the membranes of motoneurones of the frog. Pflügers Archiv. 396, 154–162.

30. Pumain, R. and Heinemann, U. (1985). Stimulus- and amino acid-induced calcium and potassium changes in the rat neocortex. J. Neurophysiol. 53, 1–16.
31. Mayer, M.L. and Westbrook, G.L. (1985). Divalent cation permeability of N-methyl-D-aspartate channels. Soc. Neurosci. Abstr. 11, 785.
32. Mayer, M.L. and Westbrook, G.L. (1987). Permeation and block by divalent cations of N-methyl-D-aspartate receptor channels in mouse spinal neurons. J. Physiol. (Lond.) 394, 501–527.
33. Ascher, P. and Nowak, L. (1986). Calcium permeability of the channels activated by N-methyl-D-aspartate (NMDA) in isolated mouse central neurones. J. Physiol. (Lond.) 377, 35.
34. Adams, D.J., Dwyer, T.M. and Hille, B. (1980). The permeability of endplate channels to monovalent and divalent cations. J. Gen. Physiol. 75, 493–510.
35. Lee, K.S. and Tsien, R.W. (1984). High selectivity of calcium channels in single dialysed heart cells of the guinea-pig. J. Physiol. (Lond.) 354, 253–272.
36. Mayer, M.L., MacDermott, A.B., Westbrook, G.L., Smith, S.J. and Barker, J.L. (1987). Agonist- and voltage-gated calcium entry in mouse spinal cord neurons under voltage clamp measured using arsenazo III. J. Neurosci., 7, 3230–3244.
37. Sladeczek, F., Pin, J.P., Récasens, M., Bockaert, J. and Weiss, S. (1985). Glutamate stimulates inositol phosphate formation in striatal neurones. Nature 317, 717–719.
38. Nicoletti, F., Meek, J.L., Iadarola, M.J., Chuang, D.M., Roth, B.L. and Costa, E. (1986). Coupling of inositol phospholipid metabolism with excitatory amino acid recognition sites in rat hippocampus. J. Neurochem. 46, 40–46.
39. Wigström, H., Gustaffson, B., Huang, Y.Y. and Abraham, W.C. (1986). Hippocampal long-term potentiation is induced by pairing single afferent volleys with intracellularly injected depolarizing current pulses. Acta. Physiol. Scand. 126, 317–319.
40. Malinow, R. and Miller, J.P. (1986). Postsynaptic hyperpolarization during conditioning reversibly blocks induction of long-term potentiation. Nature 320, 529–530.
41. Kelso, S.R., Ganong, A.H. and Brown, T.H. (1986). Hebbian synapses in hippocampus. Proc. Natl. Acad. Sci. USA 83, 5326–5330.
42. Davies, J.D. and Watkins, J.C. (1983). Role of excitatory amino acid receptors in mono- and polysynaptic excitation in the cat spinal cord. Exp. Brain Res. 49, 280–290.
43. Finkel, A.S. and Redman, S.J. (1983). The synaptic current evoked in cat spinal motoneurones by impulses in single group Ia axons. J. Physiol. (Lond.) 342, 615–632.
44. Nelson, P.G., Pun, R.Y.K., and Westbrook, G.L. (1986). Synaptic excitation in cultures of mouse spinal cord neurones: Receptor pharmacology and behaviour of synaptic currents. J. Physiol. (Lond.) 372, 169–190.
45. Thomson, A.M. (1986). A magnesium-sensitive post-synaptic potential in rat cerebral cortex resembles responses to N-methylaspartate. J. Physiol. (Lond.) 370, 531–549.
46. Wigström, H., Gustaffson, B. and Huang, Y.Y. (1985). A synaptic potential following single volleys in the hippocampal CA1 region possibly involved in the induction of long-lasting potentiation. Acta. Physiol. Scand. 124, 175–178.
47. Hablitz, J.J. and Langmoen, I.A. (1986). N-methyl-D-aspartate receptor antagonists reduce synaptic excitation in the hippocampus. J. Neurosci. 6: 102–106.
48. Dale, N. and Roberts, A. (1985). Dual-component amino acid-mediated synaptic potentials: Excitatory drive for swimming in *Xenopus* embryos. J. Physiol. (Lond.) 363, 35–59.
49. Forsythe, I.D. and Westbrook, G.L. (1986). Monosynaptic activation of NMDA receptors in mouse spinal cord cultures. Soc. Neurosci. Abstr. 12: 62.
50. Jahr, C.E. and Jessell, T.M. (1985). Synaptic transmission between dorsal root ganglion and dorsal horn neurons in culture: Antagonism of monosynaptic excitatory synaptic potentials and glutamate excitation by kynurenate. J. Neurosci. 5, 2281–2289.
51. Rothman, S.M. and Samaie, M. (1985). Physiology of excitatory synaptic transmission in cultures of dissociated rat hippocampus. J. Neurophysiol. 54, 701–712.
52. Anis, N.A., Berry, S.C., Burton, N.R. and Lodge, D. (1983). The dissociative anaesthetics, ketamine and phencyclidine, selectively reduce excitation of central mammalian neurones by N-methyl-aspartate. Br. J. Pharmacol. 79, 565–575.
53. Honey, C.R., Miljkovic, Z. and MacDonald, J.F. (1985). Ketamine and phencyclidine cause a voltage-dependent block of responses to L-aspartic acid. Neurosci. Lett. 61, 135–139.
54. Nicoll, R.A. and Alger, B.E. (1981). Synaptic excitation may activate a calcium-dependent

potassium conductance in hippocampal pyramidal cells. Science 212, 957–959.
55. Grillner, S. and Wallén, P. (1985). The ionic mechanisms underlying N-methyl-D-aspartate receptor-induced, tetrodotoxin-resistant membrane potential oscillations in lamprey neurons active during locomotion. Neurosci. Lett. 60, 289–294.
56. Dunwiddie, T. and Lynch, G. (1979). The relationship between extracellular calcium concentrations and the induction of hippocampal long-term potentiation. Brain Res. 169, 103–110.
57. Wigström, H., Swann, J.H. and Andersen, P. (1979). Calcium dependency of synaptic long-lasting potentiation in the hippocampal slice. Acta. Physiol. Scand. 105, 126–128.
58. Turner, R.W., Baimbridge, K.G. and Miller, J.J. (1982). Calcium-induced long-term potentiation in the hippocampus. Neuroscience 7, 1411–1416.
59. Collingridge, G.L., Kehl, S.J. and McLennan, H. (1983). Excitatory amino acids in synaptic transmission in the Schaffer collateral-commissural pathway of the rat hippocampus. J. Physiol. (Lond.) 334, 33–46.
60. Wigström, H. and Gustaffson, B. (1984). A possible correlate of the postsynaptic condition for long-lasting potentiation in the guinea pig hippocampus in vitro. Neurosci. Lett. 44, 327–332.
61. Harris, E.W., Ganong, A.H. and Cotman, C.W. (1984). Long-term potentiation in the hippocampus involves activation of N-methyl-D-aspartate receptors. Brain Res. 323, 132–137.
62. Choi, D.W. (1985). Glutamate neurotoxicity in cortical cell culture is calcium dependent. Neurosci. Lett. 58, 293–297.

3. CLASSIFICATION AND ALLOSTERIC MODULATION OF EXCITATORY AMINO ACID SIGNAL TRANSDUCTION IN BRAIN SLICES AND PRIMARY CULTURES OF CEREBELLAR NEURONS

E. COSTA, E. FADDA, A.P. KOZIKOWSKI,
F. NICOLETTI, AND J.T. WROBLEWSKI

Excitatory amino acid receptors have been classified into four major subclasses characterized by their high affinity binding specificity for N-methyl-D-aspartate (NMDA), quisqualate, kainate, and 2-amino-4-phosphonobutyrate (APB), none of which are the endogenous ligands for their recognition sites. This classification is based on the results of electrophysiological and radioligand binding studies [1–5], which are insufficient to express the complete profile of the transmitter receptor function. Transmitter receptor function includes the transduction of an extraneuronal chemical signal into the stimulation of intraneuronal biochemical mechanisms, leading to a change of neuronal function of variable time course. This transduction occurs at synapses and involves the activation of specific enzymes located in the membrane of the postsynaptic cells that are part of a complex receptorial system including a recognition site for the chemical signal, a coupling unit, and a catalytic unit for the production of the intracellular second messenger. Often, instead of generating a second messenger, the receptor activation gates specific ion channels. This generates ion currents that can now be recorded with patch clamp techniques. The intracellular changes induced by these ion fluxes often last longer than the detectable changes in membrane conductance associated with the activation of specific ion channels. Signal transduction might even be silent electrophysiologically when it is mediated by enzymes that form second messengers regulating membrane protein phosphorylation or releasing Ca^{2+} from intracellular stores [6–10]. In this case, as in the case of Ca^{2+} channel activation, the cellular modification ensuing could last minutes, hours, or days, depending on the substrate that is covalently modified by the enzymes

Ferrendelli, J.A., Collins, R.C. and Johnson, E.M. (eds), Neurobiology of Amino Acids, Peptides, and Trophic Factors.

that are activated during the exchange of information. These substrates may include the transmitter recognition sites, allosteric sites modulating transmitter recognition sites, or specific membrane proteins functioning as couplers (the G proteins, for instance). In this instance, the neuronal responsiveness to successive stimuli may change the threshold for the receptor activation, because an enzymatic covalent modification has changed either the recognition site for the transmitter or the recognition site for the allosteric modulator, both released from the presynaptic components of the synapse.

In light of these considerations, excitatory amino acid receptors have been characterized by studying the biochemical mechanisms operative in signal transduction and their regulation by positive and negative allosteric modulators. This approach may stimulate experimentation directed to the search for endogenous modulators of these allosteric sites. The transduction mechanisms considered include: 1) the hydrolysis of membrane inositol phospholipids (PI, PIP, and PIP_2) following the activation of receptor-coupled phospholipase C, which leads to the formation of inositol phosphates and diacylglycerol (DG) [11–18]; 2) the opening of receptor-operated Ca^{2+} channels, resulting in enhanced influx of extracellular Ca^{2+} [19–23]; 3) the increase of cyclic GMP formation due to the activation of guanylate cyclase [24–27]. Cyclic GMP, like cyclic AMP, may activate a specific kinase, although alternative mechanisms might be operative in the second messenger action of cyclic GMP. It has also been investigated whether ions participate in the regulation of these receptors in ways other than being channeled across the neuronal membrane through the opening of specific ion channels. It was found that some of the excitatory transmitter transducer systems are inhibited by Mg^{2+} (μM concentrations) and others are Mg^{2+} resistant. This was utilized as a discriminatory criterion in a provisional classification.

1. COUPLING OF EXCITATORY AMINO ACID RECOGNITION SITES WITH PI HYDROLYSIS IN RAT BRAIN

Excitatory amino acid recognition sites are coupled with PI metabolism in the early stages of postnatal development [13]. Glutamate, aspartate, quisqualate, and ibotenate greatly enhance (from 8- to 15-fold) the accumulation of ^{3}H-inositol monophosphate (IP_1) in slices prepared from the hippocampus, cerebral cortex, corpus striatum, hypothalamus, and cerebellum of 6-day old rats. In these brain slices, the efficacy of excitatory amino acids in enhancing PI hydrolysis is much greater than that of either norepinephrine (NE) or carbamylcholine (Table 3-1). The coupling of excitatory amino acid recognition sites with PI hydrolysis becomes progressively less efficient during brain maturation, and, in 2-month-old rats, only ibotenate retains the ability to stimulate PI hydrolysis [12], while glutamate and aspartate are virtually inactive [13]. In contrast, the stimulation of PI hydrolysis by NE increases postnatally (Figure 3-1) [13]. Starting from the fifteenth day of postnatal life, APB (2-amino-4-phosphonobutyrate) and the endogenous metabolite L-serine-0-

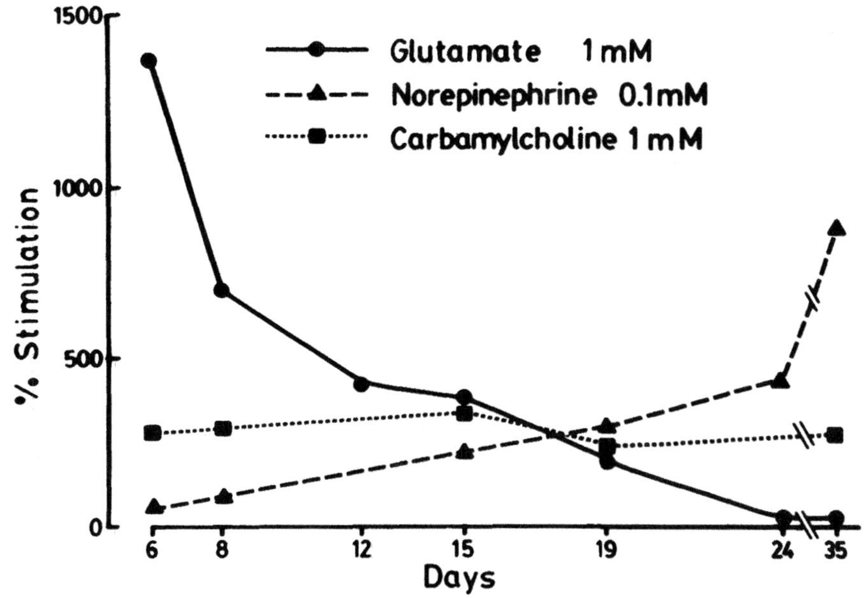

Figure 3-1. Stimulation of PI hydrolysis in rat hippocampal slices during postnatal development. Hippocampal slices prepared from rats of indicated age were incubated with 1 mM glutamate (●), 100 μM norepinephrine (▲), or 1 mM carbamylcholine (■) and the formation of ^{3}H-Ins-1-P was measured as described previously [13]. Data points are means from 4–6 slice preparations with triplicate measurements.

phosphate, two selective ligands of the Ca^{2+}/Cl^--dependent glutamate binding sites, inhibit the action of ibotenate and glutamate [12–14].

In brain slices from adult rats, a new function for glutamate and aspartate emerges: the inhibition of the NE-stimulated PI hydrolysis. This inhibition is specific, as glutamate and aspartate fail to affect the PI hydrolysis stimulated by

Table 3-1. Stimulation of PI hydrolysis in slices of newborn rats by maximal effective doses of neurotransmitters

	^{3}H-Ins-1-P (dmp/mg protein) × 10^3				
	Hippocampus	Striatum	Cerebral cortex	Hypothalamus	Cerebellum
Basal	11 ± 1.4	11 ± 1.2	7.1 ± 0.8	17 ± 1.1	3.7 ± 0.6
Glutamate 1 mM	160 ± 10*	43 ± 1.0*	33 ± 3.2*	55 ± 6.5*	16 ± 1.1*
Norepinephrine 0.1 mM	20 ± 2.6*	n.d.	36 ± 3.3*	n.d.	8.6 ± 0.9*
Carbamylcholine 1 mM	43 ± 3.8*	57 ± 7.1*	16 ± 1.1*	n.d.	7.4 ± 0.5*

Values are means ± S.E.M. from 4–6 determinations.
n.d. = not determined.
* $P < 0.01$, if compared with basal values.

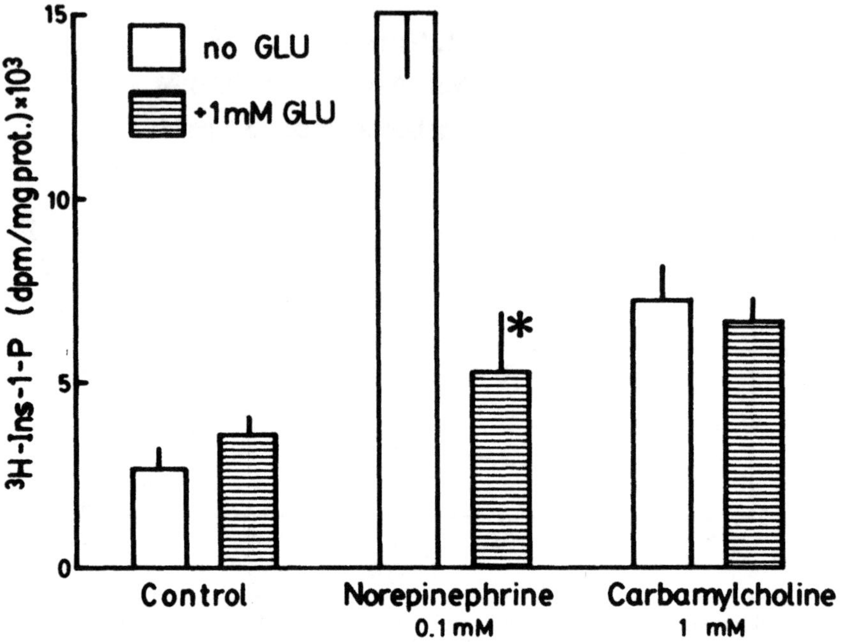

Figure 3-2. Glutamate modulates PI hydrolysis in hippocampal slices stimulated by norepinephrine. Hippocampal slices from adult rats were incubated with 0.1 mM norepinephrine or 1 mM carbamylcholine in the absence (open bars) or presence (hatched bars) of 1 mM glutamate, and the formation of ^{3}H-Ins-1-P was measured as described previously [13]. Data points are means from 4–6 slice preparations with triplicate measurements.

carbamylcholine (Figure 3-2). The interaction between excitatory amino acids and NE does not involve the receptor recognition sites since glutamate fails to modify the specific binding of NE to α_1 adrenoceptors [13]. Perhaps glutamate and NE, while acting on the specific recognition sites of their respective receptors, interact functionally, sharing some components of the signal transduction mechanism of the PI hydrolyzing mechanism of these two receptor domains.

In adult rats, the stimulation of PI hydrolysis by glutamate can be restored following specific lesions of neuronal pathways using glutamate as the putative transmitter [28]. Intrahippocampal infusion with kainate preferentially destroyed the pyramidal cells of the CA3 region [29–31], whose glutamatergic axons innervate the ipsilateral CA1 region and other regions of the contralateral hippocampus [32]. The stimulation of the PI hydrolysis by glutamate is greatly potentiated in slices from the injected or the contralateral hippocampus (Figure 3-3). A similar potentiation of glutamate action was observed in striatal slices after lesion of the corticostriatal glutamatergic fibers performed by ablation of the ipsilateral frontal cortex [33, 34]. These lesions also potentiate the stimulation of PI hydrolysis by NE without affecting that elicited by carbamylcholine (Figure 3-3).

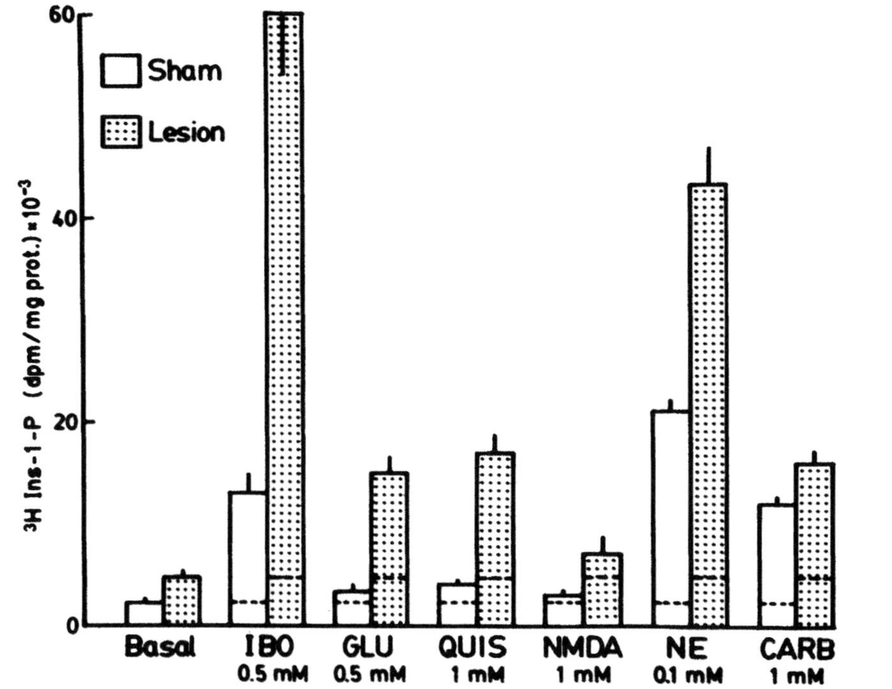

Figure 3-3. Stimulation of PI hydrolysis by transmitter receptor agonists in hippocampal slices of kainate-lesioned rats. Adult rats received intrahippocampal injections of kainate (500 ng/500 nl/2 min.) and were used for experiments 10 days later. Hippocampal slices from sham-operated and lesioned animals were incubated in the presence of the indicated concentrations of transmitter receptor agonists and the formation of ^{3}H-Ins-1-P was measured as described previously [13]. Data points are means from 4 slice preparations with triplicate measurements. IBO = ibotenate; GLU = glutamate; QUIS = quisqualate; NE = norepinephrine; CARB = carbamylcholine.

The coupling of excitatory amino acid recognition sites with PI metabolism appears to undergo plastic modification during the development of and in response to specific lesions of glutamatergic pathways. Hence, it can be speculated that stimulation of PI hydrolysis by excitatory amino acids and the consequent cascade of intracellular events might regulate growth, differentiation, and neuronal response to injuries. The molecular mechanism of this plastic modification is not entirely understood at this time.

2. EXCITATORY AMINO ACID SIGNAL TRANSDUCTION IN PRIMARY CULTURES OF CEREBELLAR NEURONS

To study the molecular nature of the mechanisms whereby excitatory amino acid recognition sites are coupled to specific signal transducing mechanisms, we have used primary cultures of cerebellar neurons prepared from 8-day old rats [15, 35, 36]. These cultures contain over 90% granule cells, 5% GABAergic neurons (Golgi and basket cells), and only 2%–3% non-neuronal cells [35]. Cerebellar neurons in culture release glutamate spontaneously; this release increases following depolarization in a Ca^{2+}-dependent manner [36], suggesting that glutamate may function as a neurotransmitter in granule cells. These cells also express specific excitatory amino acid recognition sites coupled with specific signal transducing mechanisms. The present understanding of these processes suggests that there might be four types of transducing mechanisms for excitatory amino acids. The receptors transducing the transmitter signal via PI hydrolysis are termed G_P (G_{P1} and G_{P2}). Those transducing the transmitter signal via Ca^{2+} influx are termed G_C (G_{C1} and G_{C2}).

2.1. Excitatory amino acid recognition sites coupled to PI hydrolysis

When tested in the presence of 1 mM Mg^{2+}, glutamate and quisqualate are more potent and efficacious than aspartate, kainate, and NMDA in enhancing PI hydrolysis, as measured by the accumulation of ^{3}H-inositol phosphates (Table 3-2) using LiCl as a stabilizer of inositol phosphate metabolism [2]. When 50 μM glutamate is added to the cultures, the stimulation of PI hydrolysis is independent of extracellular calcium. 2-amino-5-phosphonovalerate (APV) antagonizes the action of aspartate, NMDA, and low concentrations of glutamate (1–10 μM) but is virtually ineffective when quisqualate or higher concentrations of glutamate are used to stimulate PI hydrolysis. It can be suggested that glutamate is acting on two types of receptors: One is sensitive to APV and activated by aspartate and NMDA (G_{P1} receptor), and the other (G_{P2}) is APV resistant and is activated by quisqualate. Exposure of primary cultures of cerebellar neurons to pertussis toxin (PTX, 2 μg/16 h) reduced by 65% the stimulation of PI hydrolysis elicited by quisqualate (Table 3-3). The stimulation of PI hydrolysis by glutamate was inhibited by PTX to an extent similar to that of quisqualate if it was measured in the presence of 1 mM APV to eliminate the action of glutamate on the G_{P1} receptor. The inhibitory action of PTX is selective for the activation of G_{P2} receptors by glutamate and quisqualate but fails to affect the stimulation of PI hydrolysis elicited by carbamylcholine (Table 3-3) or by excitatory amino acids acting on G_{P1} receptors. Additionally, in membranes prepared from cultured granule cells, GTP enhances PI hydrolysis in the presence of APV and reduces the specific binding

Table 3-2. Stimulation of PI hydrolysis by excitatory amino acids in primary cultures of granule cells

Mg^{2+} = 1.2 mM	EC_{50} (μM)	Maximal stimulation (% stimulation above basal)
Glutamate	10	460
Quisqualate	20	380
Kainate	30	200
Aspartate	10	130
NMDA	200	120

Table 3-3. Pertussis toxin inhibits the stimulation of PI hydrolysis by quisqualate and gultamate in type G_{P2} receptors of primary cultures of cerebellar granule cells

	^{3}H-Ins-1-P Control	^{3}H-Ins-1P formation (dpm/mg protein × 10^{3}) PTX Treatment
Basal	31 ± 0.7	36 ± 0.2
Quisqualate 0.1 mM	140 ± 6	68 ± 1*
Glutamate 0.1 mM	190 ± 9	130 ± 10*
Glutamate + 1 mM APV	130 ± 5	67 ± 3*
Carbamylcholine 1 μM	250 ± 20	230 ± 15

Granule cells were pretreated with PTX (2μg/16 h). This treatment was shown to cause a NAD-dependent ADP ribosylation of the 41 kDa alpha subunit of GTP-binding protein in cultured granule cells [52].
* $P < 0.01$, if compared with the respective control.

of ^{3}H-glutamate. These data indicate that recognition sites for glutamate associated with G_{P2} receptors are coupled with PI hydrolysis through a PTX-sensitive GTP-binding protein.

Stimulation of PI hydrolysis mediated by the G_{P1} receptor is activated by glutamate but unlike that mediated by G_{P2}, it can be also activated by asparate and NMDA, antagonized by APV, and inhibited by micromolar concentrations of Mg^{2+}; finally, it is allosterically modulated in a negative manner by nanomolar concentrations of phencyclidine (PCP) [15–17, 22, 23, 27, 37–39].

The absence of Mg^{2+} markedly enhances the ^{3}H-IP$_1$ accumulation caused by the addition of specific agonists of G_{P1} receptor; in this condition also, the basal hydrolysis of PI can increase by 8- to 10-fold. This increase is abolished by APV (IC_{50} = 1.5 μM). Thus, in the absence of Mg^{2+}, glutamate, and/or asparate, the two endogenous excitatory amino acids spontaneously released from granule cells, activate signal transduction at G_{P1} receptors. The absence of Mg^{2+} fails to potentiate the stimulation of PI hydrolysis by quisqualate acting at G_{P2} receptors. The stimulation of PI hydrolysis occurring in the absence of Mg^{2+} is resistant to PTX, suggesting that the proteins coupling recognition sites to phospholipase C in G_{P1} receptors differ from those operative in G_{P2} receptors. The coupling of G_{P1} recognition sites with PI hydrolysis can be also differentiated by using low concentrations of Ni^{2+} and Co^{2+}. The stimulation of PI hydrolysis induced by the absence of Mg^{2+} is greatly enhanced by Ni^{2+} and Co^{2+} (Table 3-4). This effect is biphasic, since at concentrations above 100 μM both ions inhibit G_{P1} receptor signal transduction. A wide range of other divalent cations were tested, but all of them displayed only inhibitory effects. The stimulation by low concentrations of Ni^{2+} and Co^{2+} is reversed by APV, confirming that these ions potentiate signal transduction at G_{P1} receptors. When low concentrations of Ni^{2+} are applied, NMDA stimulates PI hydrolysis, even in the presence of Mg^{2+}. In contrast, the stimulation of PI hydrolysis by quisqualate (the selective agonist of G_{P2} receptors) is unaltered by Ni^{2+}. The facilitation of signal transduction by Ni^{2+} is specific for

Table 3-4. Low concentration of Ni^{2+} and Co^{2+} enhance PI hydrolysis in type G_{P1} receptors of primary cultures of cerebellar granule cells

	^{3}H-Ins-1-P (dpm/mg protein) × 10^3	
	$Mg^{2+} = 0$	$Mg^{2+} = 1$ mM
Basal	150 ± 20	14 ± 2
APV 10 μM	25 ± 6*	12 ± 2
Ni^{2+} 10 μM	440 ± 35*	18 ± 2*
Ni^{2+} 1 mM	16 ± 3*	—
Ni^{2+} 10 μM + APV 10 μM	130 ± 20*	—
Co^{2+} 25 μM	310 ± 25*	—
Co^{2+} 1 mM	17 ± 3*	—

Values are means + S.E.M. from 4–6 determinations.
* $P < 0.01$, if compared with basal values.

the stimulation of PI hydrolysis and fails to occur in the signal transduction at G_{C1} receptors. In fact, low concentrations of Ni^{2+} fail to enhance the stimulation of Ca^{2+} uptake and cGMP formation elicited by glutamate, aspartate, and NMDA added to granule cell cultures.

2.2. Excitatory amino acid recognition sites coupled with Ca^{2+} uptake and cyclic GMP formation

Ca^{2+} entry and cGMP formation stimulated by glutamate, aspartate, and NMDA is inhibited by Mg^{2+} (G_{C1} receptor) (Figure 3-4), while that mediated by kainate is not (G_{C2} receptor). Quisqualate has no specific actions on Ca^{2+} uptake and cGMP formation, irregardless of Mg^{2+} concentration. It appears that the stimulation of Ca^{2+} entry by glutamate, aspartate, and NMDA is due to the opening of specific receptor-operated cationic channels different from the voltage-sensitive Ca^{2+} channels, as they are not antagonized by organic Ca^{2+} channels antagonists [20, 22]. These channels allow a slow and sustained rate of Ca^{2+} entry, as opposed to channels activated by kainate (acting at G_{C2} receptors) or by depolarizing agents that cause a fast rate of initial Ca^{2+} entry [40]. The stimulation of cGMP formation by excitatory amino acids is probably a consequence of Ca^{2+} entry, since it cannot be observed in the absence of extracellular Ca^{2+} [27]. This evidence suggests that excitatory amino acid recognition sites may be coupled to guanylate cyclase via increase of Ca^{2+} entry, and cyclic GMP might be operative in the amplification of signal transduction.

In G_{C1} receptors, the Mg^{2+} inhibition of signal transduction can be prevented by depolarization caused by veratridine or high concentrations of K^{+}. Depolarization also abolishes the Mg^{2+} inhibition of PI hydrolysis mediated by the G_{P1} receptor. Membrane depolarization may provide a physiological mechanism whereby signal transduction at G_{P1} and G_{C1} receptors can be activated despite the presence of Mg^{2+} [41–43].

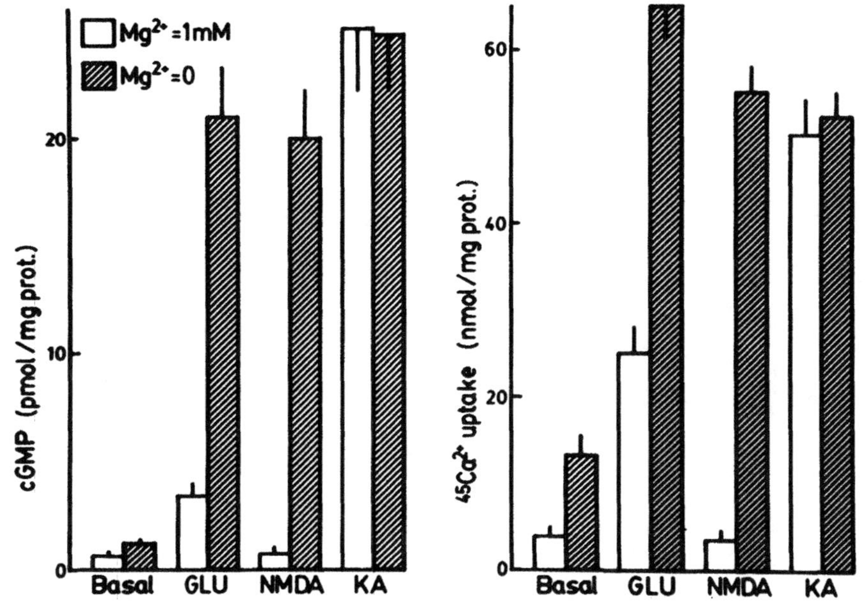

Figure 3-4. Role of Mg^{2+} ions in the stimulation of cyclic GMP formation and $^{45}Ca^{2+}$ uptake by excitatory amino acids in primary cultures of cerebellar granule cells. Cultures of cerebellar granule cells were incubated with 100 μM glutamate (GLU), NMDA, or kainate (KA) in the absence (hatched bars) or in the presence (open bars) of 1 mM Mg^{2+}. Ca^{2+} uptake and cGMP formation were measured as described previously [27, 38]. The values are means ± S.E.M. from five experiments done in triplicate.

The G_{C2} receptors are selectively activated by kainate and inhibited by 2,3-cis-piperidinedicarboxylate (PDA). Kainate stimulates strongly Ca^{2+} influx and cyclic GMP formation. The signal transduction at this receptor is mediated through the opening of specific cationic channels distinct from those activated by ligands of the G_{C1} recognition sites or by veratridine depolarization. The action of kainate at the G_{C2} receptor is neither inhibited by Mg^{2+} (Figure 3-4) nor by PCP (Table 3-5) and APV. However, in cultured cerebellar granule cells, kainate activates the release of endogenous glutamate [15], which, acting at the G_{C1} receptors, contributes to the stimulation of Ca^{2+} influx and cyclic GMP formation induced by kainate.

Quisqualate (50 μM) acts as a potent inhibitor of kainate activation of G_{C2} receptors of granule cells. The inhibition appears noncompetitive (Figure 3-5), suggesting that quisqualate recognition sites may function as allosteric sites for the modulation of signal transduction at the G_{C2} receptors. Such as interaction may occurr at the level of recognition sites, as quisqualate inhibits ^{3}H-kainate binding to membranes prepared from cerebellar granule cells (Figure 3-6). Glutamate also inhibits the stimulation of cGMP formation by kainate when

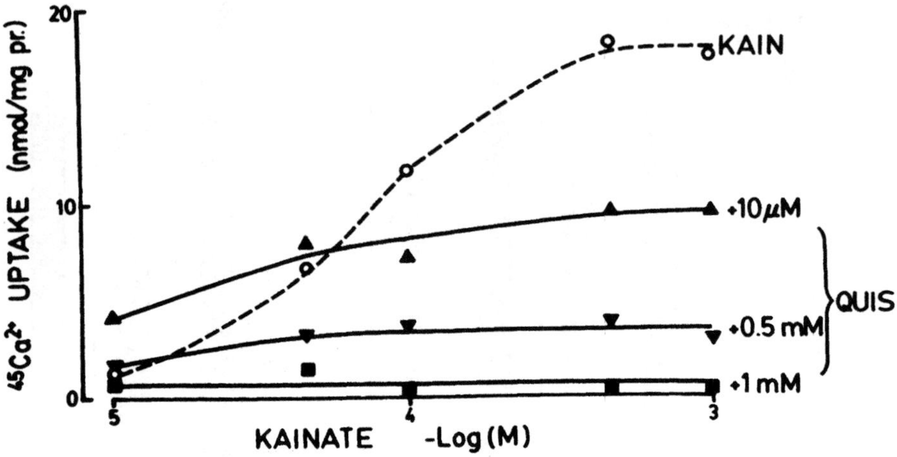

Figure 3-5. Noncompetitive inhibition of kainate-stimulated Ca^{2+} uptake by quisqualate in cerebellar granule cells. Cultured cerebellar granule cells were incubated with $^{45}Ca^{2+}$ in the presence of varying concentrations of kainate (KAIN) and with or without quisqualate (QUIS), and the uptake of $^{45}Ca^{2+}$ was measured as described previously [38]. The values are means from three experiments in triplicate.

its action is tested in the presence of high concentrations of APV in order to abolish any possible activation of the G_{C1} receptor. It is possible that glutamate, as well as quisqualate, binding at a site different from kainate recognition sites, can modulate in a negative manner signal transduction at the kainate (G_{C2}) receptor. This mechanism might have physiological implications.

3. ALLOSTERIC MODULATION OF G_{P1} AND G_{C1} RECEPTORS

Signal transduction at G_{P1} and G_{C1} receptors can be allosterically regulated by phencyclidine (PCP) and a number of its chemical analogues and pharmacological congeners [44–48]. Cerebellar granule cells in primary culture express specific recognition sites for PCP. In crude membrane preparation obtained

Table 3-5. Inhibition of PI hydrolysis by PCP and its functional analogues in primary cultures of cerebellar granule cells in the absence of Mg^{2+}

	IC_{50} (nM)
PCP	50
Dexoxadrol	150
Cyclazocine	170
(+) SKF 10047	210
Ketamine	750
Levoxadrol	Inactive

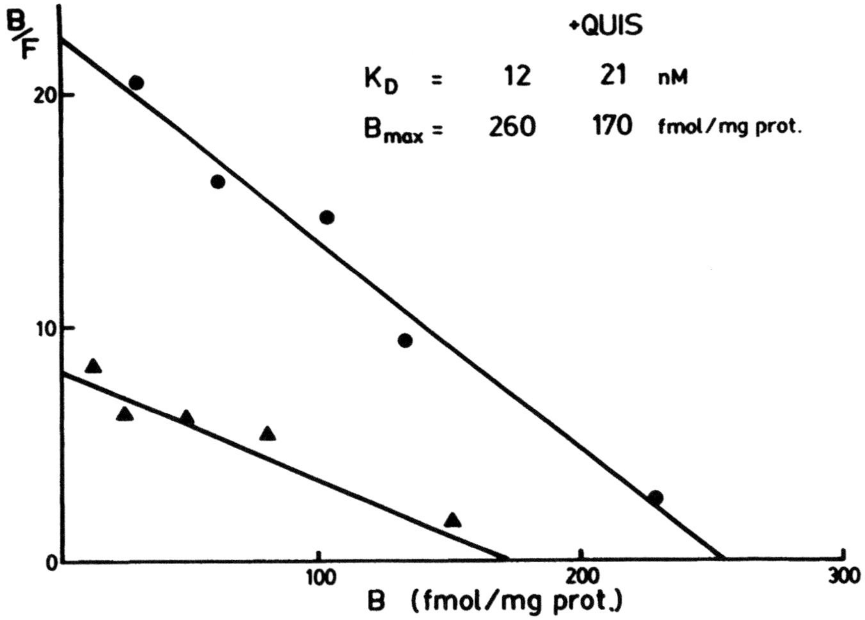

Figure 3-6. Scatchard plot of ^{3}H-kainate binding to membranes prepared from cultured cerebellar granule cells in the absence (●) or presence (▲) of 0.5 μM quisqualate (QUIS).

from these cells, the binding of ^{3}H-PCP reveals the presence of a single class of saturable sites with a K_D = 170 nM and a B_{max} = 4.2 pmol/mg protein. The specific binding of ^{3}H-PCP can be displaced by its pharmacological congeners with the following rank order of potency: PCP>(+)SKF 10047 = dexoxadrol = cyclazocine>ketamine>levoxadrol. The specific binding of PCP is affected by the ligands for the recognition sites of G_{P1} and G_{C1} receptors in such a way that an agonist (glutamate) enhances, while an antagonist (APV) inhibits, PCP binding [46]. The PCP binding sites are located within the supramolecular organization of G_{P1} or G_{C1} receptors. It can be surmised that in the supramolecular structures of G_{C1} receptor recognition sites for PCP may be located within the ionic channel and that the PCP binding to these sites occurs only after the channel is opened by glutamate, aspartate, or NMDA.

PCP and its pharmacological congeners inhibit in a dose-related manner PI hydrolysis, Ca^{2+} influx, and the cyclic GMP formation stimulated by agonists of G_{P1} and G_{C1} receptors. The order of potency of the pharmacological congeners of PCP is similar to that observed in the binding studies (Table 3-5). The PCP inhibition of excitatory amino acid transducer systems was found to be noncompetitive, in fact NMDA, even at 1 mM concentrations, could not overcome the inhibition caused by 0.5 μM PCP. PCP selectively inhibited signal transduction at G_{P1} and G_{C1} receptors (Tables 3-6 and 3-7). Perhaps,

Table 3-6. Allosteric modulation of G_{P1} receptor signal transduction by phencyclidine

Agonist	^{3}H-Ins-1-P formation (dpm/mg protein × 10^4) Without PCP	With 1 μM PCP
Control	2.9 ± 0.1	2.8 ± 0.1
Glutamate 10 μM	10.8 ± 1.0	4.0 ± 0.6*
Aspartate 100 μM	10.3 ± 0.8	3.7 ± 0.4*
NMDA 100 μM	10.4 ± 0.9	2.9 ± 0.2*
Kainate 100 μM	14.0 ± 1.1	7.7 ± 0.9*
Quisqualate 100 μM	15.9 ± 1.5	14.0 ± 0.9

* Significant decrease by PCP ($p < 0.01$) by student's t-test.
Values are means ± S.E.M. from four experiments done in triplicate.

Table 3-7. Selectivity of PCP in inhibiting the formation of cyclic GMP stimulated by excitatory amino acids

	Cyclic GMP (pmol/mg protein) Without PCP	With 1 μM PCP
$Mg^{2+} = 0$		
Basal	3.5 ± 1.0	1.4 ± 0.7*
NMDA 50 μM	38 ± 3	3.5 ± 1.5*
Aspartate 50 μM	27 ± 8	1.6 ± 0.4*
Glutamate 50 μM	35 ± 4	1.4 ± 0.6*
$Mg^{2+} = 1$ mM		
Basal	1.4 ± 0.2	1.0 ± 0.3
Kainate 50 μM	17 ± 2.5	12 ± 0.7*
Kainate + APV 0.1 mM	11 ± 0.9	11 ± 0.4

* Significant decrease by PCP ($p < 0.01$) by student's t-test.
Values are means ± S.E.M. from six to nine experiments.

G_{P1} and G_{C1} receptors are two supramolecular complexes including in their receptor domain an allosteric modulatory site for PCP.

Several structural analogues of PCP were studied in relation to their ability to modulate signal transduction at the G_{C1} receptor. Meta-amino PCP and dehydro-PCP were found to be as potent as PCP in inhibiting the Ca^{2+} uptake stimulated by asparate or NMDA; meta-nitro PCP, cycloheptyl-PCP, and metaphit were less potent. A compound chemically related to PCP (cyano PCP), which displaces ^{3}H-PCP bound to granule cell membranes, acted as a positive allosteric modulator of signal transduction at the G_{C1} receptor. Moreover, it reduced the inhibitory action of PCP (data not shown). Since an endogenous ligand of the PCP recognition site has been identified [49], the PCP recognition site may be the site where endogenous compounds act to modulate G_{P1} and G_{C1} receptor signal transduction allosterically with positive (cyano PCP-like) or negative (PCP-like) cooperativity. A similar mechanism of allosteric modulation of receptor function has been described in the case of $GABA_A$ receptor complex [50, 51].

Table 3-8. Classification of excitatory amino acid receptors in cerebellar granule cells as differentiated by signal transduction

			Allosteric modulators		Transducer		
Type	Agonist	Antagonist	Negative	Positive	Coupler or ionic modulator	Catalytic unit	Messenger
G_{P1}	GLU,ASP,NMDA	APV	PCP	cyano PCP	Mg^{2+} Ni^{2+}	Phospholipase C	IP_3,DG
G_{P2}	QUIS,GLU	?	—	—	G_o	Phospholipase C	IP_3,DG
G_{C1}	GLU,ASP,NMDA	APV	PCP	cyano PCP	Mg^{2+}	Cationic Channel	Ca^{2+},cGMP
G_{C2}	KA	PDA	QUIS,GLU	—	—	Cationic Channel	Ca^{2+},cGMP

4. CONCLUSION

The excitatory amino acid receptors of granule cells and brain slices have been characterized with respect to their signal transducing mechanisms. These results provide evidence that in slices of various structures dissected from rat brain, excitatory amino acid recognition sites are coupled with PI hydrolysis. This coupling undergoes plastic modifications during the development and in response to specific lesions of glutamatergic pathways.

In primary cultures of cerebellar granule cells, four types of receptors for excitatory amino acids have been differentiated and characterized biochemically and pharmacologically. The characteristics of these receptors are summarized in Table 3-8.

It is interesting to note that each receptor, with the only exception of the G_{P2} type, appears to have two regulatory components. This results in a binary system in which an off-on mechanism of primary transmitter action is associated with a modulatory system involving negative and positive cooperativity. An almost infinite variability would characterize signal transduction if this allosteric effect, at present delineated by pharmacological agonists, could be induced by endogenous ligands endowed with physiological function. Since PCP is a drug affecting cognition processes, one might hope that through the study of the allosteric modulation of glutamate receptor complex by PCP, one might find new therapeutic tools to alleviate the symptoms of dementia and other cognitive disorders.

REFERENCES

1. Davies, J., Francis, A.A., Jones, A.W. and Watkins, J.C. (1981). 2-amino-5-phosphonovalerate (2APV), a potent and selective antagonist of amino acid-induced and synaptic excitation. Neurosci. Lett. 21, 77–81.
2. Foster, A.C. and Fagg, G.E. (1984). Acidic amino acid binding sites in mammalian neuronal membranes: Their characteristics and relationship to synaptic receptors. Brain Res. Rev. 7, 103–164.
3. Greenamyre, J.T., Olson, M.M., Penney, J.B., Jr. and Young A.B. (1985). Autoradiographic characterization of N-methyl-D-aspartate, quisqualate and kainate sensitive glutamate binding sites. J. Pharmacol. Exp. Ther. 233, 254–263.
4. McLennan, H. (1981). On the nature of receptors for various excitatory amino acids in the mammalian central nervous system. Adv. Biochem. Psychopharmacol. 27, 253–264.
5. Watkins, J.L. and Evans, R.H. (1981). Excitatory amino acid transmitters. Ann. Rev. Pharmacol. Toxicol. 21, 165–204.
6. Berridge, M.M., Downes, C.P. and Hanley M.R. (1982). Lithium amplifies agonist dependent phosphatidylinositol responses in brain and salivary glands. Biochem. J. 206, 587–595.
7. Berridge, M.J. (1984). Inositoltriphosphate and diacylglycerol as second messengers. Biochem. J. 220, 345–360.
8. Brown, E., Kendall, D.A. and Nahorski, S.R. (1984). Inositol phospholipid hydrolysis in rat cerebral cortical slices: 1. Receptor characterization. J. Neurochem. 42, 1379–1387.
9. Michell, R.H. (1975). Inositol phospholipid and cell surface receptor function. Biochm. Biophys. Acta 415, 81–147.
10. Nishizuka, Y. (1984). Turnover of inositol phospholipids and signal transduction. Science 225, 1365–1370.
11. Iadarola, M.J., Nicoletti, F., Naranjo, J.R., Putnam, F. and Costa, E. (1986). Kindling

enhances the stimulation of inositol phospholipid hydrolysis elicited by ibotenic acid in rat hippocampal slices. Brain Res. 374, 174–178.
12. Nicoletti, F., Meek, J.L., Iadarola, M., Chuang, D.M., Roth, B.L. and Costa, E. (1986). Coupling of inositol phospholipid metabolism with excitatory amino acid recognition sites in rat hippocampus. J. Neurochem. 46, 40–46.
13. Nicoletti, F., Iadarola, M.J., Wroblewski, J.T. and Costa, E. (1986). Excitatory amino acid recognition sites coupled with inositol phospholipid metabolism: Developmental changes and interaction with alpha$_1$-adrenoceptors. Proc. Natl. Acad. Sci. USA 83, 1931–1935.
14. Nicoletti, F., Wroblewski, J.T., Iadarola, M.J. and Costa, E. (1986). Serine-o-phosphate, an endogenous metabolite, inhibits the stimulation of inositol phospholipid hydrolysis elicited by ibotenic acid in rat hippocampal slices. Neuropharmacology 25, 335–338.
15. Nicoletti, F., Wroblewski, J.T., Novelli, A., Alho, H., Guidotti, A. and Costa, E. (1986). The activation of inositol phospholipid metabolism as a signal-transducing system for excitatory amino acids in primary cultures of cerebellar granule cells. J. Neurosci. 6, 1905–1911.
16. Nicoletti, F., Wroblewski, J.T. and Costa, E. (1987). Magnesium ions inhibit the stimulation of inositol phospholipid hydrolysis by endogenous excitatory amino acids in primary cultures of cerebellar granule cells. J. Neurochem., 48, 967–973.
17. Nicoletti, F., Wroblewski, J.T., Novelli, A., Guidotti, A. and Costa, E. (1986). Excitatory amino acid signal transduction in cerebellar cell cultures. Funct. Neurol., 1, 345–349.
18. Sladeczek, F., Pin, J.P., Recasens, M., Bockaert, J. and Weiss, S. (1985). Glutamate stimulates inositol phosphate formation in striatal neurons. Nature 317, 717–719.
19. Lazarewicz, J.W., Lehman, A., Hagberg, H. and Hamberger, A. (1986). Effects of kainic acid on brain calcium fluxes studied in vivo and in vitro. J. Neurochem. 46, 494–498.
20. Riveros, N. and Orrego, F. (1986). N-methylaspartate-activated calcium channels in rat brain cortex slices. Effect of calcium channel blockers and of inhibitory and depressant substances. Neuroscience 17, 541–546.
21. Suszkiw, J.B., O'Leary, M.E., Murawsky, M.M. and Wang, T. (1986). Presynaptic calcium channels in rat cortical synaptosomes: Fast-kinetics of phasic calcium influx, channel inactivation, and relationship to nitrendipine receptors. J. Neurosci. 6, 1349–1357.
22. Wroblewski, J.T., Nicoletti, F. and Costa, E. (1988). Excitatory amino acid receptors in primary cultures of cerebellar granule cells: Two signal transducing mechanisms in receptor-modulated calcium influx. J. Neurochem., in press.
23. Wroblewski, J.T., Nicoletti, F., Fadda, E. and Costa, E. (1986). Regulation of the N-methyl-D-aspartate receptor in cultured cerebellar granule cells (abstr.). Proc. Soc. Neurosci. 16, 960.
24. Ferrendelli, J.A., Chang, M.M. and Kinscherf, D.A. (1974). Elevation of cyclic GMP levels in central nervous system by excitatory and inhibitory amino acids. J. Neurochem. 22, 535–540.
25. Foster, G.A. and Roberts, P.J. (1981). Kainic acid stimulation of cerebellar cyclic GMP levels: Potentiation by glutamate and related amino acids. Neurosci. Lett. 23, 67–70.
26. Mao, C.C., Guidotti, A. and Costa, E. (1974). The regulation of cyclic guanosine monophosphate in rat cerebellum: Possible involvement of putative amino acid neurotransmitters. Brain Res. 73, 510–514.
27. Novelli, A., Nicoletti, F., Wroblewski, J.T., Alho, H., Costa, E. and Guidotti, A. (1987). Excitatory amino acid receptors coupled with guanylate cyclase in primary cultures of cerebellar granule cells. J. Neurosci., 7, 40–47.
28. Nicoletti, F., Wroblewski, J.T., Alho, H., Eva, C. Fadda, E. and Costa, E. (1987). Lesions of putative glutamatergic pathways potentlate the increase of inositol phospholipid hydrolysis elicited by excitatory amino acids. Brain Res., 436, 103–112.
29. French, E.D., Aldinio, C. and Schwarcz, R. (1982). Intrahippocampal kainic acid, seizures and local degeneration: Relationships assessed in unanesthetized rats. Neuroscience 7, 2525–2538.
30. Nadler, J.V., Perry, B.W. and Cotman, C.W. (1978). Intraventricular kainic acid preferentially destroys hippocampal pyramidal cells. Nature (Lond.) 271, 676–677.
31. Schwob, J.E., Fuller, T., Price, J.L. and Olney, J.W. (1980). Widespread patterns of neuronal damage following systemic or intracerebral injections of kainic acid: A histological study. Neuroscience 5, 991–1014.
32. Storm-Mathisen, J. (1981). Autoradiographic and microchemical localization of high affinity glutamate uptake. In: *Glutamate: Transmitter in the Central Nervous System*, Roberts, P.J.,

Storm-Mathisen, J. and Johnston, G.A., eds., John Wiley & Sons, Chichester, New York, pp. 89–115.
33. Druce, D., Peterson, D., De Belleroche, J. and Bradford, H.F. (1982). Differential amino acid neurotransmitter release in rat neostriatum following lesions of the corticostriatal pathway. Brain Res. 247, 303–307.
34. Fonnum, F., Storm-Mathisen, J. and Divac, I. (1981). Biochemical evidence for glutamate as a neurotransmitter in corticostriatal and corticothalamic fibers in rat brain. Neuroscience 6(5), 863–873.
35. Currie, N.D. (1980). Identification of cell type by immuno-fluorescence in defined cell cultures of cerebellum. In *Tissue Culture in Neurobiology*, Giacobini E., Vernadakis A. and Shahar A., eds., Raven Press, New York, pp. 75–87.
36. Gallo V., Ciotti M.T., Coletti F., Aloisi F. and Levi G. (1982). Selective release of glutamate from cerebellar granule cells differentiating in culture. Proc. Natl. Acad. Sci. USA 79, 7919–7923.
37. Nicoletti, F., Wroblewski, J.T., Fadda, E. and Costa, E. (1986). Interactions between phencyclidine and excitatory amino acid receptors in the regulation of signal transduction in primary cultures of cerebellar granule cells (abstr.). The Pharmacologist 28, 237.
38. Wroblewski, J.T., Nicoletti, F. and Costa, E. (1985). Different coupling of excitatory amino acid receptors with Ca^{2+} channels in primary cultures of cerebellar granule cells. Neuropharmacology 24, 919–921.
39. Wroblewski, J.T., Nicoletti, F., Fadda, E., Kozikowski, A.P. and Costa E. (1986). Signal transduction at excitatory amino acid receptors in cerebellar cell cultures: Regulatory role of phencyclidine recognition sites. Clin. Neuropharmacol. 9 (suppl. 4), 494–496.
40. Carboni, E., Wojcik, W.J. and Costa, E. (1985). Dihydropyridines change the uptake of calcium induced by depolarization into primary cultures of cerebellar granule cells. Neuropharmacology 24, 1123–1126.
41. Dingledine, R. (1983). N-methyl aspartate activates voltage-dependent calcium conductance in rat hippocampal pyramidal cells. J. Physiol. (Lond.) 343, 385–405.
42. Mayer, M.L., Westbrook, G.L. and Guthrie, P.B. (1984). Voltage-dependent block by Mg^{2+} of NMDA responses in spinal cord neurones. Nature 309, 261–263.
43. Novak, L., Bregestovski, P., Ascher, P., Herbet, A. and Prochiantz A. (1984). Magnesium gates glutamate-activated channels in mouse central neurones. Nature 307, 462–465.
44. Anis, N.A., Berry, S.C., Burton, N.R. and Lodge, D. (1983). The dissociative anaesthetics, ketamine and phencyclidine, selectively reduce excitation of central mammalian neurones by N-methyl-aspartate. Br. J. Pharmacol. 79, 565–575.
45. Duchen, M.R., Burton, N.R. and Biscoe, T.J. (1985). An intracellular study of the interactions of N-methyl-DL-aspartate with ketamine in the mouse hippocampal slice. Brain Res. 342, 149–153.
46. Loo, P., Braunwalder, A., Lehmann, J. and Williams, M. (1986). Radioligand binding to central phencyclidine recognition sites is dependent on excitatory amino acid receptor agonists. Eur. J. Pharmacol. 123, 467–468.
47. Maragos, W.F., Chu, D.C., Geenamyre, J.T., Penney, J.B. and Young A.B. (1986). High correlation between the localization of [^{3}H]TCP binding and NMDA receptors. Eur. J. Pharmacol. 123, 173–174.
48. Snell, L.D. and Johnson, K.M. (1985). Antagonism of N-methyl-D-aspartate induced transmitter release in the rat striatum by phencyclidine-like drugs and its relationship to turning behavior. J. Pharmacol. Exp. Ther. 235, 50–57.
49. Quirion, R., DiMaggio, D.A., French, E.D., Contreras, P.C., Shiloach, J., Pert, C.B., Everist, H., Pert, A. and O'Donohue, T.L. (1984). Evidence for an endogenous peptide ligand for the phencyclidine receptor. Peptides 5, 967–973.
50. Costa, E. and Guidotti, A. (1979). Molecular mechanisms in the receptor action of benzodiazepines. Ann. Rev. Pharmacol. Toxic. 19, 531–545.
51. Costa, E., Guidotti, A., Mao, C.C. and Suria, A. (1975). New concepts on the mechanisms of action of benzodiazepines. Life Sci. 17, 167–186.
52. Xu, J. and Wojcik, W.J. (1986). $GABA_B$ receptor mediated inhibition of adenylate cyclase in cultured cerebellar granule cells: Blockade by islet activating protein (IAP). J. Pharmacol. Exp. Ther. 239, 568–573.

4. EXCITATORY TRANSMITTERS AND NEUROPSYCHIATRIC DISORDERS*

JOHN W. OLNEY

In recent years, the possible role(s) of excitatory amino acid (EAA) transmitters in neuropsychiatric disorders has become a topic of considerable interest. Two rather dissimilar hypotheses have evolved: 1) that excess EAA receptor stimulation might be the mechanism underlying certain neurodegenerative disorders; 2) that insufficient EAA receptor stimulation may lead to psychotic processes and/or memory dysfunction. Here evidence relevant to each of these hypotheses will be discussed.

1. EAA AND NEURODEGENERATIVE DISEASES

In recent decades, EAAs such as glutamate (Glu), aspartate (Asp), and possibly certain sulfur amino acids have become recognized as the leading neurotransmittter candidates at the majority of excitatory synapses in the mammalian central nervous system (CNS); ironically, these agents also are neurotoxins [1], and it is reasonably well established that EAA neurotoxicity is mediated through postsynaptic excitatory receptors by a depolarization mechanism. Given the high concentrations of EAA in the CNS, it follows that these endogenous excitatory neurotoxins (excitotoxins) might play a role in neurodegenerative diseases. Several possibilities have been suggested by recent findings.

* Supported in part by NIMH Research Scientist Award (MH 38894) and a grant from the Washington University/Monsanto Biomedical Research Fund.

Ferrendelli, J.A., Collins, R.C. and Johnson, E.M. (eds), Neurobiology of Amino Acids, Peptides, and Trophic Factors.

1.1. Conditions in which excitotoxins may be implicated

1.1.1. Sulfite oxidase deficiency

The first human neurodegenerative condition to receive attention as a possible excitotoxin-mediated phenomenon was sulfite oxidase deficiency, a rare metabolic disease that involves widespread degeneration of central neurons in early childhood. Cysteine-S-sulfonic acid (CSS), an abnormal metabolite structurally resembling the excitotoxin homocysteic acid, accumulates in high concentrations in body tissues in this condition. This might explain neuronal degeneration, since CSS potently induces a Glu-like lesion locally when injected directly into adult rat brain [2].

1.1.2. Seizure-related brain damage

Accumulating evidence (reviewed in Ref. 3) suggests that the brain damage associated with human epilepsy can be explained in terms of excessive seizure-mediated release and accumulation of endogenous EAA at central synapses. It has been shown, for example, that persistent focal motor seizure activity in the corticothalamic tract, a pathway that uses Glu as transmitter, results in acute Glu-like lesions in specific thalamic neurons innervated by this tract [4]. Similarly, persistent electrical stimulation of the perforant path (glutamergic tract innervating the hippocampus) results in Glu-like degenerative changes in specific hippocampal neural elements receiving perforant path afferents [5]. Recently, it was observed that ketamine, a blood-brain barrier-permeable EAA antagonist, prevents seizure-related brain damage when administered systemically to rats [6]. Presumably an anti-excitotoxic mechanism underlies such protection; whether an anticonvulsant mechanism also contributes is uncertain, since ketamine mildly suppresses, but does not prevent, seizure activity.

1.1.3. Hypoglycemic brain damage

Weiloch and colleagues [7] have presented evidence that brain damage associated with hypoglycemia may be excitotoxin-mediated; they have shown, for example, that microinjection of EAA receptor antagonists into the striatum, a region consistently damaged bilaterally by hypoglycemia in the rat, prevents such damage on the injected (but not uninjected) side of the brain.

1.1.4. Anoxic-ischemic brain damage

Several authors have recently proposed that neuronal death associated with cerebral anoxia is mediated by an excitotoxic mechanism (reviewed in Ref. 8). Cultured hippocampal neurons subjected to anoxic conditions are protected from acute neuronal necrosis by adding an EAA receptor antagonist to the culture medium [9]; endogenous excitotoxins (Glu and Asp) accumulate extracellularly in the hippocampus of rats subjected to experimental cerebral ischemia [10]. Unilateral injection of an EAA antagonist into the ischemic hippocampus protects neurons from acute necrosis in the vicinity of the injection [11]. Histologically, acute neuronal degeneration induced in immature rat brain by a combination of anoxic and ischemic circumstances appears very similar to that induced in the immature rodent hypothalamus or retina by systemic administration of exogenous Glu (Fig. 4-1). Since cerebral anoxia (stroke, cardiac arrest, perinatal asphyxia, etc.) is a common cause of irreversible brain damage, evidence implicating endogenous excitatory transmitters in these conditions is potentially of considerable importance.

1.1.5. *Huntington's chorea*

When a potent excitotoxic analog of Glu, such as kainic acid or ibotenic acid, is injected into the rat striatum, it destroys local nerve cells without damaging axons of passage. Since loss of striatal neurons with preservation of axon tracts is the type of tissue pathology observed in Huntington's chorea, excitotoxin lesioning has been used to produce an animal model for studying the human disease. In addition, it has been proposed that endogenous Glu may play a role in the pathogenesis of neuronal degeneration in Huntington's chorea, since striatal neurons are heavily innervated by corticostriatal axons that use Glu as transmitter (reviewed in Ref. 12). More recent speculation has focused on the endogenous excitotoxic tryptophan metabolite, quinolinic acid, since striatal neurons are differentially sensitive to its neurotoxic action, and it was recently demonstrated that injection of this agent into the rat striatum reproduces a unique feature of the human disease, sparing of somatostatin-containing neurons, while nearly every other type of neuron in the striatum degenerates [13]. Since quinolinic acid, unlike Glu, is ordinarily present in brain in only trace amounts, its complicity in the human disease can presumably be ruled in or out by measuring its content in the striata of Huntington's patients; however, to date no such measurements have been reported.

1.1.6. *Alzheimer's senile dementia*

Loss of basal forebrain cholinergic neurons that project to the cerebral cortex, hippocampus, and amygdala is a striking feature of the neuropathology of Alzheimer's disease, which can be reproduced in experimental animals by injection of an excitotoxin into the basal forebrain, where these cells are located. This has provided a useful animal model for studying the role of cholinergic neurons in the cognitive deficits associated with Alzheimer's disease. The fact that excitotoxins are effective in destroying cholinergic neurons implies that these neurons have EAA receptors through which endogenous excitotoxins could act pathologically to destroy these neurons; thus, it is conceivable that neuronal degeneration in Alzheimer's disease is mediated by an excitotoxic mechanism. Consistent with this hypothesis, Young and associates [14] recently demonstrated that there is a striking loss of Glu receptors in the cerebral cortex and hippocampus of brains of Alzheimer patients. This suggests a selective loss of neurons and/or dendritic processes containing EAA postsynaptic receptors, which is the expected consequence of an excitotoxic process.

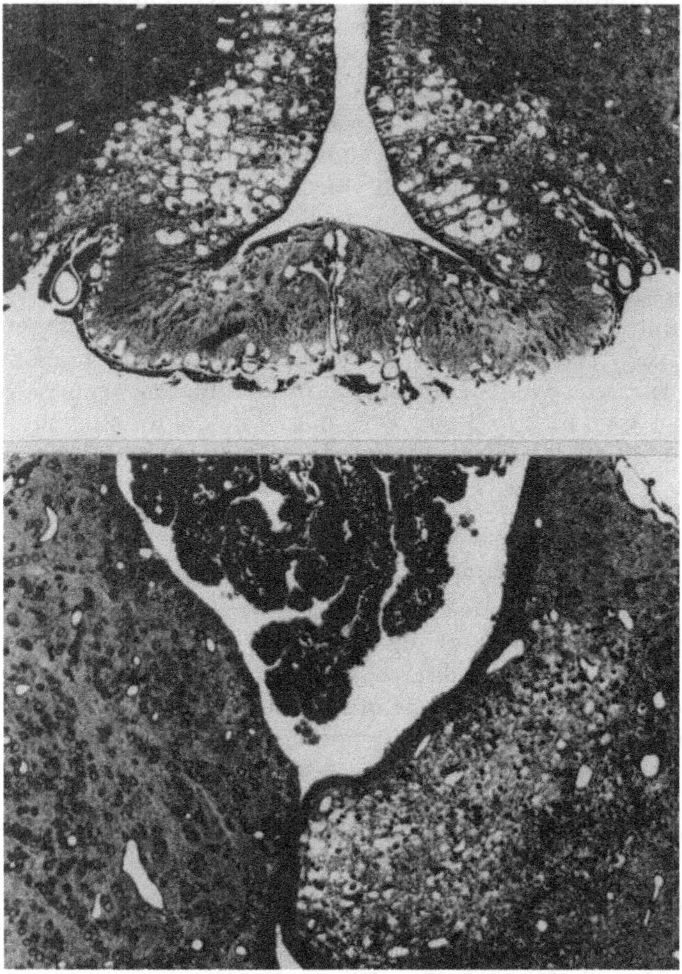

Figure 4-1. Top — light micrograph of the arcuate nucleus of the immature mouse hypothalamus 4 hours after ingestion of an aqueous solution of monosodium glutamate. Acutely degenerating neurons are readily identified as bulls eye profiles (vacuous swollen cytoplasm surrounding a dark shrunken pyknotic nucleus) distributed bilaterally in the arcuate area. This is the typical appearance of neurons undergoing acute necrosis following exposure to exogenous Glu (× 180).

Bottom — light micrograph of the medial habenular nucleus of an immature rat 16 hours following unilateral ligation of the common carotid artery and 2½ hrs of oxygen deprivation (8% O_2, balance N_2). Neuronal degeneration occurs only on the side of the brain ipsilateral to the carotid ligation and has a predilection for neocortex, striatum, hippocampus, medial habenulum, and several thalamic regions. The acutely necrotic neurons (bulls eye profiles) in the right habenular nucleus are identical to those destroyed by exogenous Glu in the photograph above, except that the habenula lesion, being of longer duration (16 hours vs. 4 hours) has a larger number of condensed dark structures that no longer display conspicuous cytoplasmic swelling (× 140).

1.2. Pathophysiology of excitotoxic phenomena

The cytopathology associated with sustained seizure activity, when examined by electron microscopy in its acute stages, is indistinguishable from the acute cytopathology resulting from direct exposure of neurons to exogenous Glu or other excitotoxic agonists [15]. Other neurodegenerative syndromes in which excitotoxins have been implicated, although not as well-studied histologically in acute stages, appear also to involve a similar type of cytopathology. For example, in a recent histopathological evaluation of the brains of infant rats subjected to unilateral carotid ligation and 2½ hour exposure to an hypoxic environment (8% oxygen, balance nitrogen), it was observed (Olney et al., unpublished) that the acute cytopathology (massive swelling of dendrites and neuronal cell bodies with pyknotic changes in the neuronal nucleus) is identical to that induced in the infant hypothalamus by systemic administration of monosodium glutamate (Figure 4-1).

Under anoxic-ischemic conditions, it has been demonstrated that there is a striking increase in Glu and Asp concentrations in the extracellular compartment of rat brain [10]. The basis for this is not clear; however, since energy-dependent transport mechanisms responsible for reuptake of Glu and Asp may be severely compromised under anoxic-ischemic conditions, failure of reuptake is likely to play an important role. A similar mechanism may be operative in seizure-related brain damage; i.e., the depolarization/repolarization process associated with persistent firing of axon terminals may diminish the energy available at the synaptic level to drive the EAA reuptake system, rendering it unable to efficiently remove endogenous EAA from the synaptic cleft. Brain damage associated with hypoglycemia also presumably entails energy deficiency and impaired reuptake of endogenous excitotoxins.

The role of depolarization as an initial step in the pathophysiology of the excitotoxic process is documented by the observation that only those analogs of Glu that mimic its depolarizing effects also mimic its neurotoxic properties and that the neurotoxic potency of each of these agents is proportional to its potency as a depolarizing agent [1]. Moreover, antagonists that block the excitatory actions of EAA display parallel blocking action against their neurotoxic effects [16]. In Table 4-1, various agents are compared for their ability to protect retinal neurons against the neurotoxic actions of the potent glutamate agonists, N-methyl aspartate (NMA), and kainic acid (KA). The anti-excitotoxic activity demonstrated for each agent is proportional to its ability to antagonize the excitatory actions of these agonists in electrophysiological studies [16, 17].

In terms of ionic events, it is thought that the depolarizing action of Glu and related EAA entails an inward Na^+ conductance; consistent with this, it appears that the neurotoxic action of EAA is Na^+-dependent, i.e., the toxic action of EAA agonists on cultured rat hippocampal neurons [18] or chick retinal neurons [19] is prevented by substituting benzoyl choline, an impermeant cation, for Na^+. The toxic action is also prevented by substituting isethionate, an impermeant anion, for Cl^- [18, 19]. Thus, in addition to an initial depolarization-related influx of Na^+, an unregulated passive influx of chloride is believed to be a critical feature of the acute neurotoxic action of EAA. Dependence on Na^+ and Cl^- and lack of dependence on Ca^{2+} has been demonstrated for the excitotoxic actions of NMA and KA as well as Glu [18].

A special situation exists with respect to the NMA receptor in that it is functionally linked to an ion channel that is subject to a voltage-dependent open channel block by Mg^{2+} [20]. High concentrations of Mg^{2+} antagonize both the excitatory [17] and neurotoxic [19] actions of NMA, and low concentrations of Mg^{2+} augment (disinhibit) these actions. Thus, the age-old practice of using $MgS0_4$ in clinical medicine to suppress CNS irritability and/or seizures may have a rational basis — the modulation by Mg^{2+} of the NMA receptor/ion channel complex. The most potent known antagonists of the excitatory [21] and neurotoxic [16] actions of NMA are not agents, such as D-aminophosphonopentanoate, that competitively inhibit binding of NMA to its EAA receptor, but rather are agents in the phencyclidine/sigma opiate category (Table 4-1) that bind at their own receptor, which is closely associated with the NMA receptor/ion channel complex. The actions of other EAA agonists such as KA and quisqualic acid are not influenced either by Mg^{2+} or by agents in the phencyclidine/sigma opiate category.

The role of Ca^{2+} in excitotoxin-induced cell death is an important issue that requires further clarification. The acute edematous degeneration that has classically been identified as an excitotoxic reaction occurs just as readily in the absence as in the presence of Ca^{2+}. This has been demonstrated both in cultured rat hippocampal neurons [18] and the ex vivo chick embryo retina [19]. Choi [22] has presented evidence, however, for a less acute form of excitotoxin-induced neuronal death that may be Ca^{2+} dependent. He found that exposing cultured rat cerebral cortical neurons to Glu for only a few minutes, then removing Glu from the medium, resulted in delayed neuronal death in 24 hours, provided Ca^{2+} was present when the culture was initially exposed to Glu. This raises the intriguing possibility that there may be two mechanisms by which excitotoxins can induce neuronal death, one being the acute fulminating reaction studied in our lab and by Rothman, which is not Ca^{2+} dependent, and the other being a slowly evolving neurotoxic process that is Ca^{++} dependent.

The distinction between fast and slow excitotoxin-induced cell death may be of greater importance than would appear at first glance. Activation of the rapid mechanism probably requires a relatively sudden change in excitotoxin homeostasis, resulting in a rapid and relatively persistent rise in extracellular excitotoxin concentrations to very high levels. Less extreme circumstances are not uncommonly encountered in clinical medicine (for example, in transient cardiac arrest, perinatal asphyxia, etc.); indeed, even in the case of a cerebral embolus or rapidly evolving stroke, the excitotoxin accumulation may be time-limited, especially at the margins of the ischemic tissue zone, since the

Table 4-1. Potencies of antagonists in blocking L-HCA, NMA, or KA neurotoxicity.

Potential antagonist	vs L-HCA (250 μM)	vs NMA (200 μM)	vs KA (25 μM)
Phencyclidine	0.5	0.5	—
Ketamine	10	5	—
(±)-SKF 10,047	10	10	—
Pentazocine	25	25	—
D-aminophosphonopentanoate	20	25	*
D-aminophosphonoheptanoate	75	75	*
D-α-aminoadipate	200	200	—
3-0H-2-quinoxaline carboxylate	200	200	2000
Kynurenate	200	200	750
(±)-cis-2,3-piperidine dicarboxylate	500	500	2000
Secobarbital	500	600	600
L-aminophosphonobutyrate	—	—	—
D-aminophosphonobutyrate	—	—	—
L-glutamic acid diethyl ester	—	—	—
Xanthurenate	—	—	—
γ-amino-n-butyrate (GABA)	—	—	—
Taurine	—	—	—

Compounds were rated according to the minimal concentration (μM) required to provide total protection against L-homocysteic acid (L-HCA) (250 μM), N-methyl-aspartate (NMA) (200 μM), or kainic acid (KA) (25 μM) toxicity. Antagonists were tested over a range of doses from 3000 μM downward and are listed in order of their potencies in blocking NMA toxicity. When no blocking was observed at 3000 μM, this is indicated by a dash (−). Partial blocking at 3000 μM is indicated by asterisk.

EAA reuptake mechanisms, although transiently impaired, may not be entirely incapacitated. Thus, many neurons may be exposed only briefly to very high concentrations of Glu (as in the Choi experiments) and might be expected to undergo a slow calcium-dependent degenerative process rather than acute fulminating cell death. If so, this may have important therapeutic implications, since the delayed nature of the neurotoxic process assures a wider time window for application of neuroprotective strategies, and the mechanism, having both an excitotoxin and calcium-dependent component, can possibly be blocked both by EAA antagonists and by pharmacological agents that act on calcium channels. Another important implication of the delayed excitotoxic concept is that it provides a plausible explanation for the involvement of excitotoxins in chronic neurodegenerative diseases such as Huntington's chorea or Alzheimer's dementia. In such cases, one might postulate a mechanism whereby pathological stimulation of EAA receptors occurs at low intensity over a protracted time course until the neuron by a calcium-dependent delayed mechanism slowly dies.

2. EAA AND PSYCHOSIS OR MEMORY DYSFUNCTION

2.1. Psychosis

Kim et al. [23] have advanced the view that schizophrenic psychoses stem from hypofunction of the EAA transmitter system. They support this proposal with evidence that cerebrospinal fluid (CSF) levels of Glu are lower than normal in schizophrenic patients, that amphetamines produce schizophrenia-like symptoms in humans and decreased CSF levels of Glu in rats, and that treatment of schizophrenics with antipsychotic agents increases CSF levels of Glu. Also consistent with the Glu hypothesis is evidence that Boclofen, which inhibits Glu release, causes a worsening of symptoms in schizophrenia [24]. Overactivity of the dopaminergic transmitter system has been hypothesized as the biochemical basis for schizophrenia. The Glu hypothesis does not compete with or contradict the dopamine hypothesis; rather, it improves its explanatory power, i.e., dopamine receptors are thought to inhibit Glu release so that excess dopaminergic activity would suppress Glu release, resulting in Glu hypofunction as the basis for schizophrenic symptoms. Amelioration of schizophrenic symptoms by dopamine receptor blockers (neuroleptics) might be explained in terms of the dopamine receptor blockade disinhibiting Glu release and correcting Glu hypofunction. Although the Glu hypothesis has not been widely accepted, it is substantially strengthened by recent evidence that certain sigma opiates and dissociative anesthetics that have potent psychotomimetic properties powerfully antagonize EAA transmission, i.e., render the EAA transmitter system hypofunctional [16, 21] (also see Table 4-1). It should be noted that these agents antagonize activity mediated through only one EAA receptor type, the N-methylaspartate (NMA) receptor.

2.2. Memory dysfunction

Lynch and colleagues [25] have proposed that stimulation of NMA receptors and, perhaps, an up-regulation of such receptors in the hippocampus (long-term potentiation) may be an integral step in the process of memory formation. These authors reported that intraventricular administration of an NMA antagonist blocks both long-term potentiation and memory (place learning). If EAA mediate memory via long-term potentiation and up-regulation of NMA receptors, hypofunction of these receptors might cause memory impairment. One can argue, however, that if hypofunction of NMA receptors underlies both memory impairment and schizophrenic psychoses, two different subsets of NMA receptors must be involved, since memory is not impaired in schizophrenia. In any event, it remains a possibility that manipulating NMA receptor systems for anti-excitotoxic purposes might impair memory unless the subset(s) of NMA receptors mediating neurodegenerative events can be differentiated from subsets mediating memory and be targeted separately by selective pharmaceutical agents.

3. THERAPEUTIC/PROPHYLACTIC CONSIDERATIONS

While it is now well established that there are several subtypes of EAA receptors, it appears that the NMA receptor subtype may comprise greater than 80% of the EAA receptors in brain [26]. In experiments showing that an EAA antagonist can prevent the neuronal necrosis associated with anoxia or hypoglycemia [7, 9, 11], it was an antagonist of the NMA receptor that was employed. Thus, of the several EAA receptor subtypes, it appears that the NMA receptor is the most logical target for therapeutic/prophylactic manipulations in either neurodegenerative conditions or psychotic processes. Fortunately, compared with other EAA receptor subtypes, greater strides have been and are being made in understanding the NMA receptor and in developing agents that antagonize this receptor or its associated Mg^{2+} sensitive ion channel (Table 4-1). It must be borne in mind, however, that to ameliorate neurodegenerative conditions one would want to decrease activity at NMA receptors, whereas to ameliorate psychotic processes one would want to increase activity at these receptors. Therefore, it is possible that efforts to treat one condition might cause serious side effects symptomatically resembling the other condition.

4. NATURAL TRANSMITTER AT NMA RECEPTOR

In view of the potential importance of the NMA receptor in CNS physiology and pathology, it is noteworthy that the natural transmitter at this receptor remains unknown. Quang Do and colleagues [27] have suggested L-homocysteic acid (L-HCA) as a possible candidate in that it is a potent excitant that is released in significant concentrations by a Ca^{2+}-dependent mechanism from K^+ stimulated brain slices and has been localized immunohistochemically to specific brain regions where NMA receptors are highly concentrated. In the ex vivo chick embryo retina, it was observed [28] that L-HCA is essentially interchangeable with NMA as a neurotoxin — the two agents are approximately equal in potency and induce cytopathological reactions affecting the same retinal cells (in contrast to kainic acid, which affects different cells). Moreover, numerous NMA antagonists were found to have the same order of potencies in blocking the neurotoxic actions of L-HCA and NMA (Table 4-1). In addition, it was shown in receptor binding experiments that L-HCA is more effective than NMA in inhibiting ^{3}H-Glu binding and that the pattern of ^{3}H-Glu displacement in receptor autoradiograms is similar for the two agents. Thus, available evidence is entirely consistent with the proposal that L-HCA may function as natural transmitter at NMA receptors. Of course, L-Glu and L-Asp, although not as potent as L-HCA, also remain potential candidates as transmitters at NMA receptors.

5. CONCLUSION

Two hypotheses pertaining to the role of EAA in neuropsychiatric disorders have been discussed: 1) that excessive stimulation of EAA receptors might give rise to neurodegenerative diseases and 2) that hypofunction of EAA transmitter systems might result in psychotic processes and/or memory dysfunction. It would be ironic if both hypotheses were proven correct, as efforts to treat or prevent one type of condition might precipitate symptoms of the other. Accumulating evidence suggests that a specific subtype of EAA receptor — the NMA receptor — may play a central role both in normal CNS physiology and the pathological phenomena mentioned above. Recent evidence suggests that, in addition to Glu and Asp, L-HCA is a logical transmitter candidate at NMA receptors. Since progress in identifying agents that block transmission through NMA receptors continues at a rapid pace, the prospects for developing successful therapies for EAA-mediated neurodegenerative disorders seems favorable, provided serious side effects of such treatment can be avoided.

REFERENCES

1. Olney, J.W., Ho, O.L. and Rhee, V. (1971). Cytotoxic effects of acidic and sulphur-containing amino acids on the infant mouse central nervous system. Exp. Brain Res. 14, 61–76.
2. Olney, J.W., Misra, C.H. and deGubareff, T. (1975). Cysteine-S-sulfate: Brain damaging metabolite in sulfite oxidase deficiency. J. Neuropathol Exp. Neurol. 34, 167–176.
3. Olney, J.W., Collins, R.C. and Sloviter, R.S. (1986). Excitotoxic mechanisms of epileptic brain damage. In *Advances in Neurology, Vol 44, Basic Mechanisms of the Epilepsies: Molecular and Cellular Approaches*, Delgado-Escueta, A.V., Ward, A.A., Woodbury, D.M. and Porter, R.J., eds., Raven, New York, pp. 857–878.
4. Collins, R.C. and Olney, J.W. (1982). Focal cortical seizures cause distant thalamic lesions. Science 218, 177–179.
5. Olney, J.W., deGubareff, T. and Sloviter, R.S. (1983). "Epileptic" brain damage in rats induced by sustained electrical stimulation of the perforant path. II. Ultrastructural analysis of acute hippocampal pathology. Brain Res. Bull. 10, 699–712.

6. Labruyere, J., Fuller, T.A., Olney, J.W., Price, M.T., Zorumski, C. and Clifford, D. (1986). Phencyclidine and ketamine protect against kainic acid-induced seizures and seizure-related brain damage. Neurosci. Abst. 12, 344.
7. Wieloch, T. (1985). Hypoglycemia-induced neuronal damage prevented by an N-methyl-D-aspartate antagonist. Science 230, 681–683.
8. Rothman, S.M. and Olney, J.W. (1986). Glutamate and the pathophysiology of hypoxic-ischemic brain damage. Ann. Neurol. 19, 105–111.
9. Rothman, S. (1984). Synaptic release of excitatory amino acid neuro-transmitter mediates anoxic neuronal death. J. Neurosci. 4, 1884–1891.
10. Benveniste, H., Drejer, J., Schousboe, A. and Diemer, N.H. (1984). Elevation of the extra-cellular concentrations of glutamate and aspartate in rat hippocampus during transient cerebral ischemia monitored by intracerebral microdialysis. J. Neurochem. 43, 1369–1374.
11. Simon, R.P., Swan, J.H. Griffiths, T. and Meldrum, B.S. (1984). Blockade of N-methyl-D-aspartate receptors may protect against ischemic damage in the brain. Science 226, 850–852.
12. Olney, J.W. (1979). Excitotoxic amino acids and Huntington's disease. In *Advances of Neurology, Huntington's Disease*, Vol. 23, Chase, T.N., Wexler, A. and Barbeau, A., eds., Raven, New York, pp. 609–624.
13. Beal, M.F., Kowall, N.W., Ellison, P.W., Mazurek, M.F., Swartz, K.J. and Martin, J.B. (1986). Replication of the neurochemical characteristic of Huntington's disease by quinolinic acid. Nature 321(6066), 168–171.
14. Young, A.B., Greenmayre, J.T. and Penney, J.B. (1986). Glutamate receptors in Alzheimer's disease. In *Excitatory Amino Acid Transmission*, Hicks, T.P., Lodge, D., McLennan, H., eds., Alan R. Liss, New York, pp. 233–240.
15. Olney, J.W. (1986). Inciting excitotoxic cytocide among central neurons. In *Excitatory Amino Acids and Epilepsy*, Schwarcz, R., Ben-Ari, Y., eds., Plenum, New York, pp. 631–646.
16. Olney, J.W., Price, M.T., Fuller, T.A., Labruyere, J., Samson, J., Carpenter, M. and Mahan, K. (1986). The anti-excitotoxic effects of certain anesthetics, analgesics and sedative-hypnotics. Neurosci. Lett. 68, 29–35.
17. Davies, J., Evans, R.H. and Jones, A.W. (1982). Differential activation and blockade of excitatory amino acid receptors in the mammalian and amphibian central nervous systems. Comp. Biochem. Physiol. 72, 211–224.
18. Rothman, S.M. (1985). The neurotoxicity of excitatory amino acids is produced by passive chloride influx. J. Neurosci. 5, 1483–1489.
19. Olney, J.W., Price, M.T., Samson, L. and Labruyere, J. (1986). The role of specific ions in glutamate neurotoxicity. Neurosci. Lett. 65, 65–71.
20. Mayer, M., Westbrook, G. and Forsythe, I. (1986). NMDA receptor function: Clues from biophysical experiments. In *Excitatory Amino Acid Transmission*, Hicks, T.P., Lodge, D. and McLennan, H., eds., Alan R. Liss, New York, pp. 27–34.
21. Anis, N.A., Berry, S.C., Burton, N.R. and Lodge, D. (1983). The dissociative anesthetics, ketamine and phencyclidine, selectively reduce excitation of central mammalian neurons by N-methyl-aspartate. Br. J. Pharmacol. 79, 565–575.
22. Choi, D.W. (1985). Two mechanisms underlying glutamate neurotoxicity in cortical cell culture. Neurosci, Abst. 11, 153.
23. Kim, J.S. (1983). Cerebral glutamate, neuroleptic drugs and schizophrenia: Increase of cerebrospinal fluid glutamate levels and decrease of striatal glutamate levels following sulpiride treatment in rats. Eur. Neurology 22, 367.
24. Simpson, G.M., Les, H., Branchey, M.H. and Shrivastavai, R.K. (1978). Boclofen in the treatment of tardive dyskinesia. Psychopharmacol. Bull. 14, 16–18.
25. Morris, R.G., Anderson, E., Lynch, G.S. and Baudry, M. (1986). Selective impairment of learning and blockade of long-term potentiation by an N-methyl-D-aspartate receptor antagonist, AP5. Nature 319(6056), 774–776.
26. Monoghan, D.T. and Cotman, C.W. (1985). Distribution of N-methyl-D-aspartate sensitive L-^{3}H-glutamate-binding sites in rat brain. J. Neurosci. 5, 2909–2919.
27. Quang Do, Mattenberger, M., Streit, P. and Cuenod, M. (1986). In vitro release of endogenous excitatory sulfur-containing amino acids from various rat brain regions. J. Neurochem. 46, 779–786.
28. Olney, J.W., Price, M.T., Shahid Salles, K., Labruyere, J., Ryerson, R. and Mahan, K. (1986). L-homocysteic acid: A potent endogenous excitotoxin and putative transmitter. Neurosci. Abst. 12, 380.

5. PHARMACOLOGY OF EXCITATORY AMINO ACID ANTAGONISTS AND THEIR POSSIBLE THERAPEUTIC USE IN NEUROLOGICAL DISEASE

B.S. MELDRUM

Excitatory amino acid antagonists are of two main types: 1) structural analogues of dicarboxylic amino acids that compete with glutamate or other agonists at the receptor site and 2) lipophilic compounds, without acidic groups, that block the excitatory action of agonists by a noncompetitive mechanism. The postsynaptic receptors at which amino acids exert an excitatory action can be classified according to their preferred agonists as kainate-, quisqualate-, and N-methyl-D-aspartate-preferring receptors [1, 2]. Referring to these receptor subtypes as kainate, quisqualate, and NMDA receptors is a convenient shorthand; it implies nothing about the nature of the endogenous neurotransmitters. Glutamate is a highly effective agonist at all three receptor subtypes. Aspartate acts preferentially on the NMDA receptor in spinal cord neurons [3]. The sulphur-containing analogues of glutamate and aspartate interact with quisqualate and NMDA receptors but not with kainate receptors [4].

1. COMPETITIVE ANTAGONISTS

Among competitive antagonists, some analogues of D-glutamate with chain elongation and a phosphono- group in the omega position show potent and selective antagonism at the NMDA receptor. The structures of leading compounds are illustrated in Figure 5-1.

The structures of some competitive antagonists with partial or minimal receptor subtype specificity are illustrated in Figure 5-2. The relative antagonist potency at the different receptor subtypes varies somewhat according to the brain region under study. Kynurenic acid appears to block all three

Ferrendelli, J.A., Collins, R.C. and Johnson, E.M. (eds), Neurobiology of Amino Acids, Peptides, and Trophic Factors.

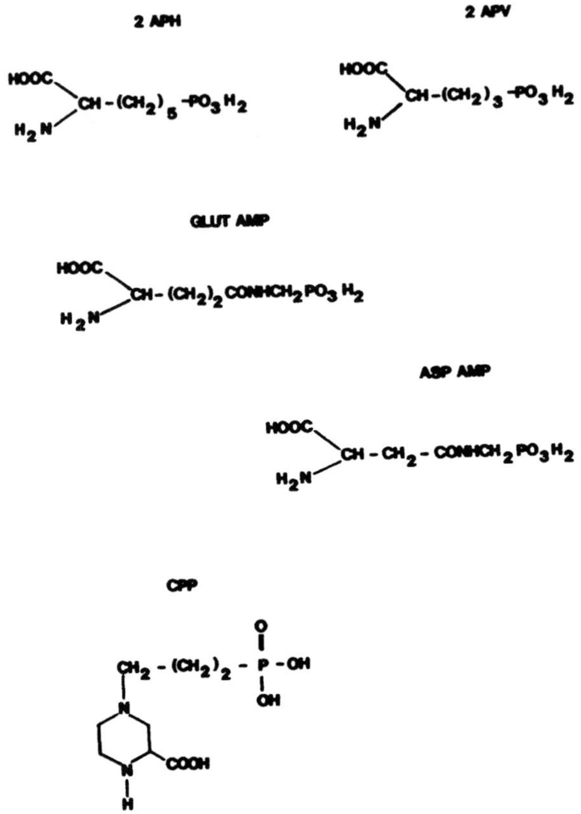

Figure 5-1. Molecular formulae of compounds acting as selective antagonists at the NMDA receptor. 2APH = 2-amino-7-phosphonoheptanoic acid; 2APV = 2-amino-5-phosphonovaleric acid; GLUT-AMP = γ-D-glutamyl-aminomethylphosphonate; ASP-AMP = β-D-aspartyl-amino-methylphosphonate; CPP = 3((+−)2-carboxypiperazin-4yl)-propyl-1-phosphonate.

receptor subtypes in the spinal cord but has a partial preferential action against NMDA and kainate receptors in the hippocampus [5].

2. NONCOMPETITIVE ANTAGONISTS

Phencyclidine and related sigma opiate antagonists, such as (−) cyclazocine and N-allylnormetazocine, the dissociative anaesthetic ketamine, and a recently identified anticonvulsant compound, MK 801, have been shown to block NMDA receptor activation by a noncompetitive mechanism [6–8]. Their structures are given in Figure 5-3.

3. PHARMACOLOGICAL STUDIES

Animal experimental studies have provided clear evidence for acute anticonvulsant effects of excitatory amino acid antagonists. These compounds, like

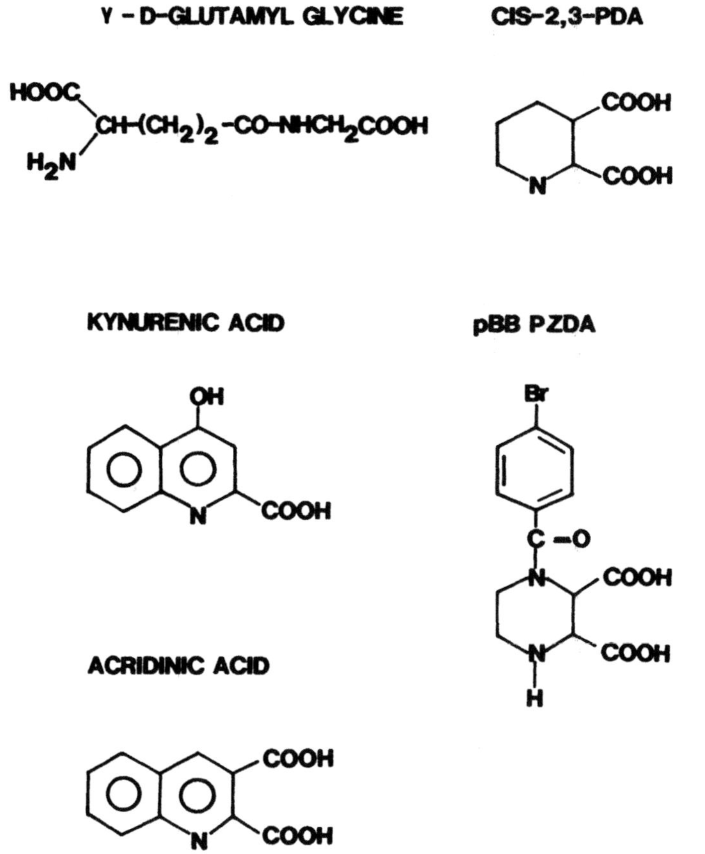

Figure 5-2. Antagonists acting at more than one receptor subtype. cis-2,3-PDA = cis-2,3-piperidine dicarboxylic acid; pBB PZDA = 1-(p-bromobenzoyl)-piperazine-2,3-dicarboxylic acid.

the benzodiazepines, also show muscle relaxant, anxiolytic, and sedative effects. Studies on cytotoxic neuropathology show a clear protective effect of the antagonists, raising the possibility of therapeutic applications in ischemic brain damage and a wide variety of neurodegenerative disorders.

4. ANTICONVULSANT EFFECTS

A potent anticonvulsant effect of compounds blocking activation at the NMDA receptor was first demonstrated in DBA/2 mice using either intracerebroventricular or intraperitoneal administration [9]. Subsequently, 2APH and 2APV were shown to be anticonvulsant in a wide variety of seizure models including chemically-induced seizures in rodents, electroshock and kindled seizures in rats, high-pressure neurological syndrome in rats, and

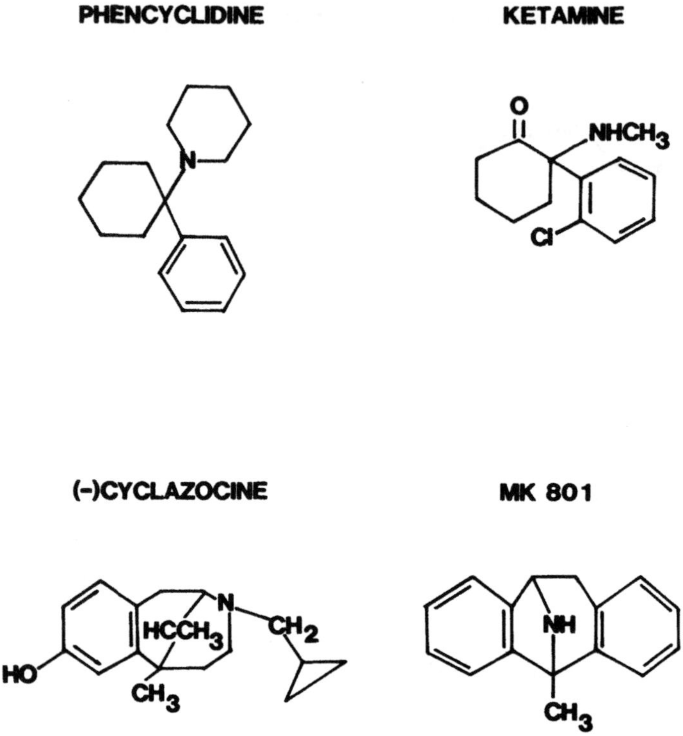

Figure 5-3. Molecular formulae of compounds that bind at the sigma opiate receptor and that decrease excitation induced at the NMDA receptor by direct agonists.

photically-induced myoclonus in baboons [10–15]. Among the compounds, there is a strong correlation between relative potency as competitive antagonists at the NMDA receptor and anticonvulsant potency, with CPP having the highest potency. The competitive antagonists are comparable in potency to the benzodiazepines when administered via the intracerebroventricular route.

When administered systemically, they are substantially less potent than the benzodiazepines (Table 5-1). The nonpolar compound MK 801 shows a potency when given i.c.v. comparable to the direct NMDA antagonists, and an i.p./i.c.v. ratio comparable to the standard anticonvulsant drugs (Chapman & Meldrum, unpublished).

5. NONSELECTIVE ANTAGONISTS

Some of the nonselective excitatory amino acid antagonists also show anticonvulsant activity in DBA/2 mice and in photosensitive baboons (see Table 5-2). Although this can be partially or wholly accounted for in terms of NMDA antagonist activity, it appears that non-NMDA antagonist activity

Table 5-1. Anticonvulsant potency of NMDA antagonists and standard anticonvulsant drugs against sound-induced seizures in DBA/2 mice: A comparison of intracerebroventricular and intraperitoneal routes of administration.

	i.c.v. nmoles	ED_{50} clonic phase i.p. μmoles/kg	i.p./i.c.v.
(−)2-APH	1.8	40	22
(±)2-APV	15.0	320	21
β-ASP-AMP	0.6	183	305
γ-D-glutamylAMP	1.8	280	156
P-BB-PDA	5.0	250	50
P-CB-PDA	15.0	530	35
(±)CPP	0.04	2.6	67
MK801	1.5	0.15	0.1
Diazepam	11	0.4	0.036
Diphenylhydantoin	300	9.1	0.030
Phenobarbital	320	9.9	0.031
Valproate	6000	1250	0.280

Table 5-2. Anticonvulsant activity of nonselective antagonists

	ED_{50} clonic phase DBA/2 mice mmoles/kg i.p.	ED_{100} myoclonus *Papio papio* mmoles/kg i.v.
Cis-2,3-PDA	0.52	3.3
Kynurenic acid	4.6	1.6
γ-D-glutamylamino methyl sulphonate	2.74	

From Ref. 70–72.

contributes significantly to the anticonvulsant activity of kynurenate and γ-D-glutamyl amino methyl-sulphonate. A potentiating effect of the combination of kainate and NMDA antagonism appears probable.

6. FOCAL SITE OF ANTICONVULSANT ACTION

The site of action of excitatory amino acid antagonists has been investigated by their focal injection in various rodent models of epilepsy. Sound-induced seizures in genetically epilepsy-prone rats can be suppressed by the focal injection of 2-APH in various midbrain sites. The lowest effective doses are found for the inferior colliculus; higher doses are required in the midbrain reticular formation and the substantia nigra, pars reticulata [16] (Figure 5-4).

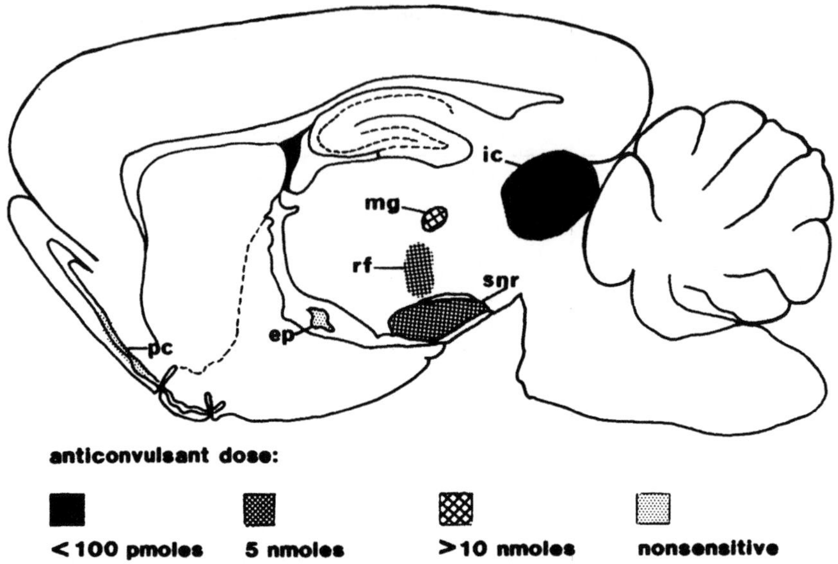

Figure 5-4. Sagittal plan of the rat brain to show regional sensitivity to the anticonvulsant action of 2-amino-7-phosphonoheptanoic acid (APH) in the genetically epilepsy-prone rat. Shading indicates the minimal dose of APH that when injected bilaterally into that structure suppresses the motor seizure sequence induced by a loud sound. i.c. = inferior colliculus; mg = medial geniculate; rf = midbrain reticular formation; snr = substantia nigra, pars reticulata; ep = entopeduncular nucleus; pc = prepyriform cortex. (Data from Ref. 16 and Millan, Patel, Faingold, and Meldrum, unpublished).

Limbic seizures induced by high intraperitoneal doses of pilocarpine can be prevented by focal injections of 2-APH in rather different brain regions. The most sensitive region is the prepyriform cortex (threshold 1 pmol); the entopeduncular nucleus and the lateral habenular nucleus are nearly as sensitive (5–10 pmol). The pedunculopontine nucleus and the substantia nigra pars reticulata are significantly less sensitive [17–19] (Figure 5-5).

The anticonvulsant action of an excitatory amino acid antagonist may depend on a diffuse action raising the threshold for induction of burst firing in the neocortex or hippocampus. Our experiments in these rodent models provide evidence for actions of two other kinds, namely, action on critical afferent trigger points (e.g., the inferior colliculus on the auditory pathway and the prepyriform cortex on the olfactory pathway) or action on basal ganglia output pathways, which modify seizure threshold within the limbic system and also control the motor expression of seizures.

7. TREMOR AND SPASTICITY

Animal models suggest possible therapeutic actions of NMDA antagonists in tremor and in spasticity.

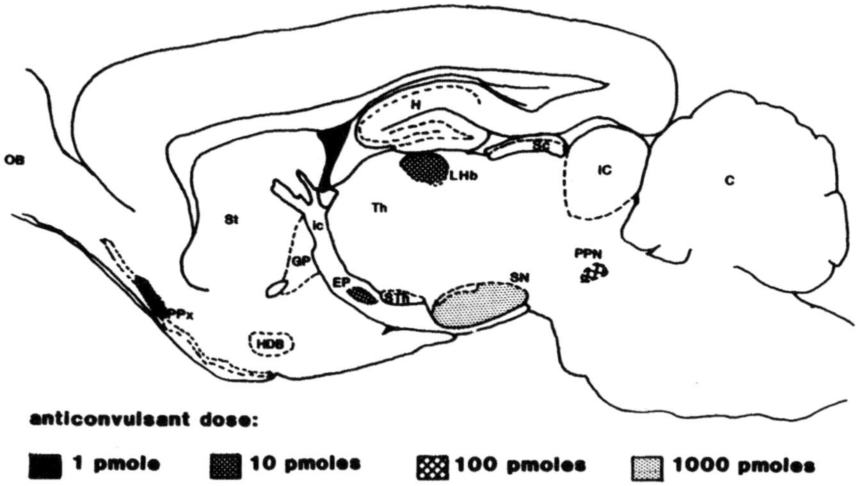

Figure 5-5. Sagittal plan of the rat brain to show regional sensitivity to the anticonvulsant action of APH against limbic seizures induced by pilocarpine (380 mg/kg, i.p.). Shading indicates the minimal dose of APH that when injected bilaterally suppresses the motor components of the seizure. LHb = lateral habenula; PPN = pedunculopontine nucleus; SN = substantia nigra, pars reticulata; EP = entopeduncular nucleus; PPx = prepyriform cortex; (Data from Refs. 14, 18, 19 and Patel, Millan and Meldrum, unpublished).

The high pressure neurological syndrome induced by increasing atmospheric pressure by the addition of an inert gas has a characteristic onset with a generalized tremor. Pretreatment of rats with 2-APH more than doubles the onset pressure for tremor [14].

A reduction in muscle tone is observed in rodents and primates receiving doses of NMDA antagonists somewhat higher than the anticonvulsant dose. In genetically spastic rats of the Ham-Wistar strain, 2-APH and other selective NMDA antagonists and kynurenate decrease the abnormal muscle tone in the hindlimbs [20].

8. ANTICONFLICT OR ANXIOLYTIC ACTIONS

NMDA antagonists have been evaluated in rodent models conventionally used to predict anxiolytic action in man. In rats, an increase in punished responding is seen after intraperitoneal administration of 2-APH or CPP [21]. Ketamine does not produce this effect. MK 801 in relatively low doses does restore shock-suppressed lever pressing or drinking [22]. In mice an "anxiolytic action" is observed in the four-plate test and the elevated plus maze after 2-APH [23]. However, 2-APH is inactive or only weakly active in several other tests in which benzodiazepines are strongly active. The anticonflict activity of MK 801 was not apparent in trained squirrel monkeys. It is at present doubtful that NMDA antagonists warrant clinical investigation as anxiolytic agents.

9. EFFECTS ON LEARNING

Long-term potentiation in some limbic pathways (e.g., the Schaffer collateral input to CA1 pyramidal neurons and the commissural input to CA3) is dependent on NMDA receptors and can be blocked by 2-APV, phencyclidine, or ketamine, whereas in others (e.g., mossy fibre input to CA3) it is not blocked by NMDA antagonists [24–26]. These observations raise the possibility that NMDA antagonists will impair learning and memory. In rats, intracerebroventricular infusion of 2-APV impairs spatial learning in a water maze but leaves the acquisition of other tasks unimpaired [16]. However, MK 801 in anticonvulsant doses does not show this effect on learning [27].

10. EXCITOTOXIC MECHANISMS AND PROTECTION BY ANTAGONISTS

Excitotoxic effects can be produced through actions at any of the three receptor subtypes. These can be demonstrated in vivo by focal injections of kainate, quisqualate, or NMDA (or ibotenate or quinolinate, which also act on the NMDA receptor). They can also be studied in vitro using tissue slices (hippocampus, cerebellum, or retina) or dissociated neuronal cultures. There is a clear correlation between the distribution of receptors and preferential vulnerability of cell types to kainate, quisqualate, or NMDA. Thus in cerebellar slices, NMDA acts selectively on inhibitory interneurons (basket, stellate, and Golgi cells), quisqualate acts on inhibitory interneurons and Purkinje cells (which lack NMDA receptors), and kainate acts additionally on granule cells [28, 29]. Excitotoxic effects of direct agonists can in general be prevented by the selective antagonists. Thus the neurotoxic effect of focal injection into the hippocampus of ibotenate (but not of kainate) is blocked by co-injection of 2-APH [30].

The acute cell loss that occurs selectively in the hippocampus and neocortex after status epilepticus appears to be excitotoxic in origin [31, 32]. The early cytological changes show the postsynaptic neuronal and focal dendritic pathology characteristic of excitotoxic lesions [33–35]. These changes can be reproduced by sustained electrical stimulation of excitatory inputs or the focal injection of glutamate or aspartate [36]. Activation of NMDA receptors on basal and apical dendrites of CA1 and CA3 pyramidal neurons, leading to massive entry of Ca^{2+}, appears to be a crucial step in the excitotoxic process [34, 35]. Similar cytological changes are seen in hippocampal pyramidal neurons during the reperfusion phase after transient forebrain ischemia [37]. There is also evidence that destroying excitatory inputs to the hippocampus protects against ischemic damage [38]. The crucial involvement of excitatory transmission at the NMDA receptor in the development of ischemic brain damage is indicated by the protective effect of specific antagonists. Focal injection of the selective antagonist 2-APH into the rat hippocampus provides protection against the early excitotoxic changes [39] and the late nerve cell loss [40]. Systemic injection of 2-APH also protects against nerve cell loss due to forebrain ischaemia in the gerbil and rat [41; Swan, Evans, Meldrum, unpublished].

Nerve cell loss in the hippocampus and striatum following profound hypoglycemia also appears to depend on an excitotoxic mechanism. Protection can be provided by destroying the glutamatergic cortical afferents to the striatum or by focal injection of 2-APH [42, 43].

To date, protective effects of excitatory amino acid antagonists have been reported only in acute degenerative syndromes in animals. These studies clearly establish the potential protective effect of antagonists against excitotoxic brain damage. If an excitotoxic mechanism is involved in chronic neurodegenerative disorders, then the possibility of a prophylactic use of excitatory amino acid antagonists exists. It is only necessary that an excitotoxic mechanism links the primary pathogenetic process to the final nerve cell loss for such therapy to be successful.

11. EXCITOTOXIC CELL LOSS IN CLINICAL CONDITIONS

Some neurodegenerative disorders in which excitotoxic mechanisms may contribute to nerve cell loss are listed in Table 5-3. The evidence for this is at present largely indirect, being derived from the animal experimental studies reviewed above. Neurolathyrism provides the clearest example of a degenerative disorder produced by an exogenous excitotoxin [44]. The principal toxin in the chick pea, *Lathyrus sativa*, is β-N-oxalylamino L-alanine, an excitotoxin of the quisqualate type [45]. There is indirect evidence that the ALS-Parkinsonism dementia complex of Guam may be caused by a toxin from *Cycas circinalis* (β-N-methyl-amino-L-alanine), which may form an NMDA-like excitotoxin in vivo.

One reason for considering that the selective loss of hippocampal neurons occurring in normal aging may be due to an excitotoxic mechanism is that cell counts show that its pattern of selectivity within the zones of the hippocampus corresponds closely to that found in patients with epilepsy [46]. In senile dementia of the Alzheimer type, postmortem brain studies provide evidence for alteration in excitatory amino acid neurotransmission in cortex and hippocampus. In one study, the content of glutamate was reported to be moderately reduced in the inferior temporal cortex [47], and in another the content of glutamate and aspartate was reported to be markedly reduced in superior frontal, orbital, and temporal cortex [48]. Sodium-dependent uptake of ^{3}H-D-aspartate is decreased, suggesting that there is a loss of specific uptake of dicarboxylic amino acids into excitatory terminals [49]. Autoradiographic studies indicate a decrease in NMDA binding in cortex and hippocampus [50]. This is probably a consequence of loss, both of neurons with NMDA receptors [51] and of apical dendrites. An increase of kainate receptors in the dentate molecular layer [52] appears to be a consequence of deafferentation. A loss of cortical inputs to the hippocampus is thought to play a crucial role in the memory impairment in Alzheimer's disease [52–54]. An NMDA-mediated excitotoxic process could explain some of these findings.

Perinatal asphyxia commonly selectively damages the globus pallidus. In

Table 5-3. Selective neuronal degeneration in which excitotoxic mechanisms may be involved.

1. Hippocampal and cortical nerve cell loss following status epilepticus or chronic epilepsy
2. Hippocampal and cortical nerve cell loss in
a. Normal aging
b. Senile dementia, Alzheimer type
3. Selective neuronal loss in hippocampus, cortex, striatum following
a. Transient forebrain ischemia
b. Profound hypoglycemia
4. Selective loss in globus pallidus and cortex following perinatal hypoxia
5. ALS-Parkinsonism-dementia complex of Guam (cortex, hippocampus, amygdala, globus pallidus, thalamus, substantia nigra, lateral spinal tract, anterior horn cells)
6. Huntington's chorea (small neurons, Golgi type II, in striatum, also thalamus-ventrobasal nucleus, cerebellar Purkinje cells, etc.)
7. Lathyrism (corticospinal tracts)
8. Olivopontocerebellar atrophy (pyramidal and posterior spinocerebellar tracts, brain stem nuclei, inferior olives, cerebellar Purkinje cells).

the neonatal period, the globus pallidus has a very high density of glutamate receptors [55], possibly making it more vulnerable to excitotoxic mechanisms.

12. HUNTINGTON'S DISEASE

The similarity between the selective loss of GABAergic and cholinergic neurons in the striatum in Huntington's disease and in rats following focal injection of kainic acid into the striatum has been considered to support an excitotoxic mechanism in the pathogenesis of Huntington's disease. However, study of peptidergic systems showed that neurons containing somatostatin and neuropeptide Y are preserved in Huntington's disease. A similar pattern of selective loss with preservation of somatostatin and NPY has been described in rats focally injected with quinolinic acid [56]. Studies in cultured cortical neurons show that neurons containing nicotinamide adenine dinucleotide phosphate diaphorase are resistant to the toxic action of quinolinate or NMDA but are vulnerable to kainate or quisqualate [57]. As these neurons are selectively spared in Huntington's disease, an endogenous excitotoxin acting on the NMDA receptor, such as quinolinate, could acount for the pattern of cell loss.

13. OLIVOPONTOCEREBELLAR ATROPHY

In the recessive form of olivopontocerebellar atrophy, there is a deficiency in one of the isoenzymes of glutamate dehydrogenase and an impaired capacity to handle an oral glutamate load [58]. The dominant form of OPCA also appears to be associated with an abnormality in the regulation of glutamate dehydrogenase activity [59]. The system degeneration might thus relate to excessive local concentrations of glutamate in the cerebellum and brain stem.

14. PSYCHOTOMIMETIC OR ANTIPSYCHOTIC POTENTIAL

Kim, Kornhuber, and their colleagues have proposed that altered glutamatergic transmission may play a key role in the pathogenesis of schizophrenia [60]. They reported that the glutamate concentration in the CSF of patients with schizophrenia was 50% lower than in controls [61]. Apparent failures to replicate this finding [62, 63] are probably not significant. One study has found an increase in kainic acid binding in the prefrontal cortex of schizophrenic patients [49]. An abnormality in glutamatergic terminals could be a cause or a consequence of altered dopaminergic activity in the basal ganglia and mesolimbic system. A presynaptic dopamine receptor controls glutamate release in the striatum. Haloperidol blocks glutamate release from amygdala synaptosomes [64], but this appears not to involve a dopamine receptor [65]. A striatal glutamate receptor, apparently of the quisqualate type, enhances release of dopamine in striatal slices [66]. There is evidence that corticostriatal glutamatergic inputs exert an important physiological control over dopamine release [67].

Phencyclidine and some other compounds that bind to the low-affinity sigma opiate receptor are psychotomimetic. This effect may or may not be related to blockade of the NMDA receptors produced by phencyclidine. Endogenous peptides (α- and β-endopsychosins) acting on the high- and low-affinity sigma opiate receptors have been purified [47, 68].

It appears that disturbance of excitatory amino acid receptor mechanisms may play a key role in schizophrenia. Antagonists could produce either therapeutic or psychotomimetic effects. Blockade of NMDA receptors may be psychotomimetic, suggesting that up-regulation of such receptors might be therapeutic in schizophrenia (but might also facilitate epilepsy). Conversely, blockade or down-regulation of the glutamate receptors enhancing dopamine release might be therapeutic.

15. CONCLUSION

15.1. Therapeutic potential

The two areas that on present evidence represent the major therapeutic application of excitatory amino acid antagonists are epilepsy (including myoclonic syndromes) and acute neuronal degeneration related to transient impairment of cerebral oxygenation or blood flow.

There can be little doubt that competitive and noncompetitive NMDA antagonists and nonselective antagonists will all show some efficacy as anticonvulsants in humans. The only compound yet in clinical trial is MK 801 [69]. This apparently produces little, if any, disturbance of cognitive function, but trials with higher doses are required to establish efficacy.

The optimal competitive NMDA antagonist for clinical trial awaits identification. Problems of pharmacokinetics need to be overcome, and the question of possible impairment of learning needs thorough investigation. This potential side effect may be no more serious than it is with benzodiazepines and barbiturates.

In the field of cerebroprotection, it is clear that early trials in transient global ischemia (post-cardiac arrest), in cardiopulmonary bypass procedures, and in stroke are indicated.

It is less clear that trials in chronic neurodegenerative disorders can be justified on the basis of available experimental data. The possibility that the compounds themselves might exacerbate some of the early cognitive dysfunctions must be borne in mind. Nevertheless, in the absence of any treatments that modify the progressive neurodegeneration in Huntington's disease or SDAT, many may consider that humanitarian considerations call for the earliest possible trials.

REFERENCES

1. Davies, J., Evans, R.H., Smith, D.A. and Watkins, J.C. (1982). Differential activation and blockade of excitatory amino acid receptors in the mammalian and amphibian spinal cord. Comp. Biochem. Physiol. 72C, 211–224.
2. Foster, A.C. and Fagg, G.E. (1984). Acidic amino acid binding sites in mammalian neuronal membranes: Their characteristics and relationship to synaptic receptors. Brain Res. Rev. 7, 103–164.
3. Mayer, M.L. and Westbrook, G.L. (1986). The physiology of excitatory amino acids in the vertebrate central nervous system. Progress in Neurobiology, 28, 197–276.
4. Murphy, D.E. and Williams, M. (1986). Interaction of sulfur-containing amino acids with quisqualate and kainate excitatory amino acid receptors in rat brain. In *Excitatory Amino Acid Transmission*, Hicks, T.P., Lodge, D. and McLennan, H., eds., Alan R. Liss, New York, pp. 63–66.
5. Peet, M.J., Curry, K., Magnuson, D.S. and McLennan, H. (1986). Conformational requirements for activation of burst firing of rat CA-1 hippocampal pyramidal neurones. In *Excitatory Amino Acid Transmission*. Hicks, T.P., Lodge, D. and McLennan, H., eds., Alan R. Liss, New York, pp. 35–42.
6. Berry, S.C., Dawkins, S.L. and Lodge, D. (1984). Comparison of σ- and K-opiate receptor ligands as excitatory amino acid antagonists. Brit. J. Pharmacol. 83, 179–185.
7. Lodge, D., Berry, S.C., Church, J., Martin, D., McGhee, A., Lai, H.M. and Thomson, A.M. (1984). Isomers of cyclazocine act as excitatory amino acid antagonists. Neuropeptides 5, 245–248.
8. Wong, E.H., Kemp, J.A., Priestley, T., Knight, A.R., Woodruff, G.N. and Iversen, L.L. (1986). The novel anticonvulsant MK 801 is a potent N-methyl-D-aspartate antagonist. Proc. Nat. Acad. Sci. USA 83, 7104–7108.
9. Croucher, M.J., Collins, J.F. and Meldrum, B.S. (1982). Anticonvulsant action of excitatory amino acid antagonists. Science 216, 899–901.
10. Czuczwar, S.J. and Meldrum, B.S. (1982). Protection against chemically-induced seizures by 2-amino-7-phosphonoheptanoic acid. Eur. J. Pharmacol. 83, 335–338.
11. Czuczwar, S.J., Cavalheiro, E.A., Turski, L., Turski, W.A. and Kleinrok, Z. (1985). Phosphonic analogues of excitatory amino acids raise the threshold for maximal electroconvulsions in mice. Neurosci. Res. 3, 86–90.
12. Meldrum, B.S., Croucher, M.J., Badman, G. and Collins, J.F. (1983). Antiepileptic action of excitatory amino acid antagonists in the photosensitive baboon, *Papio papio*. Neurosci. Lett. 39, 101–104.
13. Meldrum, B.S., Croucher, M.J., Czuczwar, S.J., Collins, J.F. Curry, K., Joseph, M. and Stone, T.W. (1983). A comparison of the anticonvulsant potency of +-2-amino-5-phosphonopentanoic acid and (+-)2-amino-7-phosphonoheptanoic acid. Neuroscience 9, 925–930.
14. Meldrum, B.S., Wardley-Smith, B., Halsey, M. and Rostain, J.C. (1983). 2-amino-7-

phosphonoheptanoic acid protects against the high pressure neurological syndrome. Eur. J. Pharmacol. 87, 501–502.

15. Peterson, D.W., Collins, J.F. and Bradford, H.F. (1984). Anticonvulsant action of amino acid antagonists against kindled hippocampal seizures. Brain Res. 311, 176–180.
16. Morris, R.G., Anderson, E., Lynch, G.S. and Baudry, M. (1986). Selective impairment of learning and blockade of long-term potentiation by an N-methyl-D-aspartate receptor antagonist, AP5. Nature 319, 774–776.
17. Millan, M.H., Faingold, C.L. and Meldrum, B.S. (1987). Intranigral 2-amino-7-phosphonoheptanoic acid protects against audiogenic seizures in genetically-epilepsy prone rats. In *Advances in Epileptology 15*, Wolf, P., ed., Raven Press, New York.
18. Patel, S., Millan, M.H., Mello, L.M. and Meldrum, B.S. (1986).2-amino-7-phosphonoheptanoic acid (2-APH) infusion into entopeduncular nucleus protects against limbic seizures in rats. Neurosci. Lett. 64, 226–230.
19. Turski, L., Cavalheiro, E.A., Turski, W.A. and Meldrum, B.S. (1986). Excitatory transmission within substantia nigra pars reticulata regulates threshold for seizures produced by pilocarpine in rats: Effects of intranigral 2-amino-7-phosphonoheptanoate and N-methyl-D-aspartate. Neuroscience 18, 61–67.
20. Turski, L., Schwarz, M., Turski, W.A., Klockgether, T., Sontag, K-H. and Collins, J.F. (1985). Muscle relaxant action of excitatory amino acid antagonists. Neurosci. Lett. 53, 321–326.
21. Bennett, D.A. and Amrick, C.L. (1986). Antagonists of N-methyl-D-aspartate (NMDA) produce anticonflict activity. In *Excitatory Amino Acid Transmission*. Hicks, T.P., Lodge, D. and McLennan, H., eds., Alan R. Liss, New York, pp. 213–216.
22. Clineschmidt, B.V., Williams, M., Witoslawski, J.J., Bunting, P.R., Risley, E.A. and Totaro, J.A. (1982). Restoration of shock-suppressed behavior by treatment with (+)-5-methyl-10,11-dihydro-5H-dibenzo[a,d]cyclohepten-5,10-imine (MK 801), a substance with potent anticonvulsant, central sympathomimetic, and apparent anxiolytic properties. Drug Develop. Res. 2, 147–163.
23. Stephens, D.N., Meldrum, B.S., Weidmann, R., Schneider, C. and Grutzner, M. (1986). Does the excitatory amino acid receptor antagonist 2-APH exhibit anxiolytic activity? Psychopharmacology 90, 166–169.
24. Collingridge, G.L., Kehl, S.J. and McLennan, H. (1983). Excitatory amino acids in synaptic transmission in the Schaffer collateral-commissural pathway of the rat hippocampus. J. Physiol. 334, 33–46.
25. Harris, E.W. and Cotman, C.W. (1986). Long-term potentiation of guinea pig mossy fiber responses is not blocked by N-methyl-D-aspartate antagonists. Brain Res.
26. Stringer, J.L. and Guynet, P.E. (1983). Elimination of long-term potentiation in the hippocampus by phencyclidine and ketamine. Brain Res. 258, 159–164.
27. Halliwell, R.F. and Morris, R.G. (1987). Anticonvulsant doses of MK 801 fail to block long-term potentiation in vivo or impair spatial memory in the rat. Abstracts, Brain Res. Assoc. March, 1987.
28. Garthwaite, G. and Garthwaite J. (1984). Differential sensitivity of rat cerebellar cells in vitro to the neurotoxic effects of excitatory amino acid analogues. Neurosci. Lett. 48, 361–367.
29. Garthwaite, G. and Garthwaite, J. (1986). Neurotoxicity of excitatory amino acid receptor agonists in rat cerebellar slices: Dependence on calcium concentration. Neurosci. Lett. 66, 193–198.
30. Schwarcz, R., Collins, J.F. and Parks, D.A. (1982). α-amino-ω-phosphonocarboxylates block ibotenate but not kainate neurotoxicity in rat hippocampus. Neurosci. Lett. 33, 85–90.
31. Meldrum, B.S. (1983). Metabolic factors during prolonged seizures and their relation to nerve cell death. In *Advances in Neurology 34, Status Epilepticus*. Delgado-Escueta, A.V., Wasterlain, C.G., Treiman, D.M. and Porter, R.J., eds., Raven Press, New York, pp. 261–275.
32. Olney, J.W. (1985). Excitatory transmitters and epilepsy-related brain damage. Int. Rev. Neurobiol. 27, 338–362.
33. Evans, M.C., Griffiths, T. and Meldrum, B.S. (1984). Kainic acid seizures and the reversibility of calcium loading in vulnerable neurons in the hippocampus. Neuropathol. Appl. Neurobiol. 10, 285–302.
34. Griffiths, T., Evans, M.C. and Meldrum, B.S. (1983). Intracellular calcium accumulation in rat hippocampus during seizures induced by bicuculline or L-allylglycine. Neuroscience 10,

385–395.

35. Griffiths, T., Evans, M.C. and Meldrum, B.S. (1984). Status epilepticus: The reversibility of calcium loading and acute neuronal pathological changes in the rat hippocampus. Neuroscience 12, 557–567.
36. Sloviter, R.S. and Dempster, D.W. (1985). "Epileptic" brain damage is replicated qualitatively in the rat hippocampus by central injection of glutamate or aspartate but not by GABA or acetylcholine. Brain Res. Bull. 15, 39–60.
37. Simon, R.P., Griffiths, T., Evans, M.C., Swan, J.H. and Meldrum, B.S. (1984). Calcium overload in selectively vulnerable neurons of the hippocampus during and after ischaemia: An electron microscopy study in the rat. J. Cereb. Blood Flow Metab. 4, 350–361.
38. Johansen, F.F., Jorgensen, M.B. and Diemer, N.H. (1986). Ischemia induced delayed neuronal death in the CA1 hippocampus is dependent on intact glutamatergic innervation. In *Excitatory Amino Acid Transmission*, Hicks, T.P., Lodge, D. and McLennan, H., eds. Alan R. Liss, pp. 245–248.
39. Simon, R.P., Swan, J.H., Griffiths, T. and Meldrum, B.S. (1984). Blockade of N-methyl-D-aspartate receptors may protect against ischaemic damage in the brain. Science 226, 850–852.
40. Evans, M.C., Swan, J.H. and Meldrum, B.S. (1987). Blockade of excitatory neurotransmission provides partial long-term protection against ischaemic brain damage. In *Fifteenth Princeton Conference on Cerebrovascular Disease*. Raichle, M.E. and Parks, W.S., eds., Raven Press, New York, 27–36.
41. Boast, C.A., Gerhardt, S.C. and Janak, P. (1986). Systemic AP7 reduces ischaemic brain damage in gerbils. In *Excitatory Amino Acid Transmission*, edited by Hicks, T.P., Lodge, D. and McLennan, H., eds., Alan R. Liss, New York, pp. 249–252.
42. Simon, R.P., Meldrum, B.S., Schmidley, J.W., Swan, J.H. and Chapman, A.G. (1987). Mechanisms of selective vulnerability: Hypoglycaemia. In *Fifteenth Princeton Conference on Cerebrovascular Diseases*, Raichle, M.E. and Parks, W.S. eds., Raven Press, New York, 27–36.
43. Westerberg, E. and Wieloch, T. (1986). Excitatory amino acids and hypoglycaemic brain damage. In *Excitatory Amino Acid Transmission*, Hicks, T.P., Lodge, D. and McLennan, H., eds., Alan. R. Liss, New York, pp. 225–232.
44. Spencer, P.S., Roy, D.N., Ludolph, A., Hugun, J., Dwived, M.P. and Schaumburg, H.H. (1986). Lathyrism: Evidence for role of the neuroexcitatory amino acid BOAA. Lancet II, 1066–1067.
45. Watkins, J.C., Curtis, D.R. and Biscoe, T.J. (1966). Central effects of B-N-oxalyl-a,e-diaminopropionic acid and other lathyrus factors. Nature 211, 637.
46. Mouritzen Dam, A. (1979). The density of neurons in the human hippocampus. Neuropathol. Appl. Neurobiol. 5, 249–264.
47. Ellison, D.W., Beal, M.F., Mazurek, M.F., Bird, E.D. and Martin, J.B. (1986). A postmortem study of amino acid neurotransmitters in Alzheimer's disease. Ann. Neurol. 20, 616–621.
48. Quirion, R., DiMaggio, D.A., French, E.D., Contreras P.C., Shiloach, J., Pert, C.B., Everist H., Pert, A. and O'Donohue, T.L. (1984). Evidence for an endogenous peptide ligand for the phencyclidine receptor. Peptides 5, 967–973.
49. Nishikawa, T., Takashima., M. and Toru, M. (1963). Increased [^{3}H]kainic acid binding in the prefrontal cortex in schizophrenia. Neurosci. Lett. 40, 245–250.
50. Greenamyre, J.T., Penney, J.B., D'Amato, C.J. and Young, A.B. (1987). Dementia of the Alzheimer's type: Changes in hippocampal L-[^{3}H]glutamate binding. J. Neurochem. 48, 543–551.
51. Geddes, J.W., Chang-Chui, H., Cooper, S.M. Lott, I.T. and Cotman, C.W. (1986). Density and distribution of NMDA receptors in the human hippocampus in Alzheimer's disease. Brain Res. 399, 156–161.
52. Geddes, J.W., Monaghan, D.T., Cotman, C.W., Lott, I.T., Kim, R.C. and Chui, H.C. (1985). Plasticity of hippocampal circuitry in Alzheimer's disease. Science 230, 1179–1181.
53. Hyman, B.T., VanHoesen, G.W., Damasio, A.R. and Barnes, C.L. (1984). Alzheimer's disease: Cell specific pathology isolates the hippocampal formation. Science 225, 1168–1170.
54. Hyman, B.T., VanHoesen, G.W., Kromer, L.J., and Damasio, A.R. (1986). Perforant pathway changes and the memory impairment of Alzheimer's disease. Ann. Neurol. 20, 472–481.
55. Greenamyre, J.T., Penney, J.B. and Young, A.B. (1987). Evidence for transient, perinatal glutamatergic innervation of globus pallidus. J. Neurosci. 7, 1022–1030.

56. Beal, M.F., Kowall, N.W., Ellison, D.W., Mazurek, M.F., Swartz, K.J. and Martin, J.B. (1986). Replication of the neurochemical characteristics of Huntington's disease by quinolinic acid. Nature 321, 168–171.
57. Koh, J-Y., Peters, S., Choi, D.W. (1986). Neurons containing NADPH-diaphorase are selectively resistant to quinolinate toxicity. Science, 234, 73–76.
58. Plaitakis A.A., Berl, S. and Yahr, M.D. (1982). Abnormal glutamate metabolism in an adult-onset degenerative neurological disorder. Science 216, 193–196.
59. Sorbi, S., Tonini, S., Giannini, E., Piacentini, S., Marini, P. and Amadulu, L. (1986). Abnormal platelet glutamate dehydrogenase activity and activation in dominant and non-dominant olivopontocerebellar atrophy. Ann. Neurol. 19, 239–245.
60. Kornhuber, H.H. (1983). Chemistry, physiology and neuropsychology of schizophrenia: Towards an earlier diagnosis of schizophrenia. I. Arch. Psychiatr. Nervenkr. 233, 415–422.
61. Kim, J.S., Kornhuber, H.H., Scmid-Burgk, W. and Holzmuller, B. (1980). Low cerebrospinal fluid glutamate in schizophrenic patients and a new hypothesis on schizophrenia. Neurosci. Lett. 20, 379–382.
62. Gattaz, W.F., Gattaz, D. and Beckmann, H. (1982). Glutamate in schizophrenics and healthy controls. Arch. Psychiatr. Nervenkr. 231. 221–225.
63. Perry, T.L. (1982). Normal cerebrospinal fluid and brain glutamate levels in schizophrenia do not support the hypothesis of glutamatergic neuronal dysfunction. Neurosci. Lett. 28, 81–85.
64. Sherman, A.D. and Mott, J. (1984). Direct effect of neuroleptics on glutamate release. Neuropharmacology 23, 1253–1259.
65. Sherman, A.D. and Mott, J. (1986). Effects of glutamine inhibition on release of endogenous glutamic acid. Neuropharmacology 25, 1353.
66. Rudolph, M.I. and Bustos, G. (1986). Search of a L-glutamate receptor related to modulation of neurotransmission in the rat corpus striatum. Neurochem. Int. 8, 481–492.
67. Cheramy, A., Romo, R., Godehu, G., Baruch, P. and Glowinski, J. (1986). In vivo presynaptic control of dopamine release in the cat caudate nucleus. II. Facilitatory or inhibitory influence of L-glutamate. Neuroscience 19, 1081–1090.
68. Contreras, P.C., DiMaggio, D.A. and O'Donohue, T.L. (1987). An endogenous ligand for the sigma opiod binding site. Synapse 1, 57–61.
69. Troupin, A.S., Mending, J.R., Cheng, F. and Risinger, M.W. (1986). MK 801. In *New Anticonvulsant Drugs*, Meldrum, B.S. and Porter, R.J., eds., John Libbey, London, pp. 191–202.
70. Croucher, M.J., Meldrum, B.S., Jones, A.W. and Watkins, J.C. (1984). γ-D-glutamylaminomethylsulphonic acid (GAMS), a kainate and quisqualate antagonist, prevents sound-induced seizures in DBA/2 mice. Brain Res. 322, 111–114.
71. Croucher, M.J., Meldrum, B.S. and Collins, J.F. (1984). Anticonvulsant and proconvulsant properties of a series of structural isomers of piperidine dicarboxylic acid. Neuropharmacology 23, 467–472.
72. Meldrum, B.S., Chapman, A.G. and Mello, L. (1987). Anticonvulsant action of kynurenic acid in reflex epilepsy in DBA/2 mice and in photosensitive baboons. Bender, D. and Joseph, M.H., eds., Progress in Tryptophan and Serotonin Research 1986. Walter de Gruyter & Co. Berlin, pp. 119–126.

II. TROPHIC FACTORS

6. EVIDENCE FOR THE ROLE OF AFFERENTS IN THE REGULATION OF NEURONAL SURVIVAL DURING NORMAL PERIODS OF DEVELOPMENTAL CELL DEATH: MOTONEURONS AND THE CILIARY GANGLION*

RONALD W. OPPENHEIM

Studies of naturally-occurring neuronal death have tended to emphasize almost exclusively the role of neuron-target interactions in the competitive events that result in the survival of a proportion of a pre-cell death population of neurons and the degeneration and death of the remainder. The reason for this restricted focus on targets, of course, is that a large number of studies examining different types of neurons in a variety of species have shown that increases or decreases in the size, volume, number, or type of targets is associated with increased or decreased survival of those neurons that innervate the altered targets [1, 2]. Consequently, there is a consensus among workers in this field that for many populations of neurons, targets are exceedingly important for regulating how many neurons will survive the cell death period. However, there is also a growing recognition that afferent influences may be involved in regulating cell death [3–5]. Ideally, in order to critically examine the relative contributions of afferent and target influences on neuronal survival and death, it would be advantageous to focus on a neuronal population that receives a single source of afferent input and projects to a single target region and in which the afferent and target cells can be independently and systematically perturbed at developmental stages prior to the onset of naturally-occurring cell death. The ciliary ganglion of the chick embryo is one of the few neuronal populations that meets these criteria. The other population of

* Supported by NIH grant NS 20402.

Ferrendelli, J.A., Collins, R.C. and Johnson, E.M. (eds), Neurobiology of Amino Acids, Peptides, and Trophic Factors.

neurons that will be focused on here are the spinal cord motoneurons (MN) that innervate the skeletal muscles in the hindlimb [4]. Although not as advantageous as the CG for studying afferent influences, the spinal motoneurons of the chick embryo have the advantage of being one of the most extensively studied systems regarding neuronal death and the role of cell-to-cell interactions.

Lumbar motoneurons are born between E2 and E4 [6]. They complete their migration to the ventral horn or lateral motor column (LMC) by E4½–E5. Innervation of the hindlimb begins between E4½–E5, and neuromuscular function begins by E5½–E6. Prior to the onset of cell death on E5½, there are approximately 20,000 motoneurons distributed throughout the eight lumbar segments on one side of the spinal cord. Between E5 and E12 roughly one-half of these cells are lost by cell death (Figure 6-1) [7]. Afferent synapses, very likely arising from rostral spinal regions, begin to form on motoneurons on E4 [8], and these synapses are functional [9]. Although afferents from supraspinal sources are present in the lumbar region by E5 [4], the time of onset of synaptogenesis and function of these afferents is not known.

Considerable evidence now exists indicating that the regulation of naturally occurring MN death in the chick embryo spinal cord occurs primarily, if not exclusively, by interactions between these neurons and their muscular targets [2]. Early limb bud ablation (target removal) results in the death of virtually all MNs during approximately the same time frame as naturally occurring cell death [10, 11]; the addition of a supernumerary limb (increased target size) prevents a significant amount of the naturally occurring loss of MNs [12]. However, both of these manipulations also induce significant numerical and other changes in the associated DRG [13, 14], which very likely leads to changes in the extent of primary afferent input to interneurons and MNs. Thus, it is not entirely clear from such studies that the only critical factor being altered that could affect MN survival is target size; changes in afferents may also be involved.

In addition to the possible influence of primary DRG afferents on the regulation of MN survival, one must also consider the role of intrinsic afferents that arise from spinal or supraspinal sources and that provide synaptic input to MNs. Previous attempts to evaluate the influence of these intrinsic afferents on MN survival in the chick have been largely negative [2] in that MN numbers were unchanged following the elimination of apparently significant amounts of such afferent input.

An important assumption, and one that is usually unstated in all of these deafferentation studies, is that the afferents in question (DRG and intrinsic) normally make synaptic contact with, or are in close apposition, to MNs during the period of naturally occurring cell death. Synapses do, in fact, begin to form on MNs during the cell death period [8], and neurons in the brain, rostral spinal cord, and DRG can be retrogradely labeled following HRP injections into the lumbar spinal cord at any time from E5½ to hatching [4]. Conse-

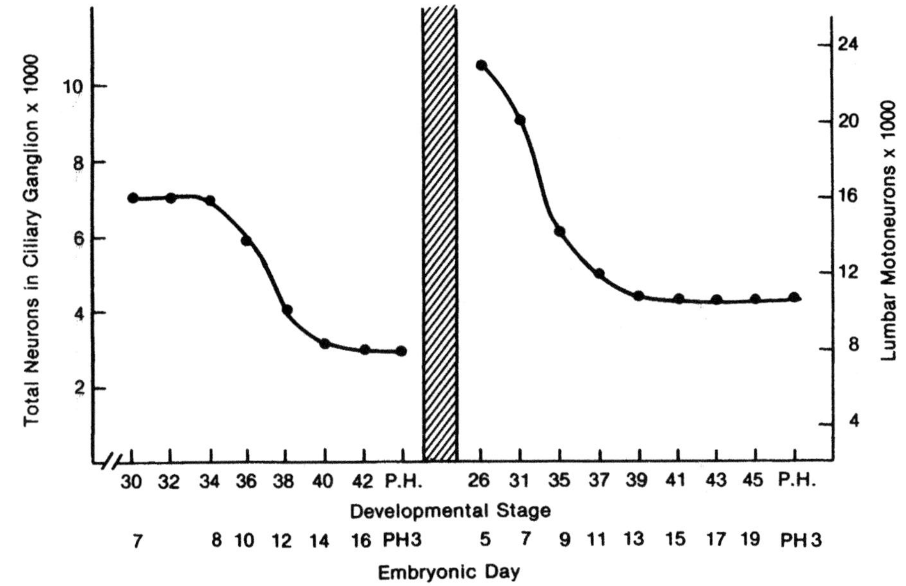

Figure 6-1. Cell loss in the chick ciliary ganglion and lumbar ventral horn.

quently, it seems plausible that afferent terminals from a variety of sources may be in a position to exert an influence upon MNs during the major period of cell death (i.e., between E5 and E10). Nonetheless, at present we do not know either the extent to which afferents form synapses on MNs at these stages or the relative contribution of afferents from various sources to the total population of synapses on either developing or adult MNs.

The chick ciliary ganglion is composed of two homogeneous populations of neurons, the small choroid cells that innervate the smooth musculature of the chroidal coat and the larger ciliary cells that innervate the striated iris and ciliary muscles (Figure 6-2). Despite these, as well as several other, anatomical and physiological differences between the ciliary and choroid cells [15], both cell types are known to be derived from the cranial neural crest [16, 17]. Beginning at stages 8–9 of Hamburger and Hamilton [18], the neural crest precursors migrate from the dorsal-lateral surface of the mesencephalon to a site behind the eye, close to the emerging optic nerve. Aggregation of the ganglion precursors is completed by about E5 (stage 25), and by E6–E7 (stages 31–33) the maximum pre-cell death population of neurons is attained. *Efferent* projections to the iris are present by E5–E6, and *afferent* projections to the ganglion from the accessory oculomotor nucleus (AON), the avian homologue of the mammalian Edinger-Westphal nucleus, are present by E3–E4 [19; own unpublished observations]. Between E7 and E15, approximately 50% of the original population of neurons in the ganglion undergo naturally occurring

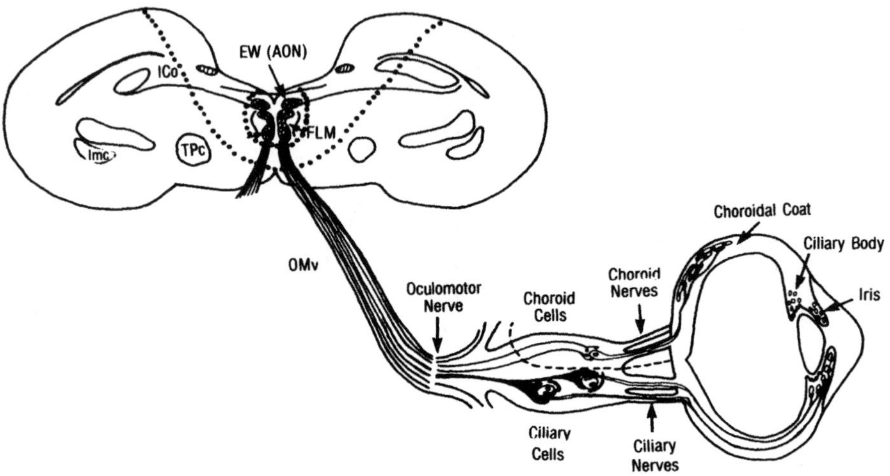

Figure 6-2. Schematic drawing of midbrain, oculomotor nerve (OMv), ciliary ganglion, and eye. Dotted lines indicate the smallest and greatest extent of the lesion following electrocautery of the mid-dorsal midbrain on E4 (Stage 25). *AON* = accessory oculomotor nucleus; *EW* = Edinger-Westphal nucleus; *ICo* = nucleus intercollicularis; *Imc* = nucleus isthmui, pars magnocellularis; *Ipc* = nucleus isthmi pars parvocellularis: *TPc* = nucleus tegmenti pedunculo-pontinus pars compacta. (Drawing of ciliary ganglion and eye modified from Landmesser and Pilar [15].)

degeneration (Figure 6-1), resulting in a final population size of about 3000 cells [20]; the ciliary and choroid populations appear to be about equally depleted by this process of cell death. Removal of the optic vesicle on E2 (target deletion), prior to target innervation, results in a greatly enhanced cell loss in the CG [21–24], whereas transplantation of a supernumerary optic vesicle on E2 rescues a significant number of ganglion cells from neuron death [25]. Finally, tissue culture media "conditioned" by heart or skeletal muscle cells has also been shown to support the survival of virtually the entire pre-cell death population of ciliary ganglion neurons in vitro [26]. Collectively, these various lines of evidence argue strongly for the important, perhaps even exclusive, role of targets and target-derived survival factors in regulating ciliary ganglion cell survival. Yet, other populations of neurons for which an equally strong case can be made for the primary role of targets have recently been shown to be significantly affected (i.e., increased cell death) by the deletion of afferents [5]. Consequently, it seems plausible that despite the obviously important role of targets in ciliary ganglion cell survival, afferents may also be involved.

1. EXPERIMENTS

1.1. Spinal cord motoneurons

In order to examine the role of supraspinal, propriospinal (intersegmental), and primary sensory afferents in motoneuron development in the lumbar

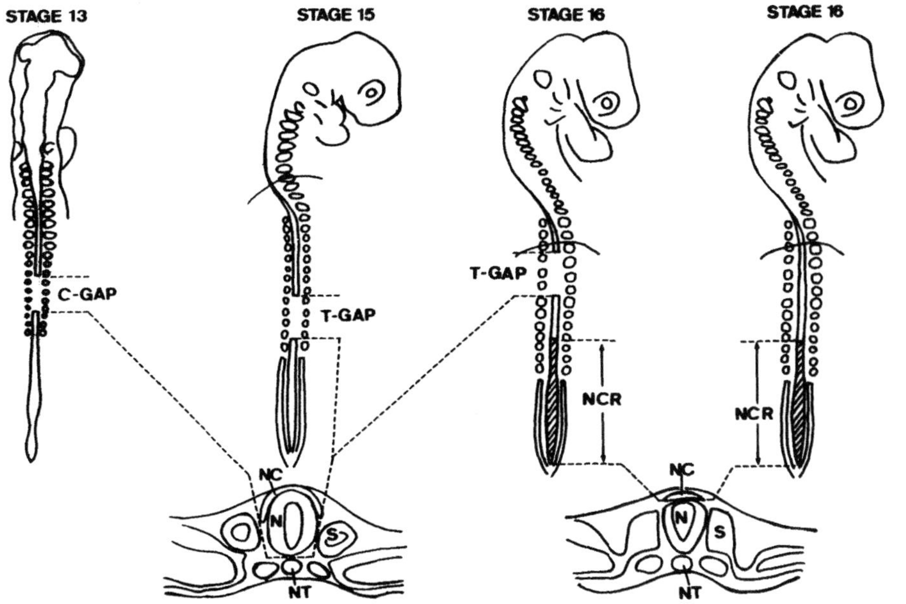

Figure 6-3. Schematic illustrations of various surgical means for the deafferentation of lumbar motoneurons. (See text and Okado and Oppenheim [4] for details.)

lateral motor column (LMC), three types of operation were carried out on E2: 1) The spinal cord was transected at the cervical (C-gap) or at the thoracic level (T-gap) in order to eliminate supraspinal (C-gap) or both supraspinal and propriospinal (T-gap) inputs to the lumbar cord (Figure 6-3); 2) The entire lumbar neural crest was removed in order to delete primary sensory input from the dorsal root ganglia (DRG); 3) A combined operation of T-gap and DRG removal was performed in order to remove all afferent inputs except those arising from intrinsic segmental interneurons within the eight lumbar segments. For each type of operation, the number of motoneurons in the lumbar LMC were counted in embryos sacrificed between E10 and E18. Dying or degenerating neurons were also evaluated over these same ages.

As summarized in Figure 6-4, we have found that spinal gap operations in which either supraspinal afferents (C-gap) or both supraspinal and propriospinal afferents (T-gap) were eliminated several days prior to the onset of naturally occurring death of lumbar MNs are without effect on the survival of these cells up to E10 to E12. Similar results were obtained following the removal of virtually all primary afferent input from the DRG. By contrast, all of these operations resulted in a significant depletion of MNs at later stages (i.e., by E16 to E18). Since a small amount of cell death occurs normally in this population after E10 (8% versus 43% before E10), one might argue that

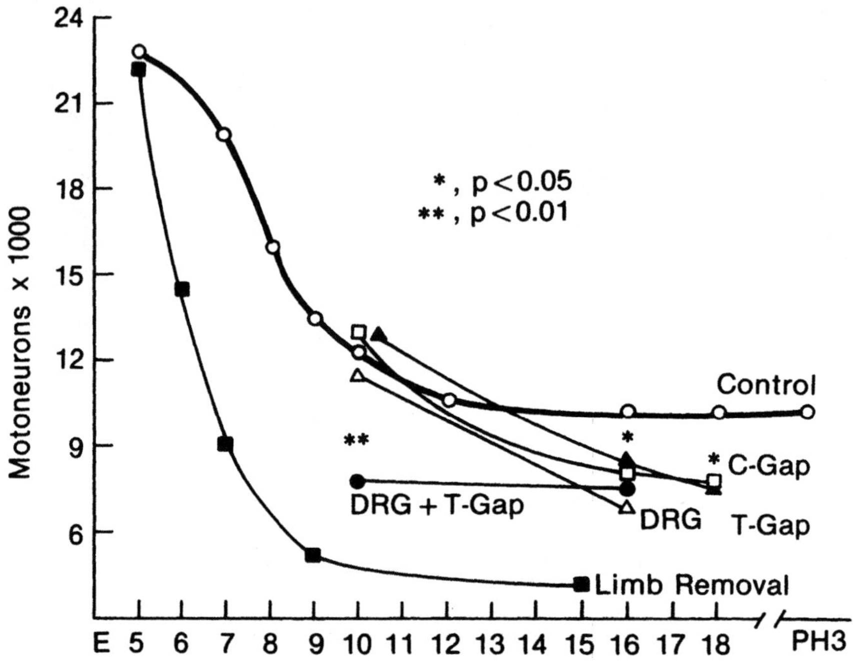

Figure 6-4. Summary of data on motoneuron survival following various types of deafferentation. (See text and Okado and Oppenheim [4] for details.)

afferents are primarily involved in maintaining MNs only during the late or terminal stages of naturally occurring cell death. The data on degenerating neurons tend to support this, in that there were significantly more dying neurons on E13 and E14, but not E10, in the T- and C-gap groups. Alternatively, afferents may only influence the later *maintenance* of MNs that have competed successfully for targets (or afferents) and thus have survived the entire period of massive cell death. Another alternative possibility, i.e., that the enhanced cell loss at late stages following spinal transection reflects the retrograde degeneration of neurons with ascending axons whose soma is located within or in close proximity to the LMC, has been ruled out here. Although we have shown that such neurons exist, they are so few in number, even at stages later than E10 [4], that they cannot account for more than a fraction of the cell loss following either type of gap operation.

The results of the combined T-gap plus DRG operation indicate, however, that it may not only be the late stages of cell death that are affected by deafferentation. In these preparations, a significant depletion of MNs was seen as early as E10. Although earlier stages were not examined, the fact that these animals had fewer degenerating MNs on E10 compared to control values indicates that the enhanced cell death did not occur only between E9 and E10. If this were the case, one would have expected to see more, not fewer, dying cells on E10. Thus, these results imply that the age of onset of a response to deafferentation may be related to the extent of the deafferentation. At stages earlier than E10, gaps or NCR alone may not remove enough afferents to influence MN survival [8]. If both are removed simultaneously, however, then many MNs may be so deprived of a putative orthograde trophic factor that even at these early stages they can no longer be sustained solely by retrograde influences from their muscular targets.

The number of MNs in a population that fall victim to deafferentation appears to be relatively fixed. The number of surviving MNs in the lumbar LMC on E16 or E18, following any of the single or combined operations, always ranged between ~6500 and 8000 (i.e., a 20%–35% decrease from control values), and none of these experimental values were statistically different from one another. Consequently, since the combined T-gap plus DRG operation probably removes considerably more (although by no means all) of the MN afferents than do the single DRG or C-gap operations, one could argue that there are a large number of MNs (~65%) that are normally sustained largely by target influences. However, until we know the actual proportion of afferents that are removed by the various operations used here, it is not possible to determine the extent to which these remaining MNs are, in fact, deafferented. Even if the operations used here do remove most of the normal afferents to MNs, it is still possible that new sources of afferents arise (e.g., from axonal sprouting of segmental interneurons) that compensate for the removed inputs [27]. Thus, the proportion of neurons that survive following deafferentation (~65%) may do so by virtue of having received enough compensating inputs.

In light of the fact that chronic neuromuscular blockade has been shown to rescue motoneurons from dying during both early and late stages of the normal cell death period [28, 29], it is of interest that the additional neurons that die after E10 following the T-gap (or C-gap) operation could not be saved by chronic curare treatment from E10 to E14, even though the neurons that normally die during this period were, in fact, saved. This result strongly implies that the induced cell loss following deafferentation is regulated differently from the normally occurring late cell loss.

In conclusion, the present results would appear to be incompatible with a model of naturally occurring MN death in which the target is thought to be the major source of information for regulating neuronal survival. Although experimental manipulations that seemingly only alter target-related factors can be shown to save virtually all neurons that would normally die [26, 28, 30], the situation in vivo during normal development may be considerably more complex. Alternatively, it must be considered whether or to what extent deletion studies such as those described above provide evidence that is pertinent to the normal biological role of afferents in vivo. Perhaps, normally, populations of neurons are buffered against small to moderate flucuations in afferent input, but following more drastic perturbations they respond in a manner (i.e., increased death) that is normally never operative. These and other issues of more general significance will be taken up in the final section, following a discussion of the results from the ciliary ganglion experiments.

1.2. Ciliary ganglion

For the deletion of afferent input to the CG, embryos were exposed via a lateral window on E4 (Stages 24–25), a small opening was made in the amnion over the head of the embryo, and using a glass probe and forceps the dorsal mesencephalic region was exposed and stabilized under this opening. Using a small, battery-operated electocautery (Storz Instruments, St. Louis) with a specially prepared fine tip, the dorsal midline region of the mesencephalon containing the AON was briefly cauterized, the head of the embryo was then replaced within the amniotic sac, the egg opening sealed, and the egg replaced in the incubator. Approximately 30%–50% of such operated embryos (total = 325) survived to between E8 and E16.

In another group of embryos, the right optic vesicle (eye primordium) was removed on E2 (Stages 11–12) using forceps and a vibrating needle [31]. In approximately one-half of these eye-removal embryos, the AON was also destroyed bilaterally on E4, as described above. Sham control operations for both AON destruction and eye removal involved all of the same procedures used for experimental embryos except for actual cauterization or eye removal [32].

Following surgery, experimental and sham-control embryos were allowed to survive to various ages, ranging from E4½ to E18. Brains were sectioned in order to assess the extent to which the AON had actually been destroyed. Only embryos with a complete unilateral or bilateral absence of the entire oculomotor nuclear complex were retained for subsequent examination of cell numbers in the deafferented CG. The numbers of both surviving as well as dying or degenerating neurons were assessed. In order to determine the extent to which deafferented CG neurons can grow and project axons to their targets in the eye, axon counts were made in the postganglionic nerves of a few embryos using the electron microscope; in other deafferented embryos, horseradish peroxidase injections were made into iris and choroid musculature in order to retrogradely label neurons in the CG. Finally, the ultrastructural changes in the CG that occur following deafferentation-induced degeneration were also examined.

1.3. Development following deafferentation

Deletion of the AON, the single source of preganglionic afferents to the CG, on E4, which is several days prior to the onset of naturally occurring cell death in the ganglion, did not have any noticeable affect on the ganglion up to E8. From the cell counts (Figure 6-5) and histology (Figure 6-6), it seems likely that the migration, proliferation, aggregation and axonal outgrowth of the deafferented CG has progressed normally in the absence of afferents [21, 22]. By E6, control and embryonic ganglia contain equal numbers of neurons. By

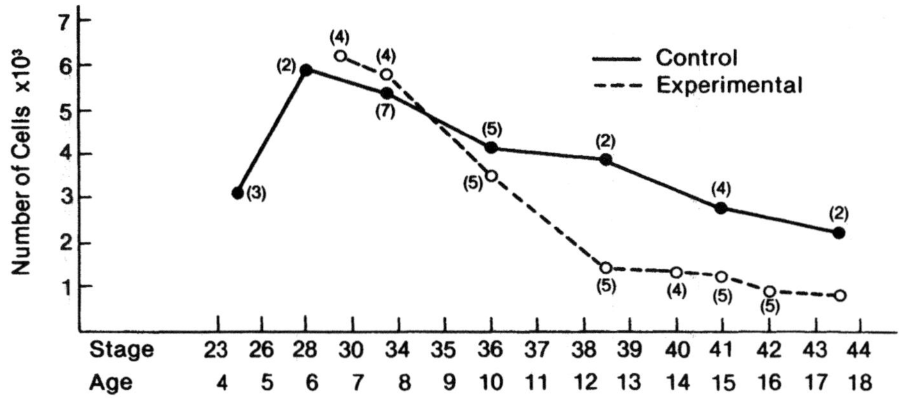

Figure 6-5. Number of ciliary ganglion cells in control and deafferented embryos; $p < 0.05$ at stages 38 to 44.

contrast, between E7 and E15, the control ganglia lose approximately 50% of their neurons (6000–2700), whereas the number of neurons in the deafferented ganglia falls from a peak of about 6200 to 900 neurons, a loss of approximately 85%. Thus, there is an enhanced cell loss in the deafferented ganglia of 35%. Most of this increased loss occurs after E10 when cell number in the control ganglia goes from 4000 to 2700 (33% loss), compared to a 75% loss (3500 to 900) in the deafferented ganglia. Although it is conceivable that this enhanced cell loss in the deafferented ganglia is due to factors other than increased cell death [5], the data on dying neurons (i.e., cells with pyknotic nuclei) makes this possibility exceedingly unlikely. There were significantly more degenerating neurons in the deafferented vs. control ganglia on E10 (57 ± 8 vs. 10 ± 3 pyknotic neurons per 1000 healthy cells, $n = 5$ per group, $p < 0.01$).

1.4 Development following eye removal and deafferentation

Consistent with prior reports [21, 23, 24], we have found that deletion of the postsynaptic targets (eye removal) of CG neurons on E2, which is several days prior to both cell death and target innervation, results in a marked reduction in the number of CG neurons at later stages. Although we have not systematically examined earlier or later stages, on E12, embryos with a complete eye removal have approximately 55% fewer CG cells than controls [24], a value that is similar to E12 embryos following deafferentation (Figure 6-7). Two embryos with eye removal that survived to E15 had 540 and 515 surviving CG neurons (i.e., 81% less than controls). By contrast, embryos with a *combined* eye removal and deafferentation have a considerably greater reduction in cell number on E12 than following either operation alone (93% fewer neurons than controls and 84% fewer than either eye or AON removal embryos, Figure 6-7); one embryo in this group that survived to E16 had few, if any,

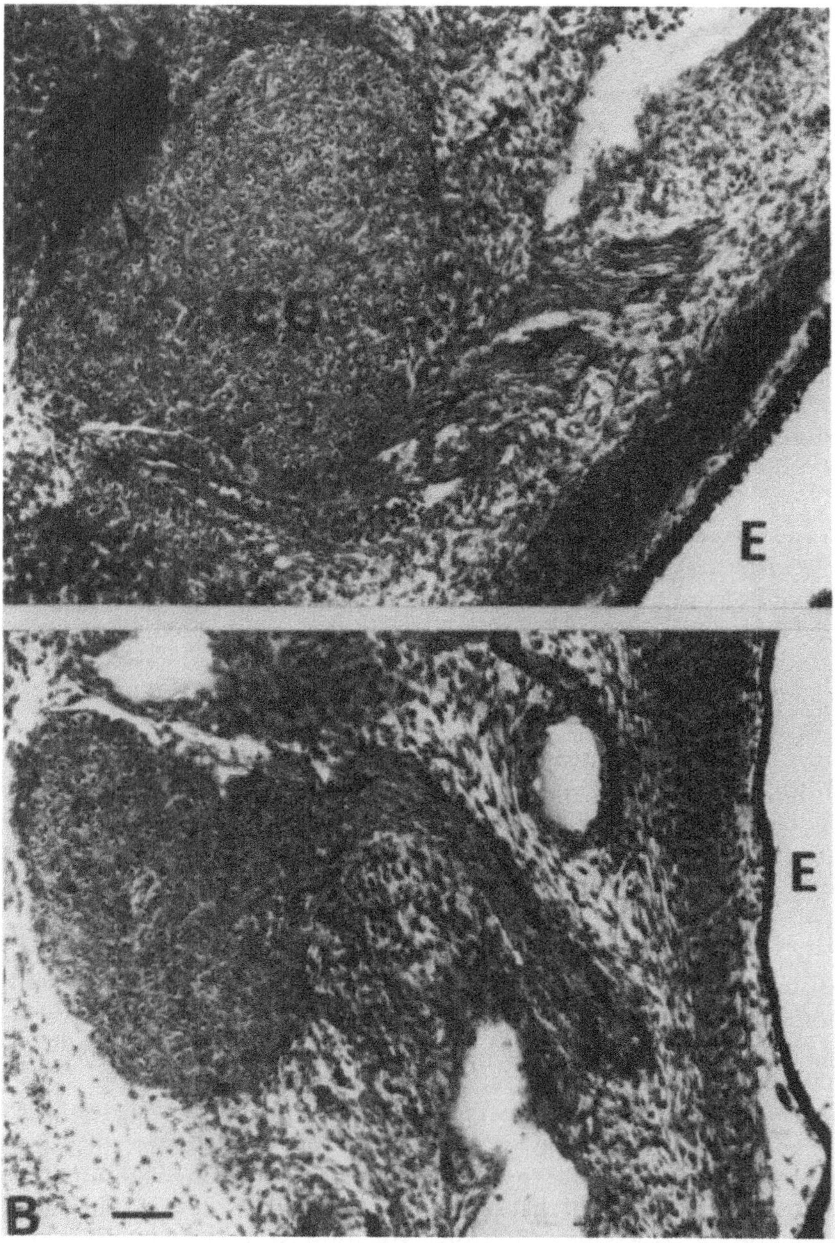

Figure 6-6. Transverse section of control (A) and deafferented (B) ciliary ganglion in the same approximate region of the ganglion on E8 (Stage 34). Note the absence of the oculomotor nerve (arrowhead) in B and the presence of the postganglionic nerve (arrows) in A and B. Silver with thionin counterstain. E = eye; bar = 30 μm.

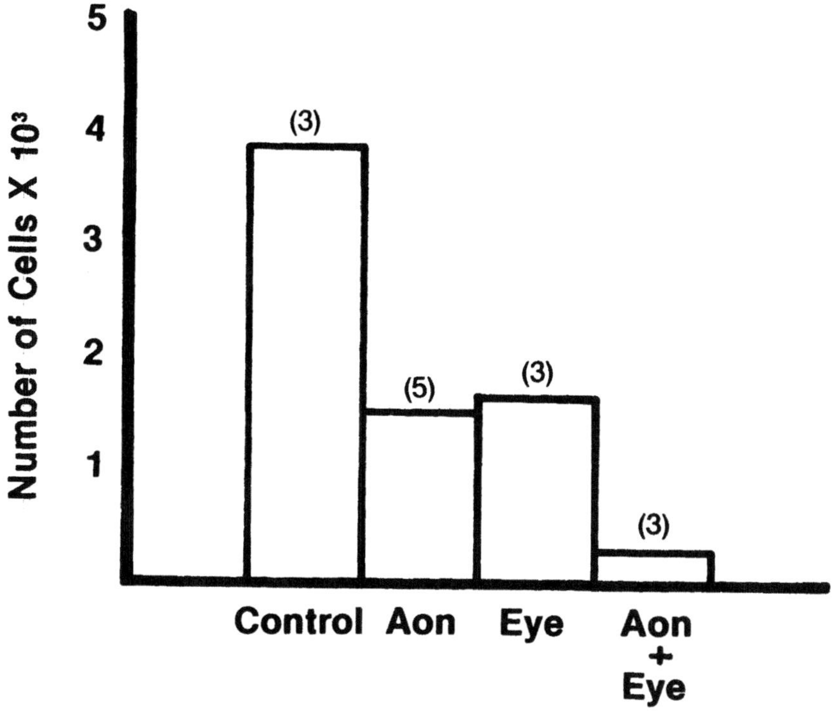

Figure 6-7. Number of ciliary ganglion cells on E12 (Stage 38) in control, deafferented (Aon), eye removal, and combined eye removal and deafferented embryos; $p < 0.05$ compared to control; $p < 0.05$ compared to *Aon* and *Eye* groups. All data depicted in this figure for control and Aon are from different embryos than shown in Figure 5-5.

discernible surviving ganglion cells on the side of the brain ipsilateral to the eye removal.

1.5. Postganglionic nerve and target innervation following deafferentation

Examination of the CG in thionin stained and silver impregnated preparations following deafferentation indicates that the deprived ganglion cells send axons towards the eye (Figure 6-6). Furthermore, postganglionic nerves could be seen running across the surface of the eye towards the ciliary musculature, as in control embryos. To confirm that all surviving ganglion cells contribute axons to the postganglionic nerves and actually innervate target structures in the eye, we have used two strategies: 1) axon counts in the postganglionic nerve immediately distal to the ganglion and 2) retrograde labeling of CG neurons following HRP injection into the target regions of the eye. Estimates of axon numbers show that virtually all of the surviving neurons have at least one axonal process in the postganglionic nerve on E12: *control* = 4336.3 axons, n = 2; *deafferented* = 2967.3 axons, n = 2. The deafferented embryos have a

32% reduction in axon number. HRP injections into the ciliary and choroidal targets of the deafferented CG neurons on E8 results in the retrograde labeling of large numbers of ganglion cells. This supports the evidence obtained from axon counts and shows, further, that many of the deafferented neurons actually innervate the eye.

In a previous study of cell death in the CG, Pilar and Landmesser [33] found that naturally-occurring cell death and cell death brought about by target deletion (eye removal) differed in the ultrastructural characteristics observed during their development and subsequent degeneration. Before the onset of degeneration, neurons in the peripherally deprived ganglia failed to develop the well-organized rough endoplasmic reticulum (RER) characteristic of normal ganglion cells. Degeneration in peripherally deprived ganglia was primarily marked by nuclear changes, followed by the breakdown of polysomes to single or free ribosomes. In contrast, naturally-occurring cell death was characterized by dilation of the previously well-organized RER, followed by cytoplasmic breakdown and, only at terminal stages, by nuclear disruption.

Although we have only made a careful study of the ultrastructure of CG neurons on E12 and E15, we have failed to detect any differences in either the development or characteristics of degeneration of control and deafferented ganglion cells. In both groups, normal (nondying) neurons exhibit all of the same ultrastructural features previously described by Pilar and Landmesser [33] for control CG neurons. Furthermore, dying cells in both groups appear to undergo the sequence of degeneratiive changes designated "cytoplasmic" by those authors in which the most notable changes involve dilation of the cisternae of the RER, mitochondrial swelling, and terminal nuclear changes.

To summarize, we have surgically destroyed the single source of afferents to the CG (the AON) on E4, several days prior to the onset of cell death in the CG. Following deafferention, the CG develops normally up to E9, after which the amount of cell death is enhanced such that the number of surviving cells on E15–E18 is reduced to less than 10%–15% of the peak number present prior to cell death. During this same period, control embryos with intact afferents lose only about 50% of the pre-cell death population. Although it is possible that at later stages (e.g., posthatching) all deafferented CG neurons may degenerate, in fact, this seems unlikely. Cell number in the deafferented CG appears to stabilize by E14–E15 and shows no further significant decrease up to E18, which is the oldest age examined by us. It is interesting that the amount of enhanced cell loss in the CG following complete *target* removal [also see Ref. 24] is quantitatively similar to that found following total deafferentation. By contrast, when *both* the targets and afferents are removed, virtually all of the CG neurons are lost by E15. Thus, neither targets nor afferents alone are able to sustain more than a small number of CG neurons (< 15%). Although it is conceivable that some of the surviving neurons in both cases are sustained by aberrant intraganglionic connections, the virtually complete degeneration of the CG following combined target and afferent removal indicates that this putative source of support is probably insignificant.

The significance of these data for normal development, as well as an examination of the possible mechanisms by which afferents may exert an influence on neuronal survival, is considered below.

2. DISCUSSION AND CONCLUSIONS

The issue raised above, regarding the biological significance of demonstrations of increased cell death following deafferentation, is one that is impossible to resolve in the absence of additional information. Ideally, one needs evidence showing that enhanced afferent input, over and above that which is normally present, can rescue a significant number of neurons that would have undergone normal cell death. In only one case is evidence of this kind available, and even here the results are not entirely unambiguous. Cunningham and colleagues [34] reported that after unilateral lesions of the visual cortex at birth, some of the remaining visual centers subsequently become "hypertrophic." The authors conclude that a lesion-induced redistribution of optic afferent fibers to these nuclei (increased afferents) act to rescue neurons that would normally have undergone natural cell death. Although this is a plausible explanation of the data, until more information is available on normal cell death in these nuclei (e.g., Does it occur?; If so, what is the time course?), it isn't possible to rule out alternative explanations.

The CG may provide a good model for increasing afferent input while holding target size constant. For instance, it should be possible to create the appropriate quantitative disparities between CG neurons and their afferents by heterospecific transplants of either the mesencephalic region containing the AON or the optic vesicle between chick, duck, and quail embryos in which cell numbers in the CNS very likely bear a close relationship to the markedly different body size of these species [35, 36]. Until such studies have been done, however, one must rely on the kind of circumstantial evidence presented in the present paper for support of the contention that afferents are biologically significant in regulating neuronal survival.

Another issue that must be discussed concerning these data is whether the enhanced neuronal loss following deafferentation is due to a secondary, transneuronally-induced abnormal target innervation. If the deafferentated neurons were impaired in their ability to project an axon and make target contacts, then the enhanced cell death could be due to the same or similar factors that lead to increased cell death following target removal (e.g., loss of trophic support from the target). The quantitative similarity in the extent of cell loss following either operation (i.e., an 80%–90% cell loss) could even be used as evidence in support of this argument. Nonetheless, several lines of evidence from the study of the CG appear to refute this notion. Silver stained preparations, axon counts, and retrograde labeling of the CG following HRP injection into the eye indicate that the deafferented ganglion cells do, in fact, project postganglionic axons to and innervate their targets in the eye. Moreover, if the cell loss following either target removal or deafferentation is actually due to a failure of

CG neurons in both situations to innervate their targets, then the combined removal of both should not result in any greater amount of cell loss than following either operation alone. But, as shown here, there is, in fact, a significantly greater cell loss in this situation. Based on these two arguments, we conclude that it is unlikely that the enhanced cell death following deafferentation is due to an induced loss of, or the failure to initiate, target contact.

In the present study, it has been found that the most prevalent type of degenerative changes observed in both the deafferented and normal CG are quite similar to the *cytoplasmic* form described by Pilar and Landmesser [33] for control ganglia. Moreover, prior to their degeneration, the deafferented ganglion cells undergo the same developmental transitions in RER and polyribosomes as seen in control ganglia. Thus, although it has been argued that deafferentation of some neuronal populations alters their differentiation in a manner similar to target deletion and also transforms the type of degeneration observed from primarily *cytoplasmic* to primarily *nuclear* [3], this is clearly not the case for the chick CG. Consequently, target influences must play some special role in *initial* CG development not shared by afferents. Except for the virtual absence of afferent input, up to E18 the *surviving* deprived CG neurons exhibit no obvious ultrastructural differences from controls. By contrast, *target* deprived CG neurons that survive to E15 continue to exhibit obvious abnormalities in ribosomes and RER [33].

Concerning their survival, one could argue that the loss of many motorneurons or CG neurons following either target removal or deafferentation should increase the availability of whatever entity (synaptic space, trophic molecules) that is needed for the survival of the remaining neurons [37, 38]. For instance, following deafferentation the initial loss of some cells might reduce the competition between the remaining cells for limited supplies of a target-derived maintenance or survival factor. If this were to occur, however, one might expect that on this basis many more neurons would survive than the 10%–15% actually observed. Nonetheless, the fact that following combined target *and* afferent removal virtually all cells die, provides some evidence that those neurons that do survive either target or afferent removal alone are supported by the remaining contacts.

Although the literature on the role of afferents in the maintenance and survival of neurons is limited, there are an increasing number of reports in support of their importance [3, 4, 5, 39–45]. Consequently, the major challenges now are to confirm the biological significance of this phenomenon by hyperinnervation experiments, to understand the mechanisms by which afferents exert this influence, and, finally, to determine how afferent inputs and target contacts interact in determining whether a given neuron will survive the period of cell death. With regard to the second question, there is evidence that in the case of the CG, chronic blockade of ganglionic transmission (activity) during the cell death period mimics the effects of surgical deafferentation [46, 47]. On the face of it, this result may seem somewhat surprising. Ganglionic blockade should also indirectly reduce the activity of the ganglionic targets in the eye, a condition which might be expected to *rescue* ciliary neurons from normal degeneration [47, 48]. Because we have not attempted to record from postganglionic nerves or targets during ganglionic blockade, we have no way of knowing the extent to which target activity is, in fact, reduced. Thus, although we can not presently shed any light on this apparent discrepancy, it serves to underscore the problems one faces in trying to sort out primary vs. secondary (transneuronal) effects of manipulations such as afferent or target perturbations during development. However, in the present case, the fact that cell survival is decreased, not increased, by ganglionic blockade supports the contention that this effect is not mediated by alteration of CG-target interactions. Afferent influences on neuronal survival in the chick auditory system are also mediated by synaptic transmission and/or postsynaptic activity [49]. If activity is the critical factor mediating afferent influences, then one might expect that the onset of this effect would coincide with the initiation of afferent synaptic transmission. Whereas this appears to be the case in the chick auditory system [39], in the CG, ganglionic input is functional 4–5 days *before* the first effects of deafferentation are observed. However, Landmesser and Pilar [20, 24] have observed that in normal control embryos there is a transient naturally-occurring failure of synaptic transmission through the CG that reaches a peak reduction of 70% at E11–E13 (stages 37–39), which is when the onset and major occurrence of deafferentation-induced cell loss is also observed. Thus, both denervation and ganglionic blockade could induce more cell death by augmenting the normal transient loss of a functional afferent input that the CG neurons may require for their survival. Alternatively, the increased cell loss following ganglionic blockade may have nothing to do with activity during normal development. Neurotransmitter receptors may be the sites at which a putative afferent-derived neurotrophic factor is bound and internalized. Ganglionic blockade would then be acting to alter the uptake of this *anterograde* factor by occupying receptors, with the resulting inactivity only being incidentally involved. Other mechanisms are also possible.

If, for the moment, however, we assume that the afferent-driven activity of ganglionic neurons is directly involved in survival, one might speculate that inactive cells are (for unknown reasons) at a competitive disadvantage in gaining access to or utilizing a putative neurotrophic factor supplied by the afferent terminals. To carry the argument one step further, in this context one would predict that if ganglionic blockade (i.e., postsynaptic inactivity) also increases the availability of a neurotrophic factor produced by the ganglion cells and if this factor is required for the survival of preganglionic neurons, then ganglionic blockade should rescue significant numbers of neurons in the AON from naturally-occurring cell death. Although this notion is presently being tested, it is worth noting that in the peripheral *sympathetic* system of the chick embryo, ganglionic blockade does, in fact, *increase* ganglion cell death [50] but *reduces* the death of preganglionic neurons in the thoracolumbar spinal cord [51].

In formulating the above arguments, the assumption has been made that neuronal survival in the CG is regulated by competition for at least two different neurotrophic factors, a retrograde factor supplied by targets and an anterograde factor associated with afferents. Recent evidence supports this assumption in showing that at least certain classes of neurons (e.g., proprioceptive neurons in the chick trigeminal mesencephalic nucleus) require at least two different factors for survival, one supplied by peripheral targets and one by central targets [52]. Furthermore, a polypeptide has recently been isolated and purified from chick brain that promotes certain aspects of myotube differentiation and that very likely acts in vivo as an anterograde trophic factor [53]. Nerve growth factor (NGF) acts as a retrograde neurotrophic survival factor for sympathetic and dorsal root ganglion cells in vivo [54–56], and there is a considerable amount of evidence for the role of target-derived survival factors in the maintenance of spinal motoneurons and ciliary ganglion neurons [57, 58]. Thus, anterograde and retrograde survival factors are plausible candidates for mediating afferent and target influences on neuronal survival in these populations.

With regard to the question of the relative roles of target and afferent influences in neuronal survival, Cunningham [3], who was the first person to focus attention on this issue, has formulated a model — the "balance" hypothesis — that attempts to explain how target contacts and afferent inputs together regulate neuronal survival. According to this hypothesis, neurons are thought to have an intrinsic requirement for a quantitative, but not necessarily one-to-one, balance or matching of afferent and target contacts. If in normal development target structures are contacted before substantial contact with afferents occurs, then the subsequent afferent contacts should be regulated so as to balance or match quantitatively with the amount of previously established target contact. In addition, of course, the converse would be true if afferent contacts occur first during development. Although there are as yet no critical tests of this hypothesis, there is some circumstantial evidence in support of certain aspects of the proposal [3]. On the other hand, one prediction of the balance hypothesis that has *not* been supported in the present study is the observation that deletion of afferent contacts does not impair the initial differentiation of CG cells in the same way that target removal does [33]. Deafferented CG cells show the same degree of initial ultrastructural differentiation and the same type of subsequent degeneration (cytoplasmic) as controls. Somewhat stronger evidence against the balance hypothesis comes from the situation in which spinal cord motoneurons are rescued from dying by chronic neuromuscular blockade [28]. In this case, target size is *reduced* (muscle atrophy) and motoneuron numbers and efferent (neuromuscular) contacts are both *increased* [29, 59], whereas the packing density of axo-dendritic and axosomatic *afferent* synapses on these motoneurons remains unchanged [60]. Furthermore, the increased supporting capacity of the targets that is assumed to occur in these curare-treated preparations is not effective in rescuing motoneurons from deafferentation-induced cell loss [4]. That is, an increased maintenance from the target cannot compensate for a depletion of afferents [5].

As noted above, the CG may provide a good model for creating anatomical and functional disparities between target and afferent contacts that will be helpful in testing the predictions of the balance hypothesis. For instance, increasing afferent input to the CG either in the presence or absence of the normal targets may be feasible using AON transplants or by forcing both AONs to innervate a single CG [61]. Similarly, target size could be increased by adding a supernumerary eye [25] in embryos that lack afferents (i.e., after AON removal). Creating size disparities by heterospecific transplants of the AON or optic vesicle between quail, chick, and duck embryos may also provide a means for altering quantitative relationships between neurons, targets, and afferents. In addition, as noted above, if activity is involved in the control of these processes, it may be possible to systematically alter the activity of either or both presynaptic and postsynaptic components.

In conclusion, there is an increasing amount of evidence indicating that the regulation of naturally-occurring neuronal death is more complex than previously suspected. In addition to the well-documented role ascribed to interactions between neurons and their targets, these new data imply that afferents are also involved in this process. Thus, many kinds of neurons may require trophic or other means of support from both their targets and afferents in order to survive during critical phases of their differentiation.

REFERENCES

1. Jacobson, M. (1978). *Developmental Neurobiology*. Plenum, New York.
2. Oppenheim, R.W. (1981). Neuronal death and some related regressive phenomena during neurogenesis: A selective historical review and progress report. In *Studies in Developmental Neurobiology: Essays in Honor of Viktor Hamburger*, W.M. Cowan, ed., Oxford, New York, pp. 74–133.
3. Cunningham, T.J. (1982). Naturally-occurring neuron death and its regulation by developing neural pathways. Int. Rev. Cytol. 74, 163–186.
4. Okado, N. and Oppenheim, R.W. (1984). Cell death of motoneurons in the chick embryo spinal cord. IX. The loss of motoneurons following removal of afferent inputs. J. Neurosci. 4, 1639–1652.
5. Clarke, P.G. (1985). Neuronal death during development in the isthmo-optic nucleus of the chick: Sustaining role of afferents from the tectum. J. Comp. Neurol. 234, 365–379.
6. Hollyday, M. and Hamburger, V. (1977). An autoradiographic study of the formation of the lateral motor column in the chick embryo. Brain Res. 132, 197–208.
7. Hamburger, V. (1975). Cell death in the development of the lateral motor column of the chick embryo. J. Comp. Neurol. 160, 535–546.
8. Oppenheim, R.W., Chu-Wang, I.W. and Foelix, R.F. (1975). Some aspects of synaptogenesis in the spinal cord of the chick embryo: A quantitative electron microscopic study. J. Comp. Neurol. 161, 383–418.
9. Provine, R. (1983). Neurophysiological aspects of behavior development in the chick embryo. In *Behavioral Embryology*, Gottlieb, G., ed., Academic Press, New York, pp. 77–102.
10. Hamburger, V. (1934). The effects of wing-bud extirpation on the development of the central nervous system in chick embryos. J. Exp. Zool. 68, 449–494.
11. Oppenheim, R.W., Chu-Wang, I.W. and Maderdrut, J.L. (1978). The differentiation of motoneurons prior to their induced degeneration following limb-bud removal. J. Comp. Neurol. 177, 87–112.
12. Hollyday, M. and Hamburger, V. (1976). Reduction of naturally-occurring motor neuron

loss by enlargement of the periphery. J. Comp. Neurol., 170, 311–320.
13. Hamburger, V. and Levi-Montalcini, R. (1949). Proliferation, differentiation and degeneration in the spinal ganglia of the chick embryo under normal and experimental conditions. J. Exp. Zool. 111, 457–502.
14. Hamburger, V. (1939). Motor and sensory hyperplasia following limb-bud transplantation in chick embryos. Physiol. Zool. 12, 268–284.
15. Landmesser, L. and Pilar, G. (1978). Interactions between neurons and their targets during in vivo synaptogenesis. Fed. Proc. 37, 2016–2022.
16. Hammond, W.S. and Yntema, C.L. (1958). Origin of ciliary ganglia in the chick embyro. J. Comp. Neurol. 110, 367–389.
17. Narayanan, C.H. and Narayanan, Y. (1978). Neuronal adjustments in developing nuclear centers of the chick embryo following transplantation of an additional optic primordium. J. Embryol. Exp. Morph. 44, 53–70.
18. Hamburger, V. and Hamilton, H.L. (1951). A series of normal stages in the development of the chick embryo. J. Morph. 88, 49–92.
19. Tello, J.F. (1922). Les differenciations neuronales dans l'embryon de poulet pendent les premiers jours de l'incubation. *Trab. Lab. Invest. Biol. Univ. Madrid.* 21:1–93.
20. Landmesser, L. and Pilar, G. (1974). Synaptic transmission and cell death during normal ganglionic development. J. Physiol. 241, 737–749.
21. Amprino, R. (1943). Correlazioni quantitative fra centri nervosi e territovi d'innevvazione peritevica durante lo sviluppo. *Arch. Ital. Anat. Embriol.* 49:261–300.
22. Levi-Montalcini, R. and Amprino, R. (1947). Recherches experimentals sur l'origine du ganglion ciliare dans l'embryon de Poulet. Arch. de Biol. 58, 265–288.
23. Cowan, W.M. and Wenger, E. (1968). Degeneration in the nucleus of origin of the preganglionic fibers to the chick ciliary ganglion following early removal of the optic vesicle. J. Exp. Zool. 168, 105–124.
24. Landmesser, L. and Pilar, G. (1974). Synapse formation during embryogenesis on ganglion cells lacking a periphery. J. Physiol. 247, 715–736.
25. Narayanan, C.H. and Narayanan, Y. (1978). On the origin of the ciliary ganglion in birds studied by the method of interspecific transplantation of embryonic brain regions. J. Embyrol. Exp. Morph. 47, 137–148.
26. Nishi, R. and Berg, D. (1979). Survival and development of ciliary ganglion neurons grown alone in cell cultures. Nature 277, 232–234.
27. Jackson, H., and Parks, T.N. (1983). An anomalous intercochlear nucleus pathway induced in chick embryos by unilateral removal of the otocyst. Soc. Neurosci. Abstr. 9, 498.
28. Pittman, R. and Oppenheim, R.W. (1979). Cell death of motoneurons in the chick embryo spinal cord: V. Evidence that a functional neuromuscular interaction is involved in the regulation of naturally occurring cell death and the stabilization of synapses. J. Comp. Neurol. 187, 425–446.
29. Oppenheim, R.W. and Chu-Wang, I.W. (1983). Aspects of naturally occurring motoneuron death in the chick spinal cord during embryonic development. In *Somatic and Autonomic Nerve Muscle Interactions*, Burnstock, G. and Vrbova, G., eds., Elsevier, Amsterdam, pp. 57–107.
30. Creazzo, T.L., and Sohal, G.S. (1979). Effects of chronic injections of α-bungarotoxin on embryonic cell death. Exp. Neurol. 66, 135–145.
31. Wenger, B. (1968). Construction and use of the vibrating needle for embryonic operations. *Bioscience* 18:226–228.
32. Furber, S., Oppenheim, R.W. and Prevette, D. (1987). Naturally occurring neuron death in the ciliary ganglion of the chick embryo following removal of preganglionic input: Evidence for the role of afferents in ganglion cell survival. *J. Neurosci.* 7:1816–1832.
33. Pilar, G. and Landmesser, L. (1976). Ultrastructural differences during embryonic cell death in normal and peripherally deprived ciliary ganglia. J. Cell Biol. 68, 339–356.
34. Cunningham, T.J., Huddelston, C. and Murray, M. (1979). Modification of neuron numbers in the visual system of the rat. J. Comp. Neurol. 184, 423–434.
35. Tanaka, H. and Landmesser, L.T. (1986). Cell death of lumbosacral motoneurons in chick, quail and chick-quail chimera embryos: A test of the quantitative matching hypothesis of neuronal cell death. J. Neurosci. 6, 2889–2899.
36. Sohal, G.S., Knox, T.S., Allen, J.C., Arumugam, T., Campbell, L.R. and Yamashita, T. (1985). Development of the trochlear nucleus in quail and comparative study of the trochlear nucleus, nerve and innervation of the superior oblique muscle in quail, chick and duck. J.

Comp. Neurol. 239, 227–236.
37. Pilar, G., Landmesser, L. and Burstein, L. (1980). Competition for survival among developing ciliary ganglion cells. J. Neurophysiol. 43, 233–254.
38. Lance-Jones, C. and Landmesser, L. (1980). Motoneuron projection patterns in embryonic chick limbs following partial deletions of the spinal cord. J. Physiol. 302, 559–580.
39. Parks, T.N. (1979). Afferent influences on the development of the brainstem auditory nuclei of the chicken: Otocyst ablation. J. Comp. Neurol. 183, 665–678.
40. Kwei, C. and Fite, K. (1985). Development of the avian accessory optic system: Effects of embryonic optic lesions. Dev. Brain Res. 20, 33–39.
41. Friedman, B. and Price, J.L. (1986). Age-dependent cell death in the olfactory cortex: Lack of transneuronal degeneration in neonates. J. Comp. Neurol. 246, 20–31.
42. Finlay, B.L., Sengelaub, D.R. and Verian, C.A. (1986). Control of cell number in the developing visual system. I. Effects of monocular enucleation. Dev. Brain Res. 28, 1–10.
43. Mouze, M. (1978). Role des fibres post-retiniennes dans la croissance du lobe optique de la larve d'*Aeshna cyanea* Mull. Roux's Arch. Dev. Biol. 184, 325–350.
44. Lopresti, V., Macagno, E. and Levinthal, C. (1973). Structure and development of neuronal connections in isogenic organisms: Cellular interactions in the development of the optic lamina of *Daphnia*. Proc. Natl. Acad. Sci. USA 70, 433–437.
45. Sohal, G.S. (1976). Effects of deafferentation on the development of the isthmo-optic nucleus in the duck. Exp. Neurol. 50, 161–173.
46. Wright, L.L. (1982). Cell survival in the chick embryo ciliary gnaglion is reduced by chronic ganglion blockade. Dev. Brain Res. 1, 283–286.
47. Maderdrut, J.L., Merchenthaler, I. and Oppenheim, R.W. (1984). Reduction and enhancement of naturally-occurring cell death in the ciliary ganglion of the chick embryo following blockade of ganglionic and neuromuscular transmission. Neurosci. Soc Abst. 10, 639.
48. Meriney, S.D., Pilar, G. and Nunez, R. (1984). The effects of chronic neuromuscular blockade and cGMP administration on differential motoneuron survival in the avian ciliary ganglion. Neurosci. Soc. Abst. 10, 640.
49. Born, D. and Rubel, E.W. (1986). Eighth nerve activity regulates protein synthesis in avian brain stem. Presented at Association for Research in Otolaryngology, Feb., 1986.
50. Maderdrut, J.L., Oppenheim, R.W. and Prevette, D. (1988). Enhancement of naturally occurring cell death in the sympathetic and parasympathetic ganglia of the chicken embryo following blockade of ganglionic transmission. *Brain Res.* (in press).
51. Oppenheim, R.W., Maderdrut, J.L. and Wells, D. (1982). Reduction of naturally occurring cell death in the thoraco-lumbar preganglionic cell column of the chick embryo by nerve growth factor and hemicholimium-3. Dev. Brain Res. 3, 134–139.
52. Davies, A.M., Thoenen, H. and Barde, Y-A. (1986). Different factors from the central nervous system and periphery regulate the survival of sensory neurons. Nature 319, 497–499.
53. Usdin, T.B., and Fischbach, G.D. (1986). Purification and characterization of a polypeptide from chick brain that promotes the accumulation of acetylcholine receptors in chick myotubes. J. Cell Biol. 103, 493–507.
54. Gorin, P.D. and Johnson, E.M. (1980). Effects of exposure to nerve growth factor antibodies on the developing nervous system of the rat: An experimental autoimmune approach. Dev. Biol. 80, 313–323.
55. Hamburger, V., Brunso-Bechtold, J. and Yip, J. (1981). Neuronal death in the spinal ganglia of the chick embryo and its reduction by nerve growth factor. J. Neurosci. 1, 60–71.
56. Oppenheim, R.W., Maderdrut, J.L. and Wells, D.J. (1982). Cell death of motoneurons in the chick embryo spinal cord. VI. Reduction of naturally occurring cell death in the thoracolumbar column of Terni by nerve growth factor. J. Comp. Neurol. 210, 174–189.
57. Berg, D.K. (1984). New neuronal growth factors. Ann. Rev. Neurosci. 7, 149–170.
58. Barde, Y.A., Edgar, D. and Thoenen, H. (1983). New neurotrophic factors. Ann. Rev. Physiol. 45, 601–612.
59. Ding, R., Jansen, J.K., Laing, N.A. and Tonnesen, H. (1983). The innervation of skeletal muscles in chickens curarized during early development. J. Neurocytol. 12, 887–919.
60. Okada, A., Furber, S., Oppenheim, R.W. and Okado, N. (1985). Synapse formation and dendritic development of spinal motoneurons in the chick embryo following chronic curare treatment. Neurosci. Soc. Abst. 11, 259.
61. O'Leary, D.D. and Cowan, W.M. (1984). Survival of isthmo-optic neurons after early removal of one eye. Dev. Brain Res. 12, 293–310.

7. THE BIOLOGY OF NERVE GROWTH FACTOR IN VIVO*

EUGENE M. JOHNSON, JR., PAMELA T. MANNING,
AND CHRISTINE WILCOX

A major theme in developmental neurobiology is the role of target tissues in the maintenance of the neurons that innervate those targets. During the development of the nervous system, more neurons are produced and send axons to targets than survive in the mature animal. Typically about 50% of the neurons projecting to a given structure will die during a restricted period. This has been termed *naturally occurring cell death.* Several lines of evidence indicate that the size of the target field is a major determinant of this cell death: Removal of the target results in greatly increased cell death, while expansion of the target decreases cell death (for reviews, see Refs. 1 and 2).

The most commonly considered mechanism by which targets exert their survival-promoting effects on neurons is the release of *trophic factors* by the target. These factors act on the neurons to promote neuronal survival. Support for the trophic factor hypothesis comes from work on nerve growth factor (NGF), the only neurotrophic factor that has been purified in sufficient quantities to allow investigation of its physiological role(s). Since its discovery three decades ago by Levi-Montalcini and Hamburger and its subsequent purification by Cohen, this molecule has been studied extensively (for reviews, see Refs. 3 and 4). A considerable body of knowledge on its function in the peripheral nervous system exists. In addition, recent evidence indicates a possible

* The authors thank our many colleagues who contributed the various studies mentioned in this paper. Work from the authors' laboratories was supported by NIH grants HL20604, NS18071, and by grants from the March of Dimes Birth Defects Foundation and from Monsanto Company.

Ferrendelli, J.A., Collins, R.C. and Johnson, E.M. (eds), Neurobiology of Amino Acids, Peptides, and Trophic Factors.

role in the central nervous system (see subsequent chapter by Hefti et al.).

In this chapter we will review our current understanding of the general mechanism by which NGF acts and the role of NGF as a survival-promoting agent in the peripheral nervous system (PNS), deduced from studies where NGF deprivation is produced by antibodies against the factor. Two unusual actions of NGF will then be discussed: 1) NGF protection against the immune-mediated destruction of sympathetic neurons caused by guanethidine and 2) the effects of NGF on herpes simplex virus infections in sympathetic neurons. These actions are not immediately obvious from its known role in development, suggesting the possibility that NGF may possess a broader range of physiological or pharmacological functions than has been considered previously.

1. GENERAL MECHANISM OF NGF ACTION

The general scheme by which NGF is thought to exert its trophic actions in maintaining responsive neurons is shown diagrammatically in Figure 7-1. NGF is made by target tissues. Assays of levels of NGF and NGF mRNA show that NGF is widely synthesized throughout the body and that these levels generally correlate with known densities of innervation of dependent neurons [5, 6]. NGF appears not to be stored, but rather to be released constitutively. NGF, elaborated by the target tissue, binds to specific NGF receptors present on the plasma membrane of nerve terminals. Subsequent to binding, NGF [7–9] and NGF receptors [10] are retrogradely transported to the cell body. The nature of the specific signal conveyed from the periphery to the cell body that produces survival or other NGF effects is not known. The signal could be one of several possibilities: For example, the message could be NGF alone, some modified form of receptor, or the NGF/NGF receptor complex [10]. Alternatively, the critical signal could be some unknown second messenger, generated by the interaction of NGF/NGF receptor at the target level, which is subsequently retrogradely transported. If this were the case, the transport of NGF and the receptor might serve as a means of regulating NGF catabolism by the cell or of regulating NGF and NGF receptor density at the terminal areas, rather than serving to carry directly the message to which the cell body responds.

The precise biochemical mechanism(s) by which the effects of NGF are mediated following signal transduction in responsive neurons in likewise unknown. It is possible that there are multiple mechanisms by which various effects such as survival, hypertrophy, enzyme induction, etc. are produced. Thus, even though general scheme of NGF action is understood, (Figure 7-1) many aspects of its mechanism of action are essentially unknown.

2. CELL TYPES DEPENDENT ON NGF IN VIVO: CHANGES WITH DEVELOPMENT

The classical approach to determining the *physiological* role of a hormone or hormone-like substance is to deprive the animal of the hormone and then to

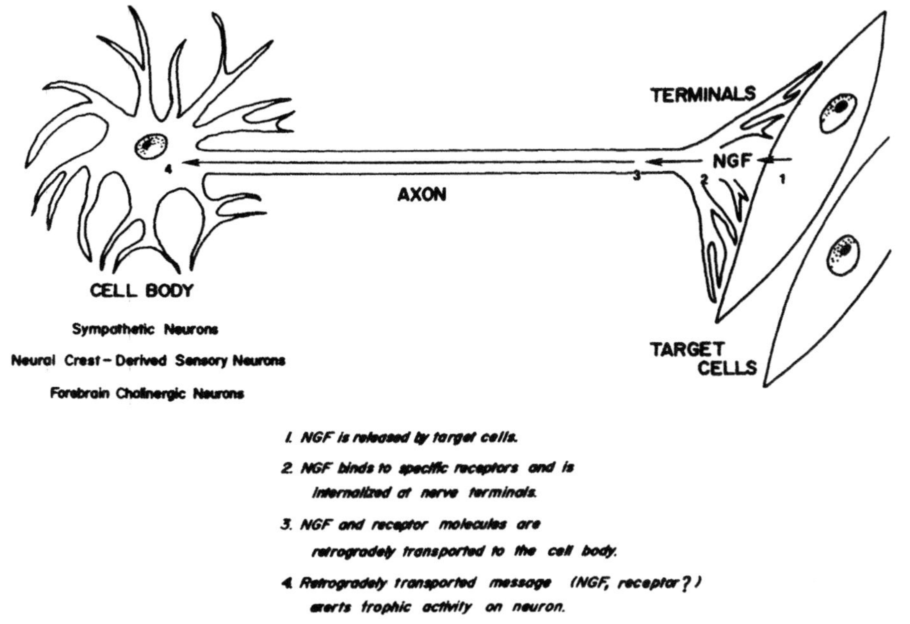

Figure 7-1. Diagram showing steps involved in the action of nerve growth factor (NGF) on responsive neurons.

observe the adverse effects of the hormone deprivation. An alternative approach is to administer exogenous hormone and to observe the effects of such administration. The latter approach suffers from the fact that administration of exogenous hormone describes the pharmacological effects of the agent but can be only suggestive of physiological function. Approaches to hormone deprivation include excision of the hormone-producing organ or tissue, administration of a specific antagonist, or the administration of antibodies to the hormone. The latter approach is the only approach available in the case of NGF, since it is made in tissues throughout the body that receive sympathetic and sensory innervation and since no antagonists to NGF have been developed. The seminal paper in the field of NGF deprivation is that of Levi-Montalcini and Booker [11] in which rabbit antibodies to partially purified mouse salivary gland NGF (anti-NGF) were administered to newborns of several species. Treatment with the antibodies resulted in destruction of the sympathetic nervous systems of these animals. In contrast to the observed NGF dependence of sensory neurons for survival in vitro, dorsal root ganglion neurons in these neonatal animals treated with anti-NGF were not obviously affected [12]. Recent studies using high doses of anti-NGF have shown that there is a modest loss (~20%) of DRG neurons when neonatal rats are treated with anti-NGF and that this loss occurs primarily among the population of small sensory neurons [13]. The fundamental observations of the early experiments of Levi-Montalcini and coworkers were, however, correct. Sympathetic neurons of neonatal rats are much more adversely affected by NGF deprivation induced by anti-NGF than are sensory neurons.

The results of Levi-Montalcini and Booker [11], supported by subsequent work in many labs, argue convincingly that anti-NGF is acting by producing NGF deprivation rather than via a direct toxic mechanism [14]. These studies established a role for NGF as a physiological factor critical for the survival of developing sympathetic neurons. Its function in the developing sensory neuron was left unresolved because of the apparently contradictory observations mentioned above. Developing mammalian sensory neurons require NGF for survival in culture but do not die following NGF deprivation in vivo as do sympathetic neurons. In addition, treatment of adult animals with comparable amounts of anti-NGF, which cause destruction of neonatal sympathetic neurons, results in no destruction of sympathetic neurons in adults. This led to the conclusion that sympathetic neurons lose their NGF requirement for survival. These experiments, however, involved short durations of treatment with anti-NGF; effects of long-term NGF deprivation were not known.

To expand the time span during which effects of NGF deprivation can be produced and, therefore, to assess the role of NGF in periods other than the neonatal period, an autoimmune approach was developed [14, 15]. This approach was predicated on the assumption that animals making antibodies against mouse NGF would also make antibodies against their own homologous NGF, thereby producing "autoimmune NGF deprivation." The feasibility of this approach was, in fact, shown in the original Levi-Montalcini and Booker paper [11], in which they demonstrated that rabbit anti-mouse NGF would produce destruction of sympathetic neurons in neonatal rabbits.

Two questions were asked. First, what are the adverse effects of chronic NGF deprivation on the mature nervous system of the immunized animal? Second, what are the adverse effects on developing fetal and neonatal animals that receive maternal anti-NGF, either transplacentally prior to parturition or postnatally via the milk?

Chronic NGF deprivation over several months by production of anti-NGF antibodies in adult animals results in destruction of the sympathetic nervous system, indicating that NGF is required for the survival of sympathetic neurons throughout the lifetime of the animal [15, 16]. Cell death in adults requires longer periods of NGF deprivation (weeks or months of exposure) than does a similar degree of neuronal death in neonatal animals (days of treatment). Thus, the dependence appears to be less acute in the adult sympathetic neuron, but qualitatively the same as in the immature neuron. Unlike sympathetic neurons, chronic NGF deprivation in adult animals produces no loss of DRG sensory neurons [17, 18]. Despite the lack of sensory neuronal death during chronic NGF deprivation, adverse effects are observed. Biochemical markers of neuronal function in DRG, such as neuropeptide levels, are reduced [17]. A generalized neuronal atrophy is also observed [18]. Thus, chronic NGF deprivation produces the same qualitative result (atrophy but no death) as does brief treatment of neonatal animals.

The effect of NGF deprivation on fetal animals produces strikingly different results. Prenatal exposure of developing animals (rats, rabbits, guinea pigs) produces destruction of sympathetic neurons in a manner similar to postnatal exposure. In addition, and in contrast to effects of anti-NGF on postnatal animals, prenatal exposure to anti-NGF produces massive destruction of DRG sensory neurons [19]. The fact that prenatal exposure to anti-NGF causes the death of DRG neurons, whereas postnatal exposure produces little or no neuronal death, indicates that these neurons go through a critical phase of dependence on NGF for survival during early development. This dependence for survival is lost later in development, even in the face of months of NGF deprivation. However, as was discussed above, NGF is required in adult animals for maintenance of normal neuronal function and morphology in DRG sensory neurons.

Several other neuronal cell types in newborn guinea pigs deprived of NGF in utero by the placental transfer of anti-NGF from their immunized mothers were also examined [20]. The results are summarized in Table 7-1. All neural crest-derived sensory ganglia examined (DRG, trigeminal, jugular) show a similar (~85%) decrease in neuronal number. In contrast, sensory ganglia derived from ectodermal placode (nodose, acoustic, vestibular) are unaffected. Therefore, only sensory neurons of neural crest origin are dependent on NGF for survival.

Despite the fact that two neuronal derivatives of neural crest, sensory and sympathetic neurons, are NGF dependent, this is not a general property of neural crest-derived neurons. Neuronal numbers in parasympathetic ganglia were counted from the same animals described above (Table 7-1). No neuronal loss was observed. Likewise, examination of the enteric nervous system of similar animals showed no apparent neuronal loss in enteric ganglia [21]. Based on these in vivo results, and in vitro experiments showing no effect of NGF on these cell types, it was concluded that parasympathetic, enteric, and placodally derived sensory neurons are not NGF dependent.

3. NGF AS A PHARMACOLOGICAL AGENT

Deficiencies in NGF and other yet unidentified trophic molecules in the development of various disease states have been proposed by many workers. However, even if a deficit of trophic molecules is shown not to have a causative role in the genesis of pathological states, their pharmacological potential may be significant. Two examples of the pharmacological potential of NGF that have been pursued in our laboratory are the prevention of an immunologically mediated destruction of sympathetic neurons induced by guanethidine treatment and the role of NGF in latent herpes viral infections of sympathetic neurons.

Table 7-1. Effects of in utero exposure to maternal antibody to NGF on neuronal numbers of ganglia of newborn guinea pigs[a]

Ganglion	Functional type	Embryonic origin	Neuronal Number (Percent control)
Superior cervical	Sympathetic	N. Crest	<1
8th cervical DRG	Sensory	Crest	15
Trigeminal	Sensory	Crest/Placode?	15
Root of IX	Sensory	Crest	15
Nodose	Sensory	Placode	100
Spiral	Sensory	Placode	100
Acoustic	Sensory	Placode	100[b]
Ciliary	Parasympathetic	Crest	100
Sphenopalatine	Parasympathetic	Crest	100

[a] Data taken from cell counts in Ref. 20.
[b] This ganglion was not counted. By visual inspection no difference from control was apparent.

3.1. Guanethidine-induced neuronal destruction

Guanethidine is an adrenergic neuron blocking agent that continues to be used clinically as an antihypertensive agent in severe cases of hypertension. Pharmacologically, guanethidine, as well as a series of structural analogs, acts to dissociate the action potential from the release of norepinephrine in the sympathetic neuron. Because of its structural similarity to catecholamines, guanethidine is taken up into sympathetic neurons by the catecholamine uptake pump and accumulates within these cells (for review, see Ref. 22). When administered chronically in high doses, in excess of those required to produce adrenergic blockade, to neonatal or adult rats [23–25], hamsters [26], or monkeys [27], guanethidine produces a selective and permanent destruction of sympathetic neurons. That monkeys are susceptible to chronic treatment with guanethidine, when using doses only slightly in excess of those used to treat hypertension (2 mg/kg/day), is significant because of its clinical usage.

The most striking morphological change that occurs in the sympathetic ganglia following chronic guanethidine treatment, prior to and during neuronal cell death, is a marked cellular infiltration. In several early papers, this cellular infiltrate was described as lymphocyte-like [23, 25]. It has recently been demonstrated that the destruction of sympathetic neurons occurs by an immunological mechanism that appears to be cellular in nature. The infiltrate is composed primarily of macrophages and lymphocytes, many of which appear to be activated. In addition, some of the lymphocytes within the infiltrate have been identified immunohistochemically as T cells by using a monospecific anti-rat T cell antisera [28]. Neuronal destruction, as well as the lymphocytic infiltration, can be prevented by a number of immunosuppressive agents, including cyclophosphamide, gamma irradiation, and azathioprine [29]; and, the capacity of an immunosuppressed animal to respond to guanethidine treatment can be restored following reconstitution with syngeneic, immune–competent spleen and bone marrow cells [28].

In 1974, prior to the demonstration that guanethidine exerted its cytotoxic effects by an immune-mediated mechanism, it was demonstrated [30] that concurrent treatment of neonatal rats with 10 mg/kg/day of mouse NGF completely prevents the neuronal destruction produced by guanethidine treatment. More recently, it has been shown that concurrent treatment of neonatal rats with a tenfold lower dose, 1 mg/kg/day, also provides complete protection against guanethidine treatment. Protection is not because of a lack of accumulation of guanethidine within treated ganglia. Also, based on a number of in vitro assays and one in vivo assay, NGF does not appear to be an immunosuppressive agent, and, in fact, if it has any immunological effect, it may stimulate antibody responses in vivo in young rats [31]. Several possible mechanisms exist to explain how NGF may protect against neuronal destruction. However, the one which is most probable is that NGF affects expression of the antigen that induces the immune response. Studies are currently underway to test this hypothesis.

Many of the experiments demonstrating that guanethidine induced an immune response directed against sympathetic neurons were conducted in 1-week-old rats, rather than in neonatal rats, which were used for the NGF protection experiments. Therefore, the protection afforded by both 1 and 5 mg/kg/day of NGF administered can currently with guanethidine to 7-day-old rats has been examined. Surprisingly, although complete protection can be achieved in the neonatal rat (starting treatment at day of birth) with 1 mg/kg/day of NGF, only incomplete protection occurs in the slightly older rats, even following treatment with fivefold higher doses of NGF (Figure 7-2). Notice that although protection is significant, it is incomplete, and neuronal destruction is more severe in animals treated with 1 mg/kg/day than with 5 mg/kg/day. This suggests that a dose-response relationship for NGF protection may exist. However, higher doses have not been tested in these animals because of the amount of NGF that would be necessary to demonstrate this relationship. Likewise, it is not feasible at the present time to conduct similar experiments in adult rats, as these results suggest that as the neuron matures, it becomes less responsive to NGF protection. An alternative explanation is that, in the more mature neurons, exogenously administered NGF may have less access to the neuronal cell bodies within the ganglion such that complete protection is difficult to achieve. Finally, it is felt that by understanding the mechanism by which pharmacological doses of NGF prevent the occurrence of an autoimmune-mediated event, insight may be gained, not only into how trophic molecules may modulate pathological processes, but also into how NGF normally maintains dependent cell types.

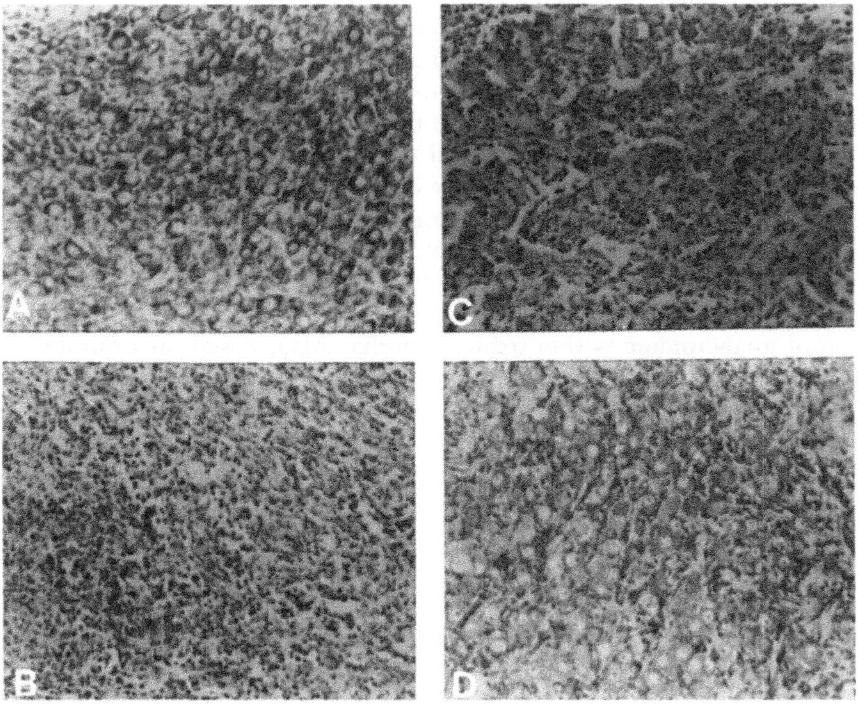

Figure 7-2. NGF protection of sympathetic neurons from guanethidine-induced destruction. One-week-old Sprague-Dawley rats were treated with 50 mg/kg/day of guanethidine sulfate alone (B) or in combination with 1 mg/kg (C) or 5 mg/kg/day (D) of NGF. Controls were untreated (A). Tissues shown are 8-μm sections of superior cervical ganglia stained with toluidine blue. Note the marked lymphocytic infiltration and lack of viable neurons following treatment with guanethidine alone (B). Partial protection occurred with both levels of concurrent NGF treatment (C, D). Neuronal hypertrophy is evident following treatment with 5 mg/kg of NGF (D).

4. NGF AND HERPES SIMPLEX VIRUS

4.1. Effects of NGF deprivation on latent HSV

Herpes simplex virus (HSV) causes diseases in humans that range in severity from the benign common cold sore to life-threatening encephalitis. HSV has the unique capability of producing latent infections in neurons of certain ganglia of the peripheral nervous system [32–34]. Other sites of latency have been suggested [35, 36], but the peripheral nervous system is the best documented and the most clinically relevant site. While HSV produces lytic infections in many cell types, the virus is neurotropic in terms of the site of latency. The virus resides in the neuron in a form that is not detectable when the ganglia are assayed for infectious virus [37]. Periodically, as the result of some signal(s)

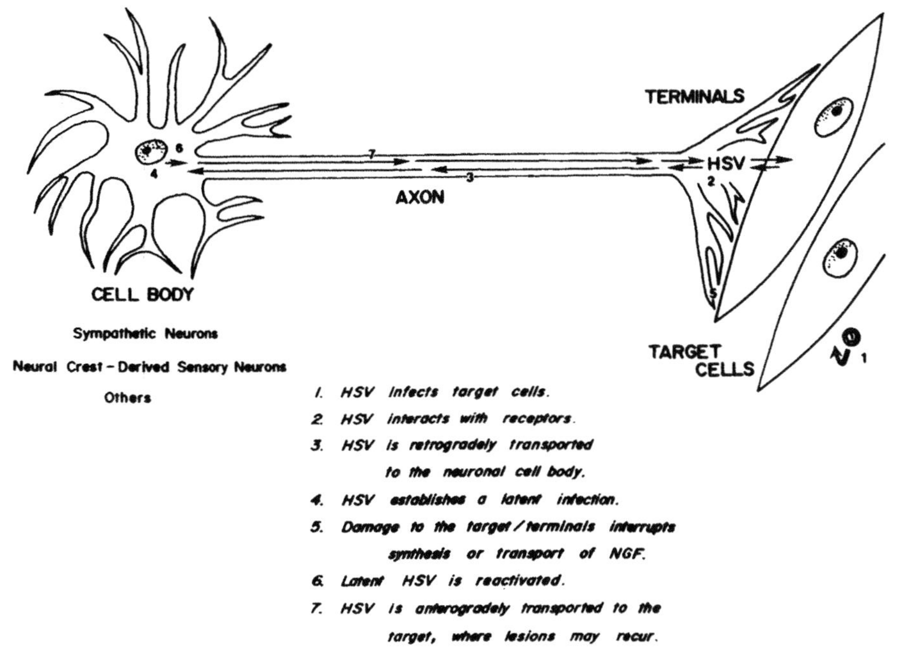

Figure 7-3. Schematic diagram showing the cycle of HSV infection, latency, and inactivation in neural crest-derived neurons.

that remains undefined, the latent virus reactivates to produce disease and transmissible virus. Extensive progress has been made in understanding the biochemistry of HSV, yet little is known about the mechanisms involved in the establishment and reactivation of latent HSV.

The study of HSV infection in the neuron, as the unique site of latency, may provide critical information for understanding the processes involved in the establishment and reactivation of latent HSV. Evidence demonstrates that certain ganglia are the predominant sites of latent HSV. Specifically, HSV becomes latent in the neurons of neural crest-derived sensory ganglia [32, 33] and sympathetic ganglia [34, 38]. These are NGF-dependent cell types (see above). Many of the stimuli reported to cause reactivation of latent HSV appear unrelated, such as UV exposure [39], fever [40], and emotional stress. However, several reactivating stimuli, e.g., central rhizotomy of trigeminal ganglia [41], and axotomy [35, 42], have in common the reduction or cessation of retrogradely transported neurotrophic support from the target. Diagrammed in Figure 7-3 are some of the events known and some suggested to be involved in the course of the HSV infection cycle. The virus is retrogradely transported, intra-axonally, to the neuronal cell body [43–45]. Whether viral DNA replication is necessary for the establishment of latency has not been clearly documented, although some evidence suggests that it is not necessary [46, 47]. The state of the viral genome during latency also has not been clearly defined; recent data suggest that the genome remains episomal [48]. Damage to the nerve terminals or target, may result in the reactivation of latent HSV via a signal that is produced by NGF deprivation.

To test the hypothesis that NGF deprivation can produce reactivation of latent HSV, HSV, type 1, infections were studied in sympathetic neurons in culture. Dissociated neuronal cultures were prepared from fetal rat superior cervical ganglia by methods described by Johnson and Argiro [49]. Enzymatically dissociated cells were plated at a density of approximately 5000 neurons per dish onto collagen-coated tissue culture dishes and maintained in Eagle's minimum essential medium with Earles salt solution, 10% fetal calf serum, 1.4 mM glutamine, and 50 ng/ml 2.5S mouse NGF. Cultures were treated with the antimitotic agent 5-fluorodeoxyuridine at 20 μM to reduce the non-neuronal cell population to less than 10%. After 10–12 days of antimitotic treatment, the drug was removed from the culture medium. The neuronal cultures were then inoculated with HSV at the multiplicity of infection (the number of infectious virus particles/cell) of HSV indicated in Table 7-2. After virus adsorption, the inoculum was removed, and standard culture media containing 1% human anti-HSV serum was added. Antiserum to HSV, which enhanced survival of the cultures, probably by limiting viral spread, was rinsed from the cultures after 10 days. Cultures infected with multiplicities of infection of 0.03 and 0.1 retained normal morphology at all times observed. Those cultures inoculated with 0.5 and 1.0 pfu/cell, 6% and 37%, respectively, developed HSV-specific cytopathology. Cultures that succumbed to lytic infection did so between 6–8 days postinoculation. Those neuronal cultures that retained normal morphology following HSV inoculation had no evidence of viral infection (no infectious virus, no virus-encoded thymidine kinase

Table 7-2. Effects of varying the multiplicity of infection (MOI) with HSV on the survival of neuronal cultures and the frequency of HSV reactivation after NGF deprivation.

MOI[a]	% Survival (no. of surviving cultures per no. of inoculated cultures)	% Reactivation (no. of HSV-positive cultures[b] per no. of cultures tested)
0.03	100 (120/120)	8 (5/60)
	100 (120/120)	10 (6/60)
0.1	100 (52/52)	19 (5/26)
0.5	93 (119/128)	26 (15/54)
	94 (120/128)	24 (15/63)
1.0	63 (38/60)	53 (10/19)

[a] MOI, multiplicity of infection with HSV (plaque-forming units/cell). HSV, type 1, F strain, used for the inoculations, was prepared and titered on Vero cells.
[b] Cultures were considered to be HSV-positive when infectious virus was demonstrated.

activity, and no viral antigens detectable by immunohistochemistry) at any of the times tested (5 weeks postinoculation was the longest time point examined). However, NGF deprivation (produced by adding antibodies to NGF to the culture medium) resulted in the production of infectious HSV, viral thymidine kinase activity, and viral antigens. Sister cultures that had also been infected with HSV were treated with nonimmune serum and did not produce any evidence of active virus infection. These data indicate that the cultures harbored latent HSV (no detectable virus), and reactivation of latent virus occurred with NGF deprivation (detectable virus). The percentage of cultures resulting in reactivation was dependent on the multiplicity of infection used for the inoculation (Table 7-2). We believe this is the first in vitro system for HSV latency in neurons that duplicates the phenomenon observed in humans. While we believe these data indicate a physiological role of NGF in the reactivation of latent HSV after, at least, certain stimuli, the method of establishing and reactivating latent HSV in the neuronal cultures will provide a useful and reproducible system to study events that have been very difficult to manipulate experimentally.

4.2. Effects of NGF on the primary HSV infection

The primary or initial HSV infection is important because it leads to the establishment of the latent infection. Understanding the events that alter the primary infection may provide information regarding the mechanism of the establishment of latent infections and may eventually lead to the prevention of latent HSV.

Previously it had been shown that the "metabolic state" of the neuron affected the primary infection at the level of the ganglia. Axotomy, after establishing an active infection in the ganglia, results in an increased production of infectious virus in the ganglia [42]. Similarly, after initiating a ganglionic HSV infection, the administration of 6-hydroxydopamine, which causes damage to sympathetic nerve terminals, results in an augmented primary HSV infection in the sympathetic ganglia [38].

On the basis that both axotomy [50] and 6-hydroxydopamine [51] result in NGF deprivation in the ganglia, it was asked whether exogenous NGF treatment during the primary HSV infection could ameliorate the infection in the ganglia. With the mouse model characterized by Price et al. [38], mice were inoculated with HSV, type 1, in the anterior eye chamber and were treated daily with either 1 mg/kg NGF or normal saline, i.p. Table 7-3 shows the results of assays of the superior cervical ganglia for infectious virus on day 5 postinoculation. Price and associates [38] showed, and we confirmed, that day 5 postinoculation was the peak time for virus replication in the ganglia. Exogenous NGF appears to prevent or significantly reduce HSV replication during the primary infection in the ganglia. The mechanism by which NGF might protect the ganglia from the primary HSV infection is not clear. We have yet to determine if NGF blocks virus entry, transport, replication, or

Table 7-3. Plaque-forming units of HSV in the homogenates of the superior cervical ganglion of mice on day 5 postinoculation with HSV.

Saline treated (n = 10)	NGF treated (n = 10)
16.2 + 5.7[a]	O[b]

Mice were treated with either normal saline or 1 mg/kg of NGF daily starting at the time of HSV inoculation. The numbers in parentheses are the number of ganglia assayed.
[a] Mean ± SEM
[b] P = 0.001

some other event(s). We also do not know if NGF treatment can affect the establishment of latency. These results in primary infections, in addition to the results in the in vitro model of latency, however, clearly suggest potential physiological and pharmacological roles for NGF in controlling HSV and perhaps other viral infections in NGF-responsive neurons.

5. CONCLUSION

The issues briefly discussed in this chapter indicate that NGF, traditionally considered a factor important during development, probably has many roles in the adult animal. In addition to issues discussed here, effects of NGF in the CNS (see the chapter by Hefti in this volume), effects of NGF in nerve injury, and others further emphasize this point. There are possibly other pharmacological, if not physiological, effects of NGF in mature animals yet to be discovered. The availability of large quantities of NGF in the future, prepared by recombinant methods, will make such investigations more practical. Such efforts will serve not only to further define the biology of NGF, but they will provide methods by which to assess the spectrum of actions of neurotrophic molecules yet to be discovered. Thus, despite the fact that it is over a quarter century since the discovery and initial description of NGF by Levi-Montalcini, Hamburger, and Cohen, the "NGF field" is probably still only in its adolescence, and the broader field of neurotrophic factors is only in its infancy.

REFERENCES

1. Oppenheim, R.W. (1981). Neuronal cell death and some related regressive phenomena during neurogenesis. In *Studies in Developmental Neurobiology: Essays in Honor of Viktor Hamburger*, Cowan, W.M., ed., Oxford U.P., New York.
2. Cowan, W.M., Fawcett, J.W., O'Leary, D.D. and Stanfield, B.B. (1984). Regressive events in neurogenesis. Science 225, 1258–1265.
3. Levi-Montalcini, R. (1982). Developmental neurobiology and the natural history of nerve growth factor. Ann. Rev. Neurosci. 5, 341–362.
4. Thoenen, H. and Barde, Y.A. (1980). Physiology of nerve growth factor. Physiol. Rev. 60, 1284–1335.
5. Korsching, S. and Thoenen, H. (1983). Nerve growth factor in sympathetic ganglia and corresponding target organs of the rat: Correlation with density of sympathetic innervation. Proc. Natl. Acad. Sci. USA 80, 3513–3516.
6. Shelton, D.L. and Reichardt, L.F. (1984). Expression of the β-nerve growth factor gene

correlates with the density of sympathetic innervation in effector organs. Proc. Natl. Acad. Sci. USA 81, 7951–7955.
7. Hendry, I.A., Stöckel, K., Thoenen, H. and Iversen, L.L. (1974). The retrograde transport of nerve growth factor. Brain Res. 68, 103–121.
8. Korsching, S. and Thoenen, H. (1983). Quantitative demonstration of the retrograde axonal transport of endogenous nerve growth factor. Neurosci. Lett. 39, 1–4.
9. Palmatier, M.A., Hartman, B.K. and Johnson, E.M., Jr. (1984). Demonstration of retrogradely transported endogenous nerve growth factor in axons of sympathetic neurons. J. Neurosci. 4, 751–756.
10. Johnson, E.M., Jr., Taniuchi, M., Clark, H.B., Springer, J.E., Koh, S., Tayrien, M.W. and Loy, R. (1987). Demonstration of the retrograde transport of nerve growth factor (NGF) receptor in the peripheral and central nervous system. J. Neurosci. 7, 923–929.
11. Levi-Montalcini, R. and Booker, B. (1960). Destruction of the sympathetic ganglia in mammals by an antiserum to the nerve growth promoting factor. Proc. Natl. Acad. Sci. USA 46, 384–391.
12. Levi-Montalcini, R. and Angeletti, P.U. (1966). Immunosympathectomy. Pharmacol. Rev. 18, 619–628.
13. Yip, H.K., Rich, K.M., Lampe, P.A. and Johnson, E.M., Jr. (1984). The effects of nerve growth factor and its antiserum on the postnatal development and survival after injury of sensory neurons in rat dorsal root ganglia. J. Neurosci. 4, 2986–2992.
14. Gorin, P.D. and Johnson, E.M., Jr. (1979). Experimental autoimmune model of nerve growth factor deprivation: Effects on developing peripheral sympathetic and sensory neurons. Proc. Natl. Acad. Sci. USA 76, 5382–5386.
15. Gorin, P.D. and Johnson, E.M., Jr. (1980). Effects of long-term nerve growth factor deprivation on the nervous system of the adult rat: An experimental autoimmune approach. Brain Res. 198, 27–42.
16. Johnson, E.M., Jr., Gorin, P.D., Osborne, P.A., Rydel, R.E. and Pearson, J. (1982). Effects of autoimmune NGF deprivation in the adult rabbit and offspring. Brain Res. 240, 131–140.
17. Schwartz, J.P., Pearson, J. and Johnson, E.M., Jr. (1982). Effect of exposure to anti-NGF on sensory neurons of adult rats and guinea pigs. Brain Res. 244, 378–381.
18. Rich, K.M., Yip, H.K., Osborne, P.A., Schmidt, R.E. and Johnson, E.M., Jr. (1984). Role of nerve growth factor in the adult dorsal root ganglia neuron and its response to injury. J. Comp. Neurol. 230, 110–118.
19. Johnson, E.M., Jr., Gorin, P.D., Brandeis, L.D. and Pearson, J. (1980). Dorsal root ganglion neurons are destroyed by exposure in utero to maternal antibody to nerve growth factor. Science 210, 916–918.
20. Pearson, J., Johnson, E.M., Jr., Brandeis, L. (1983). Effects of antibodies to nerve growth factor on intrauterine development of derivatives of cranial neural crest and placode in the guinea pig. Dev. Biol. 96, 32–36.
21. Gershon, M.D., Rothman, T.P., Sherman, D. and Johnson, E.M. (1983). Effects of prenatal exposure to anti-NGF on the enteric nervous system (ENS) of guinea pigs. Anat. Rec. 205, 62A.
22. Johnson, E.M., Jr. and Manning, P.T. (1984). Guanethidine-induced destruction of sympathetic neurons. Int. Rev. Neurobiol. 25, 1–37.
23. Jensen-Holm, J. and Juul, P. (1971). Ultrastructural changes in the rat superior cervical ganglion following prolonged guanethidine administration. Acta. Pharm. Toxicol. 30, 308–320.
24. Burnstock, G., Evans, B., Gannon, B.J., Heath, J.W. and James, V. (1971). A new method of destroying adrenergic nerves in adult animals using guanethidine. Br. J. Pharmacol. 43, 245–301.
25. Eränko, L. and Eränko, O. (1971). Effect of guanethidine on nerve cells and small intensely fluorescent cells in sympathetic ganglia of newborn and adult rats. Acta. Pharm. Toxicol. 30, 403–416.
26. Johnson, E.M., Jr., Palmatier, M.A., Rydel, R.E. and Manning, P.T. (1986). Species and structural specificity of the lipopigment accumulation and neuronal destruction induced by N-(2-guanidinoethyl)-4-methyl-1,2,5,6 tetrahydropyridine (guanacline). Brain Res. 383, 100–109.
27. Palmatier, M.A., Schmidt, R.E., Plurad, S.B. and Johnson, E.M., Jr. (1987). Sympathetic

neuronal destruction in macaque monkeys by guanethidine and guanacline. Ann. Neurol. 21, 46–52.
28. Manning, P.T., Powers, C.W., Schmidt, R.E. and Johnson, E.M., Jr. (1983). Guanethidine-induced neuronal destruction of peripheral sympathetic neurons occurs by an immune-mediated mechanism. J. Neurosci. 3, 714–724.
29. Manning, P.T., Russell, J.H., Johnson, E.M., Jr. (1982). Immunosuppressive agents prevent guanethidine-induced destruction of rat sympathetic neurons. Brain Res. 241, 131–143.
30. Johnson, E.M. and Aloe, L. (1974). Suppression of the in vitro and in vivo cytotoxic effects of guanethidine in sympathetic neurons by nerve growth factor. Brain Res. 81, 519–532.
31. Manning, P.T., Russell, J.H., Simmons, B. and Johnson, E.M., Jr. (1985). Protection from guanethidine-induced neuronal destruction by nerve growth factor: Effect of NGF on immune function. Brain Res. 340, 61–69.
32. Baringer, J. and Swoveland, P. (1973). Recovery of herpes simplex virus from human trigeminal ganglions. N. Engl. J. Med. 288, 648–650.
33. Bastian, F.D., Rabson, A.S., Yee, C.L. and Tralka, T.S. (1972). *Herpes hominis:* Isolation from human trigeminal ganglions. Science 178, 306–307.
34. Warren, K.G., Brown, S.M., Wroblewska, Z., Gilden, D., Koprowski, H. and Subak-Sharpe, J. (1978). Isolation of latent herpes simplex virus from the superior cervical and vagus ganglions of human beings. N. Engl. J. Med. 298, 1068–1069.
35. Walz, M.A., Price, R.W. and Notkins, A.L. (1974). Latent ganglionic infection with herpes simplex virus types 1 and 2: Viral reactivation in vivo after neurectomy. Science 184, 1185–1187.
36. Scriba, M. (1977). Extraneural localization of herpes simplex virus in latently infected guinea pigs. Nature 267, 529–531.
37. Walz, M.A., Price, R.W., Hayashi, K., Katz, B.J. and Notkins, A.L. (1977). Effect of immunization on acute and latent infections of vaginouterine tissue with herpes simplex virus types 1 and 2. J. Infect. Dis. 135, 744–752.
38. Price, R.W. (1979). 6-hydroxydopamine potentiates acute herpes simplex virus infection of the superior cervical ganglion in mice. Science 205, 518–520.
39. Blyth, W.A., Hill, T.J., Field, H.J. and Harbour, D.A. (1976). Reactivation of herpes simplex virus infection by ultraviolet light and possible involvements of prostaglandins. J. Gen. Virol. 33, 547–550.
40. Warren, S.L., Carpenter, C.M. and Boak, R.A. (1940). Symptomatic herpes, a sequela of critically induced fever. J. Exp. Med. 71, 155–168.
41. Carton, C.A. and Kilbourne, E.D. (1952). Activation of latent herpes simplex by trigeminal sensory-root section. N. Engl. J. Med. 246, 172–176.
42. Price, R.W. and Schmitz, J. (1978). Reactivation of latent herpes simplex virus infection of the autonomic nervous system by postganglionic neurectomy. Infec. Immun. 19, 523–534.
43. Kristensson, K. (1970). Morphological studies of the neural spread of herpes simplex virus to the central nervous system. Acta. Neuropathol. 16, 54–63.
44. Kristensson, K., Lycke, E. and Sjostrand, J. (1971). Spread of herpes simplex virus in peripheral nerves. Acta. Neuropathol. 17, 44–53.
45. Cook, M.L. and Stevens, J.G. (1973). Pathogenesis of herpetic neuritis and ganglionitis in mice: Evidence for intra-axonal transport of infection. Infec. Immunol. 7, 272–288.
46. Lofgren, K.W., Stevens, J.G., Marsden, H.S. and Subak-Sharpe, J.H. (1977). Temperature-sensitive mutants of herpes simplex virus differ in the capacity to establish latent infections in mice. Virology 76, 440–443.
47. Watson, K., Stevens, J.G., Cook, M.L. and Subak-Sharpe, J.H. (1980). Latency compentence of thirteen HSV-1 temperature sensitive mutants. J. Gen. Virol. 49, 149–159.
48. Rock, D.L. and Fraser, N.W. (1985). Latent herpes simplex virus Type I DNA contains two copies of the virion DNA joint region. Virol. 55, 849–852.
49. Johnson, M.I. and Argiro, V. (1983). Techniques in the tissue culture of rat sympathetic neurons. Methods of Enzymology 103, 334–347.
50. Hendry, I.A. (1974). The response of adrenergic neurons to axotomy and nerve growth factor. Brain Res. 94. 87–97.
51. Johnson, E.M., Macia, R.A., Andres, R.Y. and Bradshaw, R.A. (1979). The effects of drugs which destroy the sympathetic nervous system on the retrograde transport of nerve growth factor. Brain Res. 171, 461–472.

8. SCHWANN CELL CONTACT AS A FACTOR IN NEURONAL TROPHIC SUPPORT AND THE PROMOTION OF NEURITE GROWTH*

R.P. BUNGE, C.F. ELDRIDGE, M.D. ARD, AND N. KLEITMAN

During development, and in the adult organism, neurons are provided with factors from their environment that influence their survival and growth. The best known factor influencing neuronal survival, nerve growth factor (NGF), is a low molecular weight peptide that is believed to be released in minute amounts in regions innervated by specific neuronal types, taken up via receptors on the neuronal processes, and transported via axoplasmic transport to the neuronal perikaryon [1]. The limited amount of material thought to be available in target regions and the competition for this essential survival factor is considered a critical determinant of neuronal cell death during embryogenesis. This mechanism of growth factor release and uptake is generally considered a model for the action of trophic factors for other neuronal types as well [2]. Factors influencing neuronal process growth are legion; recently, particular emphasis has been placed on the efficacy of extracellular matrix materials in promoting rapid and profuse neurite growth from neurons of several types [3, 4].

This brief chapter will review several types of experiments undertaken with Schwann cells in tissue culture that have provided unexpected results related to the mechanisms by which neurons may receive trophic support and neurite growth promotion. In the instances emphasized here, direct con-

* This work was supported by NIH grants NS09923 and NS15070, NIH training grant NS07071 (CFE, NK), and a grant from the National Multiple Sclerosis Society (MDA).

Ferrendelli, J.A., Collins, R.C. and Johnson, E.M. (eds), Neurobiology of Amino Acids, Peptides, and Trophic Factors.

tact between neuron and Schwann cell appears to be critical. The first of these observations suggests that at certain stages of development rat sensory neurons grown in culture may be provided with trophic support by direct contact with Schwann cell surfaces via a mechanism that does not appear to involve the release of trophic material into the culture medium [5]. In a second set of experiments, a comparison is made between the ability of 1) Schwann cell surfaces and 2) extracellular matrix materials synthesized and assembled by Schwann cells to support neurite growth by PNS neurons. This comparison is made possible by culture techniques that allow separate (and combined) preparation of these growth substrata. The results indicate that the Schwann cell surface and the extracellular matrix deposited by the Schwann cell act separately as effective promoters of neurite growth for the PNS neurons studied [6]. A third set of tissue culture experiments designed to study the early outgrowth of retinal ganglion cell neurites in relation to Schwann cells and their extracellular matrix provides an example of neurite growth that is fostered by contact with a cell surface but not by extracellular matrix assembled by these cells [7]. Together these (and other) observations warn against ascribing common function to factors influencing neuron development; it appears that for each neuron type (and its specific stage of development), it will be necessary to separate and test specific agents for their effect on trophic support of the neuron soma, as well as for effects on neurite growth and long-term neurite survival.

The observation that Schwann cell contact may provide essential trophic support for rat sensory neurons grown in defined (serum-free) culture medium was derived from experience with preparing neuron-Schwann cell cultures for the study of PNS myelination. Several modifications of the original Wood method [8] of preparing populations of neurons and Schwann cells free of other cell types have been utilized. A particularly reproducible modification [9] has been to dissociate cells from the sensory ganglia of 15-day rat embryos and seed these in the central region of an Aclar minidish previously coated with reconstituted rat tail collagen. The cells (including about 8000 neurons, Schwann cells, fibroblasts, and other cell types) are treated alternately with 1) medium containing 10% human placental serum and NGF to promote neuron survival and growth, and 2) this same medium containing fluorodeoxyuridine to kill dividing non-neuronal cells. After three cycles (2 days each) of such treatments, essentially all non-neuronal cells have been eliminated, and the neuronal population has matured and established a substantial surrounding of outgrowing neurites. Purified populations of Schwann cells prepared by the method of either Wood [8] or Brockes and coworkers [10] can now be seeded over these cultures and allowed to populate the neurites. If complex medium (with serum and embryo extract) is provided, these cultures will progress to myelination [11]. If serum-free medium, such as the N2 medium of Bottenstein and Sato [12], is used, Schwann cell proliferation will progress but differentiation is restrained [9].

In gaining experience with these cultures, it was observed that if Schwann cell re-addition was delayed, the neurite outgrowth zone would begin a quite rapid breakdown, despite the continued presence of NGF in the culture medium. This breakdown was observed only when the cultures were maintained in serum-free medium in the absence of added Schwann cells; in medium containing serum, healthy neurites could be maintained for many weeks in the absence of Schwann cells (Figures 8-1 and 8-2). The addition of Schwann cells completely prevented the breakdown of neurites in defined medium (Figures 8-3 and 8-4). In some cultures maintained in defined medium, Schwann cells were added back focally (by transferring them on a fragment of a collagen sheet) so that some neurite outgrowth regions remained unpopulated by Schwann cells. Regions of the outgrowth populated by Schwann cells retained neurite viability; immediately adjacent neurites lacking Schwann cells exhibited fragmentation. In the absence of added Schwann cells, this regression of neurite health progressed centrally toward the region of neuronal somas, leading to a complete breakdown of the outgrowth zone. Subsequently, a portion of the neuronal somas appeared granular, and some of these neurons died. Most neuronal somas survived, however, and could re-extend neurites if Schwann cells were added. Because the medium volume in 24 mm diameter culture dishes is small (0.25 ml), one might expect factors sufficient for neuronal trophic support that are released by the Schwann cell to influence all neurons and their processes in the culture dish, but this was not observed. Neurite rescue seemed dependent on direct Schwann cell contact.

The nature of the support that could be provided by this rudimentary Schwann cell contact is not known. Moreover, this contact was adequate to convey support, even though Schwann cells do not progress to full axonal ensheathment or myelination in this serum-free medium [11]. Several mechanisms by which direct Schwann cell contact may support long-term neurite maintenance can be suggested. It has recently been established that Schwann cells separated from axonal contact express NGF receptors in substantial numbers [13], raising the possibility that surface presentation of NGF by Schwann cells may be an alternate (and in some cases, obligatory) method of NGF support of neurite health. It is known that Schwann cells are capable of altering the deposition of certain ion channels as they organize myelin internodes [14], and it is possible the correction of some ionic imbalance in the axon (such as the regulation of intra-axonal Ca^{2+} levels) may explain contact mediated support offered by Schwann cells to the developing neurite. It is known from studies of chick sensory neurons that the early dependence of these neurons on NGF is altered with development and that in later embryonic stages of chick development, other trophic factors become vital [15]. Barde and colleagues [2] have purified a growth factor from chick brain that supports cultured chick sensory neurons during this second stage of development. Whereas it has not been reported that a similar altered phase of rat sensory neuron trophic dependence occurs after an earlier dependence on NGF, our results suggest such a develop-

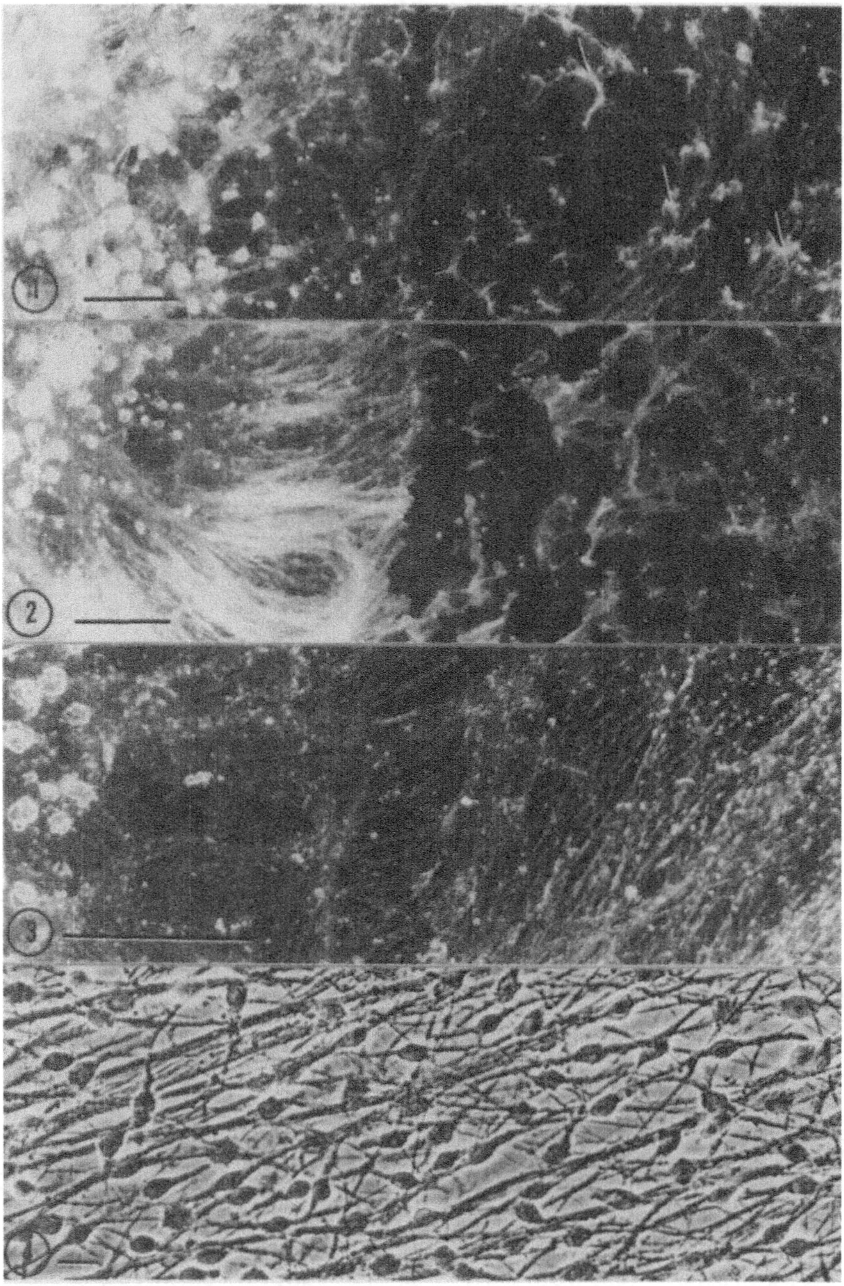
1
2
3
4

mental scenario for the rat sensory neuron. The results are not strongly parallel, however, inasmuch as the trophic support that has been observed to be provided by Schwann cell contact specifically sustains neurite health; the neuronal soma survives in the absence of Schwann cell contact, although its health is compromised.

Other experiments in which some of the neuron-Schwann cell cultures are allowed to progress to full development in culture have allowed observations comparing the ability of the Schwann cell surface and the Schwann cell extracellular matrix to promote neurite growth. In the tissue culture dish, and presumably in the animal as well, the Schwann cell is able to synthesize and deposit a basal lamina and attendant collagen fibrils around each axon-Schwann cell unit. This occurs after most Schwann cell proliferation is completed and during the period in which Schwann cells are establishing long-term relationships (myelinating or ensheathing) with a specific length of the axon(s). This basal lamina is continuous from one Schwann cell surface to the next, thus establishing a tubular cordon that retains the Schwann cells in a linear array even after axon loss, as in Wallerian degeneration. When axon regrowth occurs in peripheral nerve tissues, the growth cones are seen to progress on the inner aspect of the basal lamina [16], and in certain cases axon growth has been seen in basal lamina tubes that contain no living Schwann cells [17, 18].

For our experiments neuron-Schwann cell cultures were established by the methods of Wood [8]. Briefly, fibroblasts were eliminated from sensory ganglion explants by a combination of fluorodeoxyuridine treatment and transplantation of neurons and surviving Schwann cells to a fresh culture dish. After transplantation, a new neurite outgrowth is generated and becomes populated by large numbers of Schwann cells derived from the surviving Schwann cell population. A portion of these cultures were maintained under serum-free conditions in which Schwann cells do not deposit basal lamina but do proliferate extensively and populate the neurite outgrowth. Upon removal of the

---

Figures 8-1 to 8-4. These dark field micrographs show outgrowth regions from cultures containing a central aggregate of sensory neurons taken from 15-day rat embryos. Neuronal cell bodies are shown to the left in Figures 8-1 to 8-3 with neurites extending to the right. Bar indicates 1 mm for Figures 8-1 to 8-3. The neuronal culture in Figure 8-1 has been maintained in serum containing medium; its neurite outgrowth is intact. The air-dried collagen used as substratum in these cultures forms flocculent aggregates (examples at arrowsheads), which are emphasized in this dark field image. Figure 8-2 shows the catastrophic breakdown of neurites seen regularly at the end of the third week in cultures fed serum-free medium. This breakdown is not prevented by the presence of NGF in the culture medium but is prevented if Schwann cells are added (see text and Figure 8-3). Figure 8-3 illustrates that Schwann cells added to the periphery of the neurite outgrowth zone are effective in rescuing neurites in defined medium, even though the proximal shafts of these neurites are Schwann cell-free. Schwann cell somas are seen as light spots in the right and lower region of Figure 8-3. Figure 8-4 shows a higher magnification phase contrast picture of the Schwann cell population developing in this culture. Schwann cells are partially aligned with the bundles of axons crossing this field. Further Schwann cell functional differentiation will not occur in this defined medium (see text); the Schwann cell contact will, nonetheless, maintain the neurite outgrowth indefinitely. Bar equals 20 microns.

neuronal somas by excision of the central area, the neurite outgrowth degenerated, leaving linear arrays of Schwann cells possessing no basal lamina. Other cultures were carried in full medium to allow Schwann cell myelination and basal lamina deposition. Upon removal of the neuronal somas (by excision) from these cultures, the outgrowth retained linear arrays of Schwann cells contained within basal lamina tubes, providing an in vitro model of Wallerian degeneration. These tubes could be readily visualized by staining for characteristic basal lamina components (laminin, heparan sulfate proteoglycan, or type IV collagen). Some of these cultures were then treated with detergents to remove the cellular elements; basal lamina was retained after this treatment, as shown by immunocytochemical staining for basal lamina components.

Into the three types of preparations thus obtained (Schwann cells alone, basal lamina alone, and Schwann cells plus basal lamina), explants of autonomic or sensory neurons (freed of their own Schwann cells) were introduced. Neurites grew from these explants along the cellular/matrix constituents previously established in the dish. Analysis of results in these experiments was made by comparing neurite growth on the test substratum with growth on reconstituted type I rat tail collagen (which served as the original surface coating in these culture dishes).

Neurites grown on Schwann cells plus basal lamina were about half again as long as those on collagen, as illustrated in Figure 8-6. For eight explants of autonomic neurons cultured on this type of preparation for 3 days, median neurite length was 2.0 mm on Schwann cells plus basal lamina vs. 1.2 mm on collagen; among 20 sensory neuron explants cultured for 4 days, median neurite lengths were, respectively, 2.0 mm and 1.4 mm. Further experiments showed that this neurite promoting activity did not require the combination of both Schwann cells and their basal lamina. Very similar enhancement of neurite length was obtained when sensory neurons were added to preparations of Schwann cells alone. Alternatively, basal lamina alone promoted outgrowth from peripheral neurons (Figure 8-5). Neurites growing along oddly-shaped pathways formed by isolated basal lamina (Figure 8-7) demonstrated the pre-

Figure 8-5. Three autonomic ganglion explants have been placed near the border of extracellular matrix left on the culture dish by a previous sensory ganglion explant with its outgrowth of Schwann cells. The original sensory ganglion was excised (marks at top center), and its Schwann cells were removed by detergents. The insoluble extracellular matrix remaining guides the direction of neurite outgrowth from the new autonomic ganglion explants. Neurites growing on extracellular matrix are longer than those on the surrounding collagen. Toluidine blue stain. Bar is 1 mm.

Figure 8-6. Three autonomic ganglion explants have been placed at the border of Schwann cells plus basal lamina outgrowth from an earlier sensory ganglion explant. (Marks of the excision of the sensory neurons are seen at center.) Neurites from the autonomic ganglia, autoradiographically labeled by ^{3}H-norepinephrine uptake, extend to a much greater length on the Schwann cells plus basal lamina than on the surrounding collagen. Toluidine blue stain. Bar is 1 mm.

Figure 8-7. Neurites from a sensory ganglion explant (free of non-neuronal cells) follow invisible pathways of extracellular matrix left after detergent-extraction of a previous culture on this dish. Bar is 100 microns.

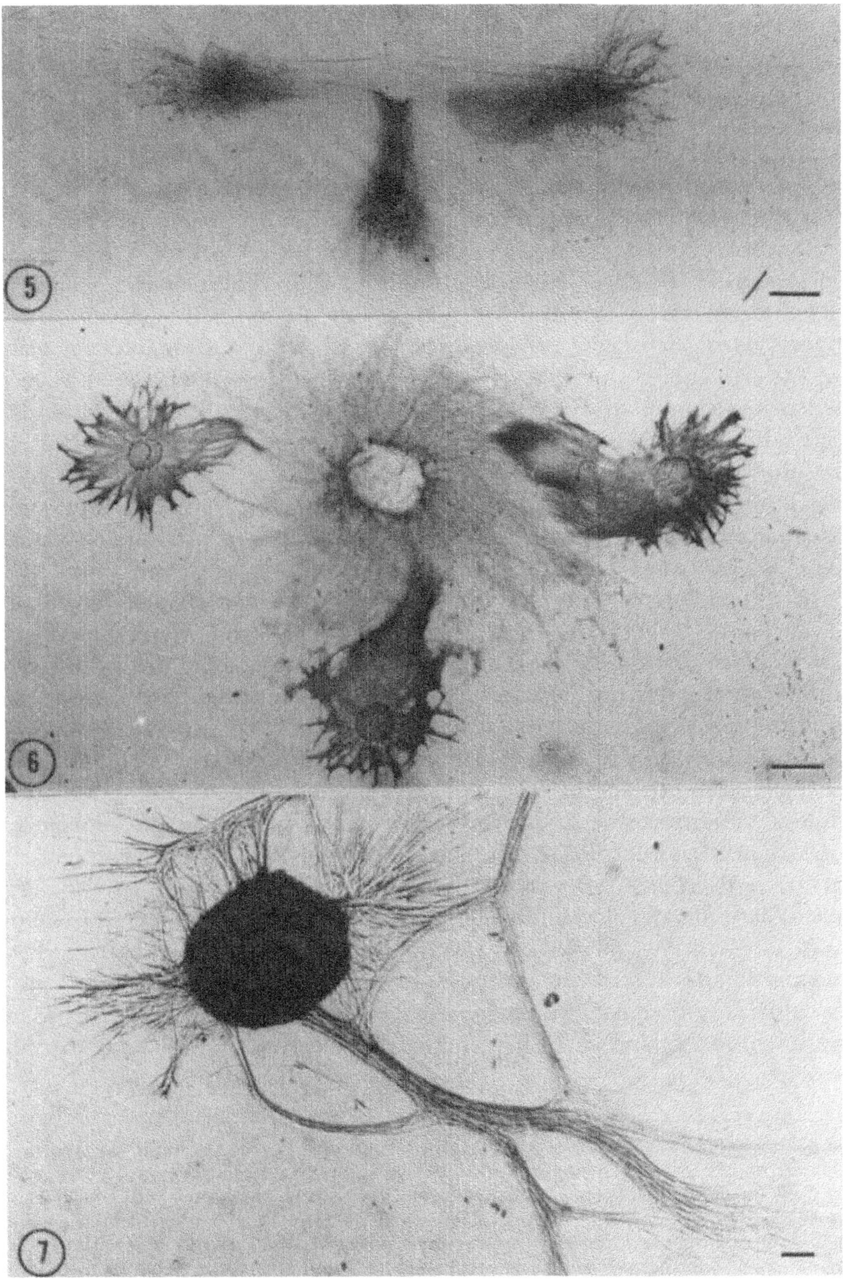
5
6
7

ference for basal lamina over rat tail collagen as a growth substratum (Figure 8-7).

These experiments clearly showed that *both* Schwann cell surfaces and basal lamina accelerated growth of regenerating neurites from adrenergic autonomic and sensory peripheral neurons. Both isolated Schwann cells and the basal lamina preparations contain laminin, because isolated Schwann cells express some laminin on their surfaces even though they do not organize a basal lamina [19]. However, recent work using antibodies that functionally block laminin receptors indicates that laminin is not the only neurite promoting molecule on the Schwann cell surface [20]. These antibodies blocked neurite outgrowth on extracellular matrix but not on cell surfaces.

The types of Schwann cell-produced basal lamina preparations utilized in the experiments on peripheral neurite growth described above have also proved instructive in studying influences on central nerve growth in culture. The growth of several types of central neurites has been tested on isolated Schwann cell basal lamina, and it has been observed that embryonic cortex [6], olfactory bulb [21], and locus coeruleus (Kleitman and Johnson, unpublished) explants extend neurites when confronted with tracks of previously deposited matrix.

Of particular interest were recent experiments in which 1) Schwann cells alone, 2) basal lamina alone, and 3) Schwann cells plus Schwann cell basal lamina were compared for their ability to promote neurite growth in retinal ganglion cells taken from 15-day embryonic rats (Figures 8-8, 8-9, 8-10). Considering our previous experience with peripheral neurite growth summarized above, and various reports that laminin may promote neurite growth of chick retinal cells [22–24], the observed results were unexpected. Under our experimental conditions, neurites grew vigorously on Schwann cell surfaces but not on isolated basal lamina synthesized and deposited by Schwann cells. The neurite growth in this case was not faster or slower, it was all or none. Antibodies to laminin did not influence this cell mediated promotion of neurite growth. Growth was also vigorous on Schwann cell plus Schwann cell basal lamina preparations. Ultrastructural studies revealed that retinal neurites in these cultures contacted only Schwann cell surfaces or other neurites, not Schwann cell basal lamina. In fact, neurite fascicles were surrounded by Sch-

---

Figure 8-8 to 8-10. Comparison of growth promoting capability of Schwann cells and/or their extracellular matrix for retinal ganglion cells. Bar in Figure 8-10 equals 1 mm. Retinal explants were grown on different substrata for 6 days, then fixed, osmicated, and Sudan black stained. **Figure 8-8**. Extensive neuritic growth from an embryonic retinal explant in a culture containing Schwann cells and Schwann cell extracellular matrix. **Figure 8-9**. Isolated Schwann cell extracellular matrix did not support retinal neurite extension. Underlying extreacellular matrix debris (arrowheads) extended across the culture. (Some non-neuronal cells have migrated out of the retinal explant.) **Figure 8-10**. Neurite fascicles extended from two hemiretinas plated in a culture of Schwann cells alone. Schwann cells in the vicinity of growing neurites migrated onto and enhanced the fasciculation of retinal neurites.

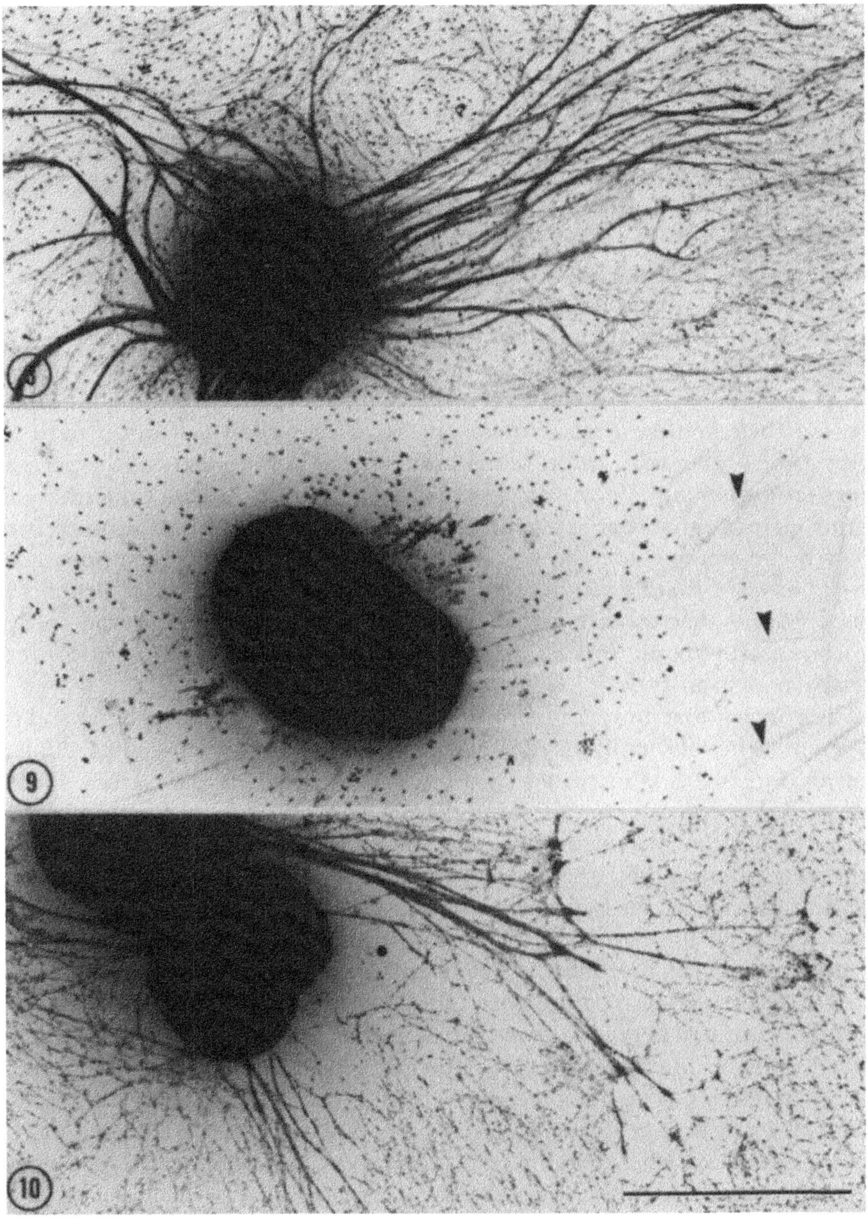
9
10

wann cell processes which were, in turn, surrounded by a basal lamina. It is clear that neurite promotion in these cultures must be attributed entirely to the presence of Schwann cells, because no neurite growth was seen on the ammoniated rat tail collagen used as the original surface on which Schwann cell cultures were prepared. The results of retinal ganglion cell neurite growth on Schwann cell surfaces were remarkably consistent from culture series to culture series in these experiments and the all-or-none nature of the response made analysis of results quite definitive.

The issue of cellular vs. extracellular matrix promotion of neurite extension of retinal ganglion cell axons is a particularly interesting one because of the demonstration that retinal ganglion cell neurite extension can occur in adult mammals after optic nerve section if retinal ganglion cell neurites are given access to the environment of a peripheral nerve trunk [25]. Our own experiments may be only indirectly relevant to this situation in the adult animal, because they involve observations on retinal ganglion cell outgrowth from embryonic (rather than adult) retina into isolated components of the peripheral nerve environment. We would emphasize, in light of the data presented earlier in this chapter, that this Schwann cell surface mediated promotion of neurite growth did not include the subsequent provision of trophic support. After 10–12 days of rapid growth, the Schwann cell-related neurites degenerated; it is apparent that other experimental approaches will be required to define neuron health-promoting vs. neurite extension-promoting agents for this particular neuron type.

The concept that emerges from our own studies summarized here, and from the many other observations now accumulating (for review, see Ref. 20) is that neurite outgrowth is mediated by a remarkable diversity of factors. Here the role of direct cell-cell contact in mediating trophic support for some neurons and in tutoring neurite growth for others is emphasized. When considered in light of the homophilic interactions known to be involved in mediating fasciculation of neurites during growth, the array of extracellular matrix materials known to influence neurite growth, and the soluble factors released by target or supporting cells that influence neuron survival, neurite health, and neurite growth, the substantial complexity of the ways in which neurons interact with their environment begins to come into focus. Furthermore, it is clear that rules and equipment differ for different neuronal types. In the same culture system, retinal ganglion cell neurites require Schwann cell surfaces for growth, whereas sensory ganglion cell neurites grow on both Schwann cell surfaces and basal lamina deposited by Schwann cells. Certainly, the type of detailed analysis of components undertaken recently by Tomaselli and associates [20] will be necessary to sort out the reasons why neurite extension occurs in certain instances and not others. These efforts will hardly be exercises in esoteric biology. The clear demonstration that central neurites can extend processes in segments of degenerating peripheral nerve shows that the lack of CNS regeneration in adult higher vertebrates may result from a failure of the CNS milieu to provide the particular ingredient that these neurites need for a regenerative effort. It will not be an easy task to define precisely what the essential tutorial and trophic factors are for each of the many kinds of neurons in the adult mammalian nervous system, but it surely will be a worthwhile effort.

REFERENCES

1. Thoenen, H. and Barde, Y. (1980). Physiology of nerve growth factor. Physiol. Inv. 60, 1284–1335.
2. Barde, Y.-A., Davies, A.M., Johnson, J.E., Lindsay, R.M. and Thoenen, H. (1987). Brain derived neurotrophic factor. In *Proceedings of the International Symposium on Neural Regeneration*, Progress in Brain Research, Vol. 71, F.J. Seil, E. Herbert, B.M. Carlson, eds., Elsevier, pp. 185–190.
3. Chiu, A.Y., Matthew, W.D. and Patterson, P.H. (1986). A monoclonal antibody that blocks the activity of a neurite regeneration-promoting factor: Studies on the binding site and its localization in vivo. J. Cell Biol. 103, 1383–1398.
4. Davis, G.E., Varon, S., Engvall, E. and Manthorpe, M. (1985). Substratum-binding neurite-promoting factors: Relationships to laminin. Trends in Neurosci. 8, 528–532.
5. Eldridge, C.F. and Bunge, R.P. (1987). Schwann cell-axon contact as a mechanism of neuronal trophic support, in preparation.
6. Ard, M.D., Bunge, R.P. and Bunge, M.B. (1987). Comparison of the Schwann cell surface and Schwann cell extracellular matrix as promoters of neurite growth. J. Neurocytol. 16, 539–555.
7. Kleitman, N., Wood, P., Johnson, M.I. and Bunge, R.P. (1988). Schwann cell surfaces but not extracellular matrix support neurite outgrowth from cultured embryonic rat retina. J. Neurosci. 8, 653–663.
8. Wood, P.M. (1976). Separation of functional Schwann cells and neurons from normal peripheral nerve tissue. Brain Res. 115, 361–375.
9. Eldridge, C.F., Bunge, M.B. and Bunge, R.P. (1987). Differentiation of axon-related Schwann cells in vitro. I. Ascorbic acid regulates basal lamina assembly and myelin formation. J. Cell Biol. 105, 1023–1034.
10. Brockes, J.P., Fields, K.L. and Raff, M.C. (1979). Studies on cultured rat Schwann cells. I. Establishment of purified populations from cultures of peripheral nerve. Brain Res. 165, 105–118.
11. Moya, F., Bunge, R.P. and Bunge, M.B. (1980). Schwann cells proliferate but fail to differentiate in defined medium. Proc. Natl. Acad. Sci. USA 77, 6902–6906.
12. Bottenstein, J.E. and Sato, G.H. (1979). Growth of a rat neuroblastoma cell line in serum-free supplemented medium. Proc. Natl. Acad. Sci. USA 76, 514–517.
13. Taniuchi, M., Clark, H.B. and Johnson, E.M. (1986). Induction of nerve growth factor receptor In Schwann cells after axotomy. Proc. Natl. Acad. Sci. USA 83, 4094–4098.
14. Waxman, S.G. and Ritchie, J.M. (1985). Organization of ion channels in the myelinated nerve fibers. Science 228, 1502–1507.
15. Barde, Y.-A., Edgar, D. and Thoenen, H. (1980). Sensory neurons in culture: Changing requirements for survival factors during embryonic development. Proc. Natl. Acad. Sci. USA 77, 1119.
16. Scherer, S.S. and Easter, S.S. (1984). Degenerative and regenerative changes in the trochlear nerve of goldfish. J. Neurocytol. 13, 519–565.
17. Ide, C., Tohyama, K., Yokota, R., Nitatori, T. and Onodera, S. (1983). Schwann cell basal lamina and nerve regeneration. Brain Res. 288, 61–75.
18. Hall, S.M. (1986). Regeneration in cellular and acellular autografts in the peripheral nervous system. Neuropath. Appl. Neurobiol. 12, 27–46.
19. Cornbrooks, C.J., Carey, D.J., McDonald, J.A., Timpl, R. and Bunge, R.P. (1983). In vivo and in vitro observations on laminin production by Schwann cells. Proc. Natl. Acad. Sci. USA 80, 3850–3854.
20. Tomaselli, K.J., Reichardt, L.F. and Bixby, J.L. (1986). Distinct molecular interactions mediate neuronal process outgrowth on non-neuronal cell surfaces and extracellular matrices.

J. Cell Biol. 103, 2659–2672.
21. Kleitman, N. and Johnson, M.I. (1986). Olfactory bulb neurite extension in cultures is age and substrate dependent. Soc. Neurosci. Abstr. 12, 1112.
22. Manthorpe, M., Engvall, E., Ruoslahti, E., Longo, F.M., Davis, G.E. and Varon, S. (1983). Laminin promotes neuritic regeneration from cultured peripheral and central neurons. J. Cell Biol. 97, 1882–1890.
23. Rogers, S.L., Letourneau, P.C., Palm, S.L., McCarthy, J. and Furcht, L.T. (1983), Neurite extension by peripheral and central nervous system neurons in response to substratum-bound fibronectin and laminin. Dev. Biol. 98, 212–220.
24. Adler, R., Jerdan, J. and Hewitt, A.T. (1985). Responses of cultured neural retinal cells to substratum-bound laminin and other extracellular matrix molecules. Dev. Biol. 112, 100–114.
25. So, K.-F. and Aguayo, A.J. (1985). Lengthy regrowth of cut axons from ganglion cells after peripheral nerve transplantation into the retinal of adult rats. Brain Res. 328, 349–354.

9. ROLE OF NERVE GROWTH FACTOR IN THE CENTRAL NERVOUS SYSTEM*

FRANZ HEFTI, JUKKA A. HARTIKKA, CLAUDIA N. MONTERO and EMMANUEL O. JUNARD

In recent years, the concept has evolved that survival of neurons during development is influenced by "neurotrophic factors." Paradigmatic studies were those on nerve growth factor (NGF), which affects survival and function of peripheral sympathetic and sensory neurons [1–4]. Other neurotrophic factors have been characterized that affect the survival and function of parasympathetic neurons [5], of cholinergic motorneurons [6], of retinal cells, and of a subpopulation of sensory neurons [7, 8]. These findings have been taken to suggest that populations of neurons require the presence of specific neurotrophic factors for survival during development, during differentiation, and for maintenance of function [9, 10].

The best characterized neurotrophic factor, NGF, is a protein of known amino acid sequence and structure [1, 4]. In this chapter NGF is used synonymously with beta-NGF, the active molecule, which in some tissues occurs as part of a larger protein complex [11]. The gene coding for NGF has been sequenced and cloned, and its organization has been elucidated [12–16]. NGF has been extensively characterized in its role as a specific neurotrophic factor for peripheral sympathetic neurons. It is synthesized by target tissues of sympathetic neurons and acts on specific receptors located on the sympathetic neurons. These receptors mediate local actions of NGF and its internalization,

* These studies were supported by the National Parkinson Foundation, Miami, Florida, the Alzheimer's and Related Disorders Association, Chicago Illinois, NIH Grant NS22933, and NSF Grant BNS-8708049.

Ferrendelli, J.A., Collins, R.C. and Johnson, E.M. (eds), Neurobiology of Amino Acids, Peptides, and Trophic Factors.

which initiates retrograde transport to the cell bodies of sympathetic neurons. In the cell body, NGF stimulates the synthesis of proteins essential for survival and expression of transmitter-specific properties by sympathetic neurons. Administration of NGF to rodents produces a hypertrophic reaction of sympathetic ganglia and results in selective stimulation of the synthesis of key enzymes for the production of norepinephrine, the transmitter of sympathetic neurons. Administration of antibodies to these animals results in atrophy of the sympathetic ganglia. The crucial role played by NGF in the function of sympathetic neurons is best demonstrated in cell culture experiments. Sympathetic neurons, isolated and placed in culture dishes, require NGF for survival, fiber growth, and for the expression of transmitter-specific enzymes. (For review of NGF's role in sympathetic function see Refs. 1, 3, 4, 9.)

Besides being a neurotrophic factor for catecholaminergic peripheral sympathetic neurons, NGF also affects peptidergic neurons of the peripheral sensory system [17, 18]. Other neurons of the peripheral mammalian nervous system do not seem to be influenced [9, 19]. Given the fact that peripheral catecholaminergic neurons are affected, several studies attempted to characterize the influence of NGF on central noradrenergic and dopaminergic neurons. The findings clearly demonstrated that NGF fails to affect central catecholaminergic neurons. Intracerebral injections of NGF did not promote development of central catecholaminergic neurons [20]. NGF did not affect central catecholaminergic neurons in culture [21 and Hefti et al., unpublished findings). NGF injected into target areas of catecholaminergic neurons was not taken up by these cells and transported retrogradely to their cell bodies, as occurs in peripheral catecholaminergic neurons [22]. The negative findings obtained with central catecholaminergic neurons have led many investigators to believe that NGF has no functional role in the CNS. However, in recent years evidence has accumulated that NGF acts as neurotrophic factor for central cholinergic neurons in a manner similar to its influence on peripheral sympathetic neurons. These findings were surprising and unexpected, because cholinergic neurons of the peripheral autonomous nervous system and cholinergic motor neurons are not affected by NGF [9, 23].

1. NGF: A NEUROTROPHIC FACTOR FOR FOREBRAIN CHOLINERGIC NEURONS

The evidence indicating that NGF is a selective neurotrophic factor for forebrain cholinergic neurons includes the following points. First, NGF, as well as the mRNA coding for NGF, is present in the rat brain [24–27]. The levels of both protein and its mRNA correlate with the anatomical distribution of cholinergic neurons of the rat brain [25–28]. NGF levels are highest in hippocampus, cortex, septum, and nucleus basalis, i.e., in target areas and areas of origin of ascending cholinergic neurons of the basal forebrain, and are lowest in optic tectum, cerebellum, and medulla, i.e., in areas not receiving an input from forebrain cholinergic neurons [28]). The corresponding mRNA is present at maximal levels in hippocampus and cortex [24, 26, 27]. Both, mRNA (NGF) and NGF levels in the hippocampus change in relation to the development of the cholinergic septo-hippocampal projection [30]. These findings suggest that NGF in the brain is produced by target cells of forebrain cholinergic neurons in a similar way as target cells provide peripheral sympathetic neurons with NGF.

A second group of findings indicates that central cholinergic neurons contain receptors for NGF. When NGF is injected into target areas of forebrain cholinergic neurons (i.e., hippocampus and cortex), it is taken up by nerve terminals and is transported in a retrograde fashion to the cholinergic cell bodies located in the basal forebrain, but not to other cell bodies projecting to these areas [22, 31]. These findings provide indirect evidence for the existence of NGF receptors on cholinergic neurons. NGF receptors have been directly demonstrated in the rat brain by immunoprecipitation with a monoclonal antibody to the NGF receptor protein [32]. Using autoradiographic techniques, NGF receptors have been located in the septum and nucleus basalis of the rat brain [33]. Using monoclonal antibodies against NGF receptors [34, 35], NGF receptors have recently been visualized in the rat and human brain. In the basal forebrain, NGF receptors were exclusively localized in areas containing cell bodies of cholinergic neurons (medial septal nucleus, diagonal band of Broca, nucleus basalis). These findings are presented in more detail in a subsequent section of this chapter.

A third group of findings provides evidence that the stimulation of NGF receptors on cholinergic neurons mediates trophic influences on these cells. In studies in vivo and in cell culture, NGF has been found to elevate the activity of choline acetyltransferase (CAT), the key enzyme in the synthesis of acetylcholine. NGF injected into the brain of newborn rats results in an increase in CAT activity in the septal area, hippocampus, and cortex [36–38]. In transplantation experiments in which cholinergic cells derived from fetal rats were injected into the brain of adult animals, the transplanted neurons expressed a higher CAT activity when they were treated with NGF [19]. Repeated intraventricular injections of NGF into adult rats with fimbrial transection elevated hippocampal and septal CAT activity [39]. In the septal area, elevated CAT activities were found to reflect increased survival of cholinergic neurons due to the NGF treatment (see below). In vitro, NGF-mediated increases in CAT activity were found in cultures of dissociated neurons obtained from the septal area of fetal rat brains [40, 41]. Initial experiments with cell cultures suggested that NGF elevates CAT activity without affecting survival or fiber growth of cholinergic neurons [40]. However, in more recent studies with a modified cell culture system, NGF was found to strongly promote the survival and fiber growth of cholinergic neurons (see below).

A fourth group of findings supporting the notion that NGF acts as a neurotrophic factor for cholinergic neurons of the basal forebrain is derived from results of transplantation studies. When the cholinergic fibers innervating the hippocampus are destroyed by a fimbrial lesion and parts of embryonic sympathetic ganglia are implantated at the site of the lesion, sympathetic fibers innervate the hippocampus and occupy the same anatomical sites that were previously occupied by cholinergic fibers [42, 43]. In the absence of implanted sympathetic ganglia, sympathetic fibers associated with brain blood vessels grow into the hippocampus at the sites previously occupied by the cholinergic fibers, whereas lesions of other neuronal systems do not elicit a similar response. These findings suggest that peripheral sympathetic neurons and cholinergic neurons of the basal forebrain react to the same neurotrophic factor. Since sympathetic neurons react to NGF, it was concluded that central cholinergic neurons also react to NGF [44].

2. VISUALIZATION OF NGF-RECEPTORS USING IMMUNOHISTOCHEMICAL PROCEDURES WITH MONOCLONAL ANTIBODIES

Monoclonal antibodies recognizing NGF receptors have been produced in recent years. A first antibody [34] binds to NGF receptors on PC12 cells, a second one recognizes the NGF receptor in human tissue [35]. We have developed immunohistochemical methods using these antibodies with which NGF receptors were successfully visualized in rat and human brains. In the brains of adult rats, the immunohistochemical procedure resulted in visualization of cell bodies and fibers in the septum, the diagonal band of Broca, and the nucleus basalis. Some NGF receptor-positive fibers were observed in the hippocampus. In the basal forebrain, the morphology, number, and distribution of NGF receptor-positive cells closely corresponded to that of cholinergic cell bodies in this area [45, 46], suggesting that NGF receptors are selectively located on ascending cholinergic neurons of the basal forebrain (Figure 9-1). Results of these studies obtained with the immunohistochemical procedure are in line with those obtained in a recent study in which NGF receptors were located in the basal forebrain using receptor autoradiography [33].

Similar results were obtained in the human brain as in the rat brain [47]. In the areas of the basal forebrain, the monoclonal antibody against NGF receptors visualized cells in the nucleus basalis, the diagonal band of Broca, and the medial septal nucleus. The areas studied included the caudate nucleus, internal and external segments of the globus pallidus, putamen, preoptic area, anterior nuclei of thalamus and hypothalamus, parts of the amygdala, anterior commissure, internal capsule, column of the fornix, and the olfactory tubercle. None of these additional structures contained positively stained cells for NGF receptors. The localization of NGF receptor-positive cells corresponds very closely to the location of cholinergic neurons of the basal forebrain in the human brain [45, 46], suggesting that NGF receptors are located on cholinergic neurons but not on other neurons in the same area. Number, morphology, and localization of NGF receptor-positive cells matched that of AChE-positive cells visualized in adjacent sections. Furthermore, costaining for NGF recep-

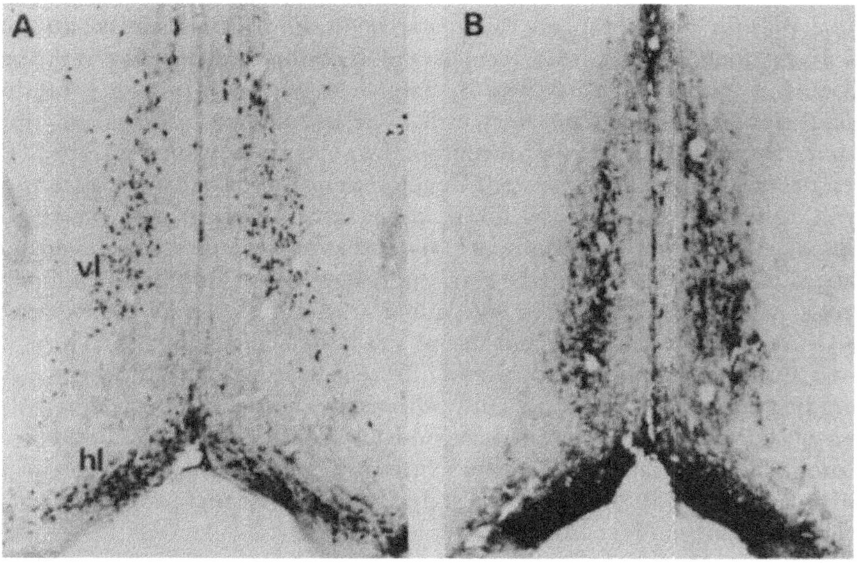

Figure 9-1. Localization of CAT-positive and NGF receptor-positive cells in the septal area of adult rat brains. CAT and NGF receptors were visualized using monoclonal antibodies and an avidin-biotin-peroxidase procedure. A. Section of the septal area stained for CAT. B. Adjacent section stained for NGF receptors. hl = horizontal limb; vl = vertical limb of the diagonal band of Broca.

tors and acetylcholinesterase (AChE) directly confirmed that NGF receptors are exclusively located on the cholinergic neurons of the basal forebrain [47].

In both rat and human brain sections, the reaction product visualizing NGF receptors was located on the outer membrane of the cell body and proximal processes. Furthermore, intracellular staining was heavily concentrated in the perinuclear area of the cell body [47]. This latter finding strongly suggests that NGF receptors are synthesized within cholinergic neurons. This notion is further supported by findings obtained in lesion studies. Transection of the septohippocampal pathway by a knife-cut through the fimbria resulted in a loss of NGF receptor-positive cells in the medial septal nucleus and the diagonal band of Broca. The effects of the lesion became apparent 3–5 days after fimbrial transection and were complete 14 days thereafter. Furthermore, 2–5 days after lesioning, accumulation of NGF receptor immunoreactivity was observed on the septal but not on the hippocampal side of the fimbrial transection.

NGF receptor histochemistry revealed no positively labeled cells in the corpus striatum of the rat and nucleus caudate and putamen of the human brain. This is surprising, since cholinergic interneurons of the striatum have been shown to react to NGF in a way similar to the cholinergic neurons of the basal forebrain [37, 38, 48]. Furthermore, NGF receptors were recently visualized in the rat striatum using receptor autoradiography and iodinated NGF [33]. Several reasons might explain this negative finding. First, striatal interneurons might contain fewer NGF receptors than cholinergic neurons of the basal forebrain, resulting in an inability to stain them with the present procedure. Second, striatal tissue contains very little NGF in contrast to cortex and hippocampus, the terminal areas of forebrain cholinergic neurons [27, 29]. This difference might result in different development of striatal interneurons and projecting neurons of the basal forebrain. Striatal interneurons express NGF receptors during early development only and stop the expression of this protein because of lack of NGF in the striatum. In contrast, forebrain cholinergic neurons, which project to NGF containing areas, might retain the expression of NGF receptors because of continuous availability of the ligand. Third, immunohistochemistry might visualize a different subtype of NGF receptor than autoradiography [33]. Receptor autoradiography visualized only slow, high-affinity NGF receptors, whereas the monoclonal antibody IgG 192 used for the immunohistochemical procedure was shown to bind to the fast, low-affinity NGF receptors [34]. It has not been established whether this antibody is able to recognize slow type receptors.

3. EFFECTS OF NGF ON FOREBRAIN CHOLINERGIC NEURONS IN CULTURES

Cell cultures represent ideal experimental systems to study the effects of neurotrophic factors on a given neuronal population. To establish the role of NGF in the function of cholinergic neurons of the basal forebrain, culture systems for these cells were developed and used for the study of the effects of NGF. Neurons were dissociated from the septal area of fetal rat brain and were grown in culture. Cholinergic neurons were identified by immunocytochemical visualization of CAT and cytochemical demonstration of acetylcholinesterase. CAT immunocytochemistry stained cell bodies and proximal processes of cholinergic neurons, while AChE cytochemistry visualized the entire neuron. All of the CAT-positive neurons were double-stained for AChE, while only 6% of the AChE-positive cells were CAT-negative in these cultures, indicating that CAT and AChE can be used to identify cholinergic cells in these cultures. The culture methods were described in detail elsewhere [40].

In initial studies, high-density cultures were used in which the growth of non-neuronal cells was suppressed by adding cytostatic compounds to the medium. In these "pure neuronal cultures," addition of NGF to the medium did not affect the number of surviving cholinergic neurons. Furthermore, NGF and anti-NGF failed to influence the general morphological appearance and the number of processes of these neurons. However, NGF elevated the biochemically measurable activity of CAT approximately twofold. This NGF-mediated increase in CAT activity was dose-dependent, with an ED_{50} of 0.4 nM. The increase was highly specific for NGF and was blocked by anti-

Table 9-1. Effects of NGF on survival and fiber growth of cholinergic neurons in culture. Neurons of the septal region of fetal rats were dissociated and grown in low density culture. NGF (100 ng/ml) was present during the entire culture time. After 14 days of growth, cultures were fixed and stained for AChE. Neurons were counted and their morphology was analyzed using a computerized image analysis system.

	Controls	NGF	% increase
Number of cells per dish	25.2 ± 3.1	61.7 ± 1.6	144.8% ★
Total fiber length of single neuron (mm)	4.65 ± 0.69	7.83 ± 0.85	68.4% ★
Branching points per neuron	54.3 ± 7.1	76.8 ± 9.9	41.4% ★
Length between branching points (mm)	0.083 ± 0.004	0.108 ± 0.006	30.1% ★

m ± S.E.M. Four control dishes and 4 dishes grown in the presence of NGF were analyzed. 100% of the area was counted to establish cell number, and the area was taken from all cells. The other parameters were measured from 20 randomly chosen neurons in each group. ★-significantly different from control value ($p < 0.05$).

NGF. Other growth factors and control proteins failed to exert a similar influence. These findings indicate that NGF is able to elevate CAT activity in cultured cholinergic neurons taken from fetal rat brain. However, in the pure neuronal cultures, NGF apparently does not influence survival of cholinergic neurons. These findings have been reported in detail elsewhere [40].

In more recent experiments, septal neurons were cultured at low density and in the presence of glial cells. In these cultures, NGF increased the number of cholinergic neurons (Table 9-1). The stimulatory effect of NGF was prevented by the addition of antisera to NGF, indicating that the effect was specific for NGF. Cultures grown in the presence of both NGF and anti-NGF or in the presence of anti-NGF alone contained significantly fewer AChE-positive cells than control cultures. These findings suggest that NGF is formed by neurons or glial cells growing in the cultures in sufficient quantities to support the survival of an intermediate number of cholinergic cells. The ED_{50} of NGF's effect on survival of cholinergic neurons was found to be approximately 0.4 nM. This concentration is in the range of concentrations necessary to stimulate NGF receptors on sympathetic and sensory neurons [1, 9]. The low-density cultures were furthermore taken for morphometric analysis of cholinergic neurons using a computerized image analysis system. The total length of fibers of a single cell, the total number of branching points, and the average length between two branching points were found to be elevated by 30%–70% in neurons grown in the presence of NGF as compared to control neurons (Table 9-1). These findings suggest that NGF is able to promote survival and fiber growth of cholinergic neurons in culture in addition to its well-established elevation of CAT activity.

4. EFFECTS OF NGF ON SURVIVAL OF LESIONED CHOLINERGIC NEURONS

Neurons studied in cell cultures are taken from embryonal animals, and findings obtained with these systems are mainly relevant for the development aspects. NGF injected into the brain of adult animals failed to trophically influence forebrain cholinergic neurons [39]. However, such effects became apparent when NGF was injected chronically into the ventricles of adult rats with unilateral partial lesions of the cholinergic septohippocampal pathway. The septohippocampal pathway was chosen for lesioning because it represents the best characterized part of the ascending cholinergic projection of the basal forebrain, which innervates the cortex and hippocampus [45, 46]. The septohippocampal pathway was lesioned by making a transection of the fimbria. Such transections resulted in a pronounced, but not total, reduction of the cholinergic input to the hippocampus, the reduction being maximal at the temporal pole. NGF was injected over 4 weeks into the ventricles of lesioned animals and was found to significantly elevate hippocampal and septal CAT activity.

The NGF-mediated elevations of septal CAT activity observed in these studies led to the hypothesis that NGF might affect survival of septal cholinergic neurons. This hypothesis was tested using histochemical procedures. The fimbrial transections were found to reduce the number of large cell bodies, as visualized by Nissl staining in the medial septal nucleus and in the vertical limb of the diagonal band of Broca. Furthermore, in the same nuclei, they reduced the number of cell bodies positively stained for CAT, AChE (after pretreatment with diisopropylfluorophosphate; a method known to result in reliable identification of cholinergic neurons in the septal area [49, 50]), and NGF receptors. These results strongly suggest that the fimbrial transections resulted in a retrograde degeneration of cholinergic neurons in the spetal area. NGF-treatment antagonized the effect of the lesion. On lesioned sides, the number of cholinergic cells in the medial septal nucleus and the vertical limb of the diagonal band was reduced by 50% as compared to that on contralateral sides; whereas on lesioned sides of animals chronically treated with NGF, the number of AChE-positive cells in these areas was only reduced by 12%. These findings suggest that NGF-treatment strongly attenuated the lesion-induced degeneration of septal cholinergic neurons. These findings were described in detail elsewhere [51].

5. IMPLICATIONS FOR ALZHEIMER'S DISEASE

Findings indicating that NGF acts as a neurotrophic factor for cholinergic neurons of the basal forebrain and that NGF is able to prevent lesion-induced degeneration of these neurons have implications for the understanding of Alzheimer's disease. This disease is characterized by progressive loss of memory and other cognitive functions, resulting in permanent and irreversible disability. Alzheimer's disease is associated with characteristic neuropathological changes. There is an increase in the number of neuritic plaques and neurofibrillary tangles, mainly in the neocortex and hippocampus [52, 53]. Furthermore, there are degenerations of specific neuronal systems, mainly of cholinergic, noradrenergic, and somatostatin-containing neurons [33]. The loss of cholinergic neurons represents one of the most consistent finding in neuropathological analysis of Alzheimer's brains [33, 54–56]. The pathways affected are those forming the ascending cholinergic pathways of the basal forebrain. The decrease in cholinergic parameters correlates with both the number of plaques and the clinical assessement of dementia [57–59]. The loss of cholinergic neurons is therefore regarded by many investigators as being an important factor responsible for the memory loss characteristic of Alzheimer's disease [54, 55, 60]. This notion draws further support from many studies which demonstrate that manipulation of cholinergic transmission affects memory function [61–63].

The hypothesis that the selective loss of cholinergic neurons in Alzheimer's disease might be caused by a lack of NGF available to the cholinergic neurons was formulated earlier and attention was drawn to the possibility that NGF or drugs mimicking NGF's actions might be useful in the treatment of the disease [64]. So far, no supportive evidence has been found for a causative involvement of NGF in the pathophysiology of Alzheimer's disease [25]. Furthermore, recent findings on the pathology of the disease have revealed that the degeneration of cholinergic neurons may represent a secondary degenerative event only (for discussion of this point see Ref. 65). Nevertheless, given the close correlation between cholinergic loss and decrease in memory function and the findings indicating that cholinergic neurons are involved in memory function [63], it seems probable that the cholinergic deficit is responsible for some of the major symptoms of the disease, and compounds mimicking NGF's actions might be beneficial in the treatment of the disease.

REFERENCES

1. Greene, L.A. and Shooter, E.M. (1980). The nerve growth factor: Biochemistry, synthesis, and mechanism of action. Ann. Rev. Neurosci. 3, 353–402.
2. Levi-Montalcini, R. (1982). Developmental neurobiology and the natural history of nerve growth factor. Ann. Rev. Neurosci. 5, 341–362.
3. Thoenen, H. and Barde, Y.A. (1980). Physiology of nerve growth factor. Physiol. Rev. 60, 1284–1335.
4. Yankner, B.A. and Shooter, E.M. (1982). The biology and mechanism of action of nerve growth factor. Ann. Rev. Biochem. 51, 845–868.
5. Barbin, G., Manthorpe, M. and Varon, S. (1984). Purification of the chick eye ciliary neuronotrophic factor. J. Neurochem. 43, 1468–1478.
6. Hill, M.A. and Bennett, M.R. (1983). Cholinergic growth factor from skeletal muscle elevated following denervation. Neurosci Lett. 35. 31–35.
7. Barde, Y.A., Edgar, D. and Thoenen, H. (1982). Purification of a new neurotrophic factor from mammalian brain. EMBO J. 1, 549–559.
8. Johnson, J.E., Barde, Y.A., Schwab, M. and Thoenen, H. (1986). Brain-derived neurotrophic factor supports the survival of cultured rat retinal ganglion cells. J. Neurosci. 6, 3031–3038.
9. Thoenen, H. and Edgar, D. (1985). Neurotrophic factors. Science 229, 238–242.
10. Varon, S. and Adler, R. (1980). Nerve growth factors and control of nerve growth. Curr. Top. Dev. Biol. 16, 207–252.
11. Murphy, R.A., Landis, S.C., Bernanke, J. and Siminoski, K. (1986). Absence of the alpha and gamma subunits of 7S nerve growth factor in denervated rodent iris: Immunocytochemical

studies. Develop. Biol. 114, 369–380.
12. Edwards, R.H., Selby, M.J. and Rutter W.J. (1986). Differential RNA splicing predicts two distinct nerve growth factor precursors. Nature 319, 784–787, 1986.
13. Francke, U., DeMartinville, B., Coussens, L. and Ullrich, A. The human gene for the beta-subunit of nerve growth factor is located on the proximal short arm of chromosome 1. Science 222, 1248–1250, 1983.
14. Huebner, K., Isobe, M., Chao, M., Bothwell, M., Ross, A.H., Finan, J., Hoxie, J.A., Sehgal, A., Buck, C.R., Lanahan, A., Nowell, P.C., Koprowski, H. and Croce, C.M. (1986). The nerve growth factor receptor gene is at human chromosome region 17q12–17q22, distal to the chromosome 17 breakpoint in acute leukemias. Proc. Natl. Acad. Sci. USA 83, 1403–1407.
15. Scott, J., Selby, M., Urdea, M., Quiroga, M., Bell, G.I. and Tutter, W.J. (1983). Isolation and nucleotide sequence of cDNA encoding the precursor of mouse nerve growth factor. Nature 302, 538–540.
16. Ullrich, A., Gray, A., Berman, C. and Dull, T.J. (1983). Human beta-nerve growth factor gene sequence highly homologous to that of mouse. Nature 303, 821–825.
17. Johnson, E.M., Gorin, P.D., Brandeis, L.D. and Pearson, J. (1980). Dorsal root ganglion neurons are destroyed by exposure in utero to maternal antibody to nerve growth factor. Science 210, 916–918.
18. Yip, H.K., Rich, K.M., Lampe, P.A. and Johnson, E.M. (1984). The effects of nerve growth factor and its antiserum on the postnatal development and survival after injury of sensory neurons in rat dorsal root ganglia. J. Neurosci. 4, 2986–2992.
19. Toniolo, G., Dunnett, S.B., Hefti, F. and Will, B. (1985). Acetylcholine-rich transplants in the hippocampus: Influence of intrinsic growth factors and application of NGF on choline acetyltransferase activity. Brain Res. 345, 141–146.
20. Kaufman, L.M., Barry, S.R. and Barrett, J.N. (1985). Characterization of tissue-derived macromolecules affecting transmitter synthesis in rat spinal cord neurons. J. Neurosci. 5, 160–166.
21. Dreyfus, C.F., Peterson, E.R. and Crain, S.M. (1980). Failure of nerve growth factor to affect fetal mouse brain catecholaminergic neurons in culture. Brain Res. 194, 540–551.
22. Schwab, M., Otten, U., Agid, Y. and Thoenen, H. (1979). Nerve growth factor (NGF) in the rat CNS: Absence of specific retrograde axonal transport and tyrosine hydroxylase induction in locus coeruleus and substantia nigra. Brain Res. 168, 473–483.
23. Dribin, L.B. and Barrett, J.N. (1980). Conditioned medium enhances neuritic outgrowth from rat spinal cord explants. Dev. Biol. 74, 184–195.
24. Crutcher, K.A. and Collins, F. (1982). In vitro evidence for two distinct hippocampal growth factors: Basis of neuronal plasticity? Science 217, 67–70.
25. Goedert, M., Fine, A., Hunt, S.P. and Ullrich, A. (1986). Nerve growth factor mRNA in peripheral and central rat tissues and the human central nervous system: Lesion effects in the rat brain and levels in Alzheimer's disease. Molec. Brain Res. 1, 85–92.
26. Konkol, R.J., Mailam, R.B., Bendeich, E.G., Garrison, A.M., Mueller, R.A. and Breese, G.R. (1978). Evaluation of the effects of nerve growth factor and anti-nerve growth factor on the development of central catecholaminergic neurons. Brain Res. 144, 277–285.
27. Shelton, D.L. and Reichardt, L.F. (1986). Studies on the expression of the beta nerve growth factor (NGF) gene in the central nervous system: Level and regional distribution of NGF mRNA suggest that NGF functions as a trophic factor for several distinct populations of neurons. Proc. Natl. Acad. Sci. USA 83, 2714–2718.
28. Whittemore, S.R., Ebendal, T., Larkfors, L., Olson, L., Seiger, A., Stromberg, I. and Persson, H. (1986). Developmental and regional expression of beta nerve growth factor messenger RNA and protein in the rat central nervous system. Proc. Natl. Acad. Sci. USA 83, 817–821.
29. Korsching, S., Auburger, G., Heumann, R., Scott, J. and Thoenen, H. (1985). Levels of nerve growth factor and its mRNA in the central nervous system of the rat correlate with cholinergic innervation. EMBO J. 4, 1389–1393.
30. Large, T.H., Bodary, S.C., Clegg, D.O., Weskamp, G., Otten, U. and Reichardt, L.F. (1986). Nerve growth factor gene expression in the developing rat brain. Science 234, 352–355.
31. Seiler, M. and Schwab, M.E. (1984). Specific retrograde transport of nerve growth factor (NGF) from neocortex to nucleus basalis in the rat. Brain Res. 300, 33–36.

32. Taniuchi, M., Schweizer, J.B. and Johnson, E.M. (1986). Demonstration of nerve growth factor receptor in the rat brain. Proc. Natl. Acad. USA 83, 4094–4098.
33. Richardson, P.M., Verge Issa, V.M. and Riopelle, R.J. (1986). Distribution of neuronal receptors for nerve growth factor in the rat. J. Neurosci. 2312–2321.
34. Chandler, C.E., Parsons, L.M., Hosang, M. and Shooter, E.M. (1984). A monoclonal antibody modulates the interaction of nerve growth factor with PC12 cells. J. Biol. Chem. 259, 6882–6889.
35. Ross, A.H., Grob, P., Bothwell, M., Elder, D.E., Ernst, C.S., Marano, N., Ghrist, B.F., Slemp, C.C., Herlyn, M., Atkinson, B. and Koprowski, H. (1984). Characterization of nerve growth factor receptor in neural crest tumors using monoclonal antibodies. Proc. Natl. Acac. USA 81, 6681–6685.
36. Gnahn, H., Hefti, F., Heumann, R., Schwab, M. and Thoenen, H. (1983). NGF-mediated increase of choline acetyltransferase (ChAT) in the neonatal forebrain; evidence for a physiological role of NGF in the brain? Dev. Brain Res. 9, 45–52.
37. Mobley, W.C., Rutkowski, J.L., Tennekoon, G.I., Buchanan, K. and Johnston, M.V. (1985). Choline acetyltransferase activity in striatum of neonatal rats increased by nerve growth factor. Science 229, 284–286.
38. Mobley, W.C., Rutkowski, J.L., Tennekoon, G.I., Buchanan, K., Gemski, J. and Johnston, M.V. (1986). Nerve growth factor increases choline acetyltransferase activity in developing basal forebrain neurons. Molec. Brain Res. 1, 53–62.
39. Hefti, F., Dravid, A. and Hartikka, J. (1984). Chronic intraventricular injections of nerve growth factor elevate hippocampal choline acetyltransferase activity in adult rats with partial septohippocampal lesions. Brain Res. 293, 305–309.
40. Hefti, F., Hartikka, J., Eckenstein, F., Gnahn, H., Heumann, R. and Schwab, M. (1985). Nerve growth factor (NGF) increases choline acetyltransferase but not survival or fiber growth of cultured septal cholinergic neurons. Neuroscience 14, 55–68.
41. Honegger, P. and Lenoir, D. (1982). Nerve growth factor (NGF) stimulation of cholinergic telencephalic neurons in aggregating cell cultures. Dev. Brain Res. 3, 229–238.
42. Bjorklund, A. and Stenevi, U. (1977). Experimental reinnervation of the rat hippocampus by grafted sympathetic ganglia I. Axonal regeneration along the hippocampal fimbria. Brain Res. 138, 259–270.
43. Bjorklund, A. and Stenevi, U. (1979). Regeneration of monoaminergic and cholinergic neurons in the mammalian central nervous system. Physiol. Rev. 59, 62–100.
44. Crutcher, K.A. and Davis, J.N. (1981). Sympathetic noradrenergic sprouting in response to central cholinergic denervations. Trends Neurosci. 4, 70–72.
45. Mesulam, M.M., Mufson, E.J., Wainer, B.H. and Levey, A.I. (1983). Central cholinergic pathways in the rat: An overview based on an alternative nomenclature (Ch1–Ch6). Neuroscience 10, 1185–1201.
46. Wainer, B.H., Levey, A.I., Mufson, E.F. and Mesulam, M.M. (1984). Cholinergic systems in mammalian brain identified with antibodies against choline acetyltransferase. Neurosci. Int. 6, 163–182.
47. Hefti, F., Hartikka, J., Salvatierra, A., Weiner, W.J. and Mash, D.C. (1986). Localization of nerve growth factor receptors in cholinergic neurons of the human basal forebrain. Neurosci. Lett. 69, 37–41.
48. Martinez, H.J., Dreyfus, C.F., Jonakait, G.M. and Black, I.B. (1985). Nerve growth factor promotes cholinergic development in brain striatal cultures. Proc. Natl. Acad. Sci. USA 82, 7777–7781.
49. Eckenstein, F. and Sofroniew, M.W. (1983). Identification of central cholinergic neurons containing both choline acetyltransferase and acetylcholinesterase and of central neurons containing only acetylcholinesterase. J. Neurosci. 3, 2286–2291.
50. Levey, A.I., Wainer, B.H., Mufson, E.J. and Mesulam, M.M. (1983). Co-localization of acetylcholinesterase and choline acetyltransferase in the rat cerebrum. Neuroscience 9, 9–22.
51. Hefti, F. (1986). Nerve growth factor (NGF) promotes survival of septal cholinergic neurons after fimbrial transections. J. Neurosci. 6, 2155–2162.
52. Price, D.L., Struble, R.G., Whitehouse, P.J., Kitt, C.A. and Cork, L.C. (1985). Neuropathological processes in Alzheimer's disease. Drug Develop. Res. 5, 59–67.
53. Wisniewski, H.M. and Merz, G.S. (1983). Neuritic and amyloid plaques in senile dementia of the Alzheimer type. In *Banbury Report 15: Biological Aspects of Alzheimer's Disease*, Katzman, R., ed., Cold Spring Harbor Laboratory, Cold Spring Harbor, pp. 145–153.

54. Coyle, J.T., Price, D.L. and DeLong, M.R. (1983). Alzheimer's disease: A disease of cortical cholinegic innervation. Science 219, 1184–1190.
55. Davies, P. (1985). Is it possible to design rational treatment for the symptoms of Alzheimer's disease? Drug Develop. Res. 5, 69–75.
56. Wilcock, G.K., Esiri, M.M., Bowen, D.M. and Smith, C.C. (1983). The nucleus basalis in Alzheimer's disease: Cell counts and cortical biochemistry. Neuropathol. Appl. Neurobiol. 9, 175–179.
57. Arendt, T., Bigl, V., Tennstedt, A. and Arendt, A. (1984). Correlation between cortical plaque count and neuronal loss in the nucleus basalis in Alzheimer's disease. Neurosci. Lett. 48, 81–85.
58. Francis, P.T., Palmer, A.M., Sims, N.R., Bowen, D.M., Davison, A.N., Esiri, M.M., Neary, D., Snowden, J.S. and Wilcock, G.K. (1985). Neurochemical studies of early-onset Alzheimer's disease. Possible influence on treatment. Lancet, July 4, 7–11.
59. Perry, E.K., Tomlison, B.E., Blessed, G., Perry, R.H., Cross, A.J. and Crow, T.J. (1978). Correlation of cholinergic abnormalities with senile plaques and mental test scores in senile dementia. Brit. Med. J. 2, 1457–1459.
60. Bartus, R.T., Dean, R.L., Beer, B. and Lippa, A.S. (1982). The cholinergic hypothesis of geriatric memory dysfunction. Science 217, 408–417.
61. Flicker, C., Dean, R.L., Watkins, D.L., Fisher, S.K. and Bartus, R.T. (1983). Behavioral and neurochemical effects following neurotoxic lesions of a major cholinergic input to the cerebral cortex in the rat. Pharmacol. Biochem. Behav. 18, 973–981.
62. Hepler, D.J., Olton, D.S., Wenk, G.L. and Coyle, J.T. (1985). Lesions in nucleus basalis magnocellularis and medial septal area of rats produce qualitatively similar memory impairments. J. Neurosci. 5, 866–873.
63. Russell, R.W. (1982). Cholinergic system in behavior: The search for mechanisms of action. Ann. Rev. Pharmacol. Toxicol. 22, 435–463.
64. Hefti, F. and Weiner, W. J. (1986). Nerve growth factor and Alzheimer's disease. Ann. Neurol. 20, 275–281.
65. Mesulam, M.M. (1986). Alzheimer plaques and cortical cholinergic innervation. Neuroscience 17, 275–267.

III. NEUROPEPTIDES

10. NEUROPEPTIDES: GENERAL ASPECTS

FLOYD E. BLOOM

Neuropeptides remain everyone's favorite transmission factors. Not only does a new one appear nearly every week, but their picturesque and occasionally informative names are complemented by esthetically pleasing photomicrography of the cells containing the newly recognized substance. When the molecular identification of a new peptide even partially aligns with peptides already discovered, the family portraits of the major groups of brain, gut, and endocrine peptides readily enlarge. As shown by the accompanying reports, these peptides are also often quickly found to possess potent ability to influence whole animal physiological events or behaviors, including those central or visceral disorders that affect humans. While all this is indeed quite exciting, the key puzzles surrounding the nature of neuropeptides and their verified functional roles remain unanswered [1, 2].

There are three major neurobiological distinctions of neuropeptides: 1) They can only be synthesized in cellular compartments that contain rough endoplasmic reticulum, 2) the propeptide must be actively transported to sites of secretion and processed to the active forms while en route, and 3) there is no known form of neuronal conservation of the secreted peptide. These unique signal attributes all conspire to make it difficult to convert normal peptide biology into the sorts of changes in the amounts of peptide that are generally employed as links to pathophysiology. Thus, the finding that a specific neuropeptide may be decreased in concentration in spinal fluid or in postmortem brain tissue could reflect either increased rates of release; decreased rates of

Ferrendelli, J.A., Collins, R.C. and Johnson, E.M. (eds), Neurobiology of Amino Acids, Peptides, and Trophic Factors.

transport, synthesis, processing, or overall catabolism; or actual damage to the neurons that make and secrete that peptide.

In addition to the potentially ambiguous interpretation of tissue assay values, other medically relevant aspects need recognition. Attempts to make nonpeptide analogs of peptides that can act within the brain after conventional routes of administration to simulate or to antagonize perceived deficiencies or excesses of peptide signals have so far had very limited successes outside the opioid peptide family. Furthermore, the existence of multiple closely related peptide structures in many widely distributed central and peripheral neuronal systems suggests that peptide receptor characterization will need very careful scrutinization to develop selective treatment tools against peptides in those places where they may be misfunctioning.

However, the most perplexing aspect of neuropeptides may well be the increasingly clear trait of "coexistence" [3]. Neurons that contain peptides also contain 10- to 1000-fold higher amounts of nonpeptide transmitters. One could presently take the position that no neuron is truly "peptidergic." Rather, the peptide or peptides within a neuron may be considered as chemical embellishments to the more conventional monoamine and amino acid transmitters. Exactly what these embellishments are and where and when they are expressed is of course part of the mystique of brain peptides, the emerging puzzles of what it is that transmitters do, and the general issue of how many forms of synaptic transmitter signals are used by our brains.

Philosophizing over the criteria by which the effects of transmitter substances can be classified and compared, not simply as "factors" assessed in vitro for biochemical regulatory actions, but rather as physiological regulators operating within the context of their circuit anatomy and their overall signaling value, is an occasional pastime of mine [4, 5]. With the accelerated progress of present-day science developments, one recognizes that we have been blessed with an enormous richness of factual information. For this communication, remarks will be concentrated on three accumulations of our recent data. First, some recent insight from applications of molecular biological methods to the diversity of peptides made by brain neurons will be reviewed. Next, one excellent functional example of a peptide in action will be analyzed in reviewing the ability of vasoactive intestinal polypeptide (VIP) to influence responsiveness, both biochemically and electrophysiologically, to noradrenaline in the cerebral cortex through their interactive regulation of neocortical adenylate cyclase. Finally, some recent studies will be examined that were undertaken to examine the interplay between the neuropeptide somatostatin and the classical amine transmitter, acetylcholine, on common target neurons in the cerebral cortex and hippocampal formation.

From these data, it is inferred that the interactions between neuropeptides and other transmitters on their shared target cells may represent regulatory mechanisms that are "conditional" and that such conditional signaling mechanisms will set the scales on which other spatial and temporal signals between neurons are ultimately manifested as purposeful. The general conclusion is one that has special relevance to the present conference: *Many visceral systems, even sparsely innervated ones, use peptides as signals; thus the study of peptides in all these systems has revealed general properties of intercellular communication that, while not previously recognized, are probably elicitable by nonpeptide signals as well.*

1. IDENTIFYING NEUROPEPTIDES BY GENE CLONING

The catalog of neurotransmitters, including neuropeptides, is far from completely compiled. Many important genetic and non-genetic disorders may only be amenable to comprehension, diagnosis, treatment, and ultimate prevention when the remaining new transmitters are available as probes of the pathology. Looking back upon the growing list of neuropeptides proposed as consensus transmitters [4, 5], some have functional names (somatostatin, endorphin, enkephalin, cholecystokinin) and others have largely chemical names (substance P. neuropeptide Y, PHI-27). The development of a bioassay for an unknown regulatory factor was the traditional starting point for the early gastrointestintal and endocrine regulatory peptides and for most of the neuropeptides to emerge from the hypophysiotrophic era: gastrin, cholecystokinin, angiotensin, oxytocin, vasopressin, the ever popular endogenous opioid peptides, and all of the specific pituitary hormone releasing hormones, including the last two of the originally postulated hypophysiotrophic factors predicted, corticotropin releasing factor [6] and growth hormone releasing factor [7], the totally unexpected inhibitory regulator somatostatin, the atriopeptides, and a possible endogenous benzodiazepine ligand (see Costa, Chapter 3).

2. TWO MODERN STRATEGIES OF PEPTIDE DISCOVERY

Two series of developments over the past half decade have further expanded the emerging list of peptides with agents whose functional role is scarcely even acknowledged. Mutt and colleagues [8, 9] looked at the frequent occurrence of C-terminally amidated peptides that functioned as messengers. Using chemical methods that detect C-terminally amidated peptide fragments, they were able to identify other important molecules with this common structure. Using this approach they found new peptide members of the glucagon-VIP family and the pancreatic polypeptide family, using the biochemical test as the primary assay for their isolation and classical structural determination.

A second new approach is based on the central dogma of molecular biology — all peptides are synthesized under the direction of a specific messenger RNA (mRNA) encoded by the gene for that peptide. With the emergence of recombinant DNA technologies, restriction endonucleases, and nucleotide sequencing, and a new opportunity for molecular discovery became available. Nakanishi and colleagues [10] were the first to use molecular biological methods to determine the sequence of an mRNA that encodes the expression of a neuropeptide. With the mRNA purified from 40 bovine pituitaries, they were able to analyze a cDNA library and identify the specific mRNA for the common precursor of corticotropin, determine its nucleotide sequence, and deduce the amino acid sequence of the gene product. In addition to revealing the contiguous encoding of corticotropin and β-lipotropin, their mRNA sequence deductions also revealed a third possible biologically relevant peptide, termed *gamma-melanocyte stimulating hormone* (MSH). Subsequently, the recombinant DNA approach has been employed to obtain the prohormone structural sequences, and some of the genomic sequences for almost every one of the previously identified neuropeptides (see Ref. 11 for review).

These studies have directly contributed to the degree of diversity at the molecular level. Potentially new, previously unsuspected coexpressed peptides were also suggested strictly from mRNA sequences to predict new forms of VIP [12] and substance P [13]. Moreover, pursuit of the prohormone for calcitonin, led Rosenfeld and Evans and their collaborators to the recognition that rearrangements of parts of the mRNA domains of procalcitonin could give rise to a "calcitonin-gene related peptide" [14], which, in fact, was found in special segments of the rat CNS and had unsuspected biological activity. In fact, the recombinant approach has yielded so many new molecules, all roughly equivalent candidates for consideration as neurotransmitters, that the next major phases of the investigation, localization, and assessment of function have lagged far behind.

3. A GENERAL MOLECULAR DISCOVERY STRATEGY

Our approach has been to attack the molecular specificity of the mature rat and primate brain with a direct examination of the complexity of the genetic messages being expressed there. Every protein product being expressed in brain, as in all cells, depends for its synthesis on the transcription of a specific piece of genetic information into a messenger RNA that guides synthesis of the gene product. Using the powerful tools of recombinant DNA technology, we have embarked on a long-term study aimed at characterizing the messenger RNA molecules that are specific to brain. Our results suggest that, on average, the mammalian brain derives its complexity through only 30,000 or so messenger RNAs enriched in brain and not detectable in other major organ systems.

Among the more interesting of these highly specific, chemically determined marker molecules, we have found both neuron-specific and glia-specific examples. Our most intensively studied system has satisfied some, but not yet all, of the cellular, subcellular, and biochemical criteria of a neurotransmitter peptide prohormone. Thus, a genetic analysis of brain complexity and functional specificity is a potent and efficient strategy for molecular discovery.

Our examination of one apparently "brain-specific" protein product, as defined by our criteria, seems especially relevant to complete our documentation of the powers of neuropeptide localization. The clone 1B236 hybridizes to two brain specific mRNAs, one 2500 nucleotides in length, and the other 3000.

Both mRNAs show parallel regional heterogeneity across rat brain, with the 2500 nucleotide form predominant, and regions such as thalamus, midbrain, and pons-medulla higher than cortical regions. The complete open reading frame of the full length mRNA encodes 626 amino acids, including a prototypic N-terminal signal peptide, several potential glycosylation sites, and three C-terminal peptide-like fragments, (peptides 5, 6, and 7) separated by pairs of basic amino acids, following a presumptive transmembrane domain of 21 hydrophobic amino acids. Further genomic analysis of 1B236 exons suggests that although there is only one 1B236 gene, there are at least two forms of mRNA splicing. In the major alternative to the originally encountered form, an additional exon is spliced 3' to that encoding peptide 5, with the result that the most N-terminal of the three presumptive peptides, peptide 5, is C-terminally extended with loss of translation of peptides 6 and 7.

Antisera raised against peptides 5, 6, and 7 of the deduced amino acid sequence have localized this presumptive gene product in pontine, cerebellar, cortical, and limbic structures [15, 16] and provide strong support for the interpretation that this protein corresponding to an mRNA cloned and selected as brain-specific [15, 17] is expressed in the brain, and that this gene product is shared by a select number of neuronal systems. The cytochemical and subcellular fractionation data are consistent with the view that a large precursor form of the protein is processed during its transit through the perikaryal cytoplasm en route to nerve terminals. At least one form of the molecule is best described as a presumptive membrane-bound glycoprotein [18] capable of being processed under as yet undetermined conditions to three or more neuropeptide-like fragments. The N-terminal glycoprotein domains may have functional properties akin to other cell surface macromolecules, including certain very interesting relationships to immunoglobulins [19].

Nevertheless, while it seems clear to me that the advent of molecular biological methods will greatly accelerate the pace and breadth of molecular hunting expeditions, the major functional problems of what peptides do is not aided by compounding the profusion of peptide molecular complexity.

4. INTERACTIONS BETWEEN VASOACTIVE INTESTINAL POLYPEPTIDE AND NORADRENALINE IN RAT CEREBRAL CORTEX

Several lines of evidence support a role for vasoactive intestinal polypeptide (VIP) as a neuronal messenger in cerebral cortex, and study of this peptide has suggested some possible general principles of peptide function. Biochemical data support its presence, release, binding, and, at best, one possible action. Immunocytochemical data have localized VIP to cortical bipolar neurons. Single unit recording studies show that iontophoretically applied VIP inconsistently excites some cortical neurons. Other cellular actions reported for VIP in cortex include the ability to stimulate cyclic AMP formation somewhat more potently than noradrenaline (NA) [20, 21, 22 for further references].

Cytochemically, VIP and NA containing circuits show a contrasting but complementary cortical anatomy [20]: VIP neurons are intrinsic, bipolar, radially-oriented, intracortical neurons [23]; the NA innervation arises only from locus ceruleus and innervates a broad expanse of cortex in a horizontal plane. The two fiber systems may, however, have the same targets, the pyramidal cells. Identified cortical pyramidal neurons are depressed in spontaneous firing by iontophoresis of either NA or cyclic AMP [24]. The recent findings of Magistretti and Schorderet [22] suggest that VIP and NA can act synergistically to increase cyclic AMP in cerebral cortex. Therefore, Ferron and colleagues [25] tested VIP and NA on rat cortical neurons and found definitively that there are significant interactions: Iontophoretic application of VIP during subthreshold NA administration causes pronounced inhibitions of cellular discharge regardless of the effect of VIP prior to NA [25]. To examine for possible interactions between VIP and NA effects on single neurons, ejection currents of NA were reduced until they had little or no direct effect on neuronal firing. Ejection of VIP during subthreshold NA administration now produced consistent inhibition of firing. Such synergistic inhibitions were seen in more than half the cells, regardless of whether VIP alone had elicited excitatory, inhibitory, or negligible effects on the test neuron [25].

Magistretti and Schorderet [22] showed that the synergism of VIP by NA was blocked by phentolamine, an alpha adrenergic receptor antagonist, and mimicked by phenylephrine, an alpha receptor agonist. Therefore, we also examined the effect of phenylephrine as well as NA pretreatment on neuronal responses to VIP. In cells showing an interaction between VIP and NA, nine revealed equivalent interactive synergisms of depressant responses with phenylephrine [25]. Thus, the interaction of VIP and NA at the cellular level may also involve alpha receptor activation, although further testing is required.

Our electrophysiological indications of a VIP-NA interaction at the cellular level may arise from their biochemical effects in vitro on cyclic AMP generation. Such parallel findings strengthen the suggestions that cAMP may mediate both NA and VIP evoked depressions of neuronal firing in cortex. The reported enhancement by NA of synaptic and other transmitter responses (including inhibitory ones) may be related phenomena [4, 24]. An apparently similar, cAMP-mediated, enhancement by beta receptors of noradenergic target cell responsiveness to alpha adrenergic agonists has been reported for pineal [26, 27]. Furthermore, in rat hepatocytes, increased cAMP levels induced by glucagon enhance binding of alpha adrenergic agonists to these cells [28]. If NA and VIP-containing fibers do indeed converge on the same cortical target cell, it is feasible that cAMP is the intracellular mediator of their synergistic interaction.

5. INTERACTIONS BETWEEN SOMATOSTATIN AND ACETYLCHOLINE

The tetradecapeptide somatostatin was originally isolated from extracts of ovine hypothalamus as an inhibitor of anterior pituitary growth hormone release. Subsequently, it has become evident that this peptide has a widespread distribution throughout the central, peripheral, and gastrointestinal nervous systems, and the endocrine pancreas. Somatostatin has become a leading candidate for a neurotransmitter peptide based on its extensive cellular localizations in the brains of all species of mammals, where it is prominent in neocortex (see Ref. 5 for references). In hippocampus and cerebral cortex, SS-14 was first reported to depress neuronal activity in vivo, as have more recent studies in vivo and in vitro in many regions [29].

Recently, in the course of evaluating the effects of ethanol on the responses of hippocampal pyramidal cells to several neurotransmitters [30], we noticed that SS-14 had inhibitory effects on spontaneous firing unless acetylcholine (ACh) was included in the multibarrel iontophoresis assembly. In this case, leakage of ACh was noted to favor excitatory responses to SS-14. Therefore, the responses of pyramidal cells were explored in vivo to the iontophoretic application of either substance alone or together.

These studies [31] confirm that SS-14, when applied alone, directly depresses spontaneous discharge rate, with a slow onset and offset of its effects. However, when tested concurrently with either brief pulses or small amounts of ACh continuously leaked from an iontophoretic pipette, SS-14 caused a dose-dependent enhancement of ACh-induced facilitations but not those produced by glutamate. Our data could explain the apparent contradictory or inconsistent effects of SS-14 reported by others (see 29 for further references). Our results further indicate that iontophoretic application of somatostatin-14 can yield different, but consistent, effects on postsynaptic cell activity, depending on what other neurotransmitters are being tested simultaneously. For example, SS-14 enhances excitatory actions of ACh but not those of glutamate. This interaction appears to be selective for SS-14 and ACh, as there was no enhancement of responses to glutamate, another putative excitatory transmitter. In addition, the qualitative effect produced by SS-14 on neuronal activity in the presence of ACh depends on the relative dose of the peptide and the test history of the neuron being monitored.

The molecular or cellular mechanisms that underlie the interactions between SS-14 and ACh are not yet understood. It is recognized that the two SS-14 actions could arise from any of several sites (e.g., presynaptic and postsynaptic) where ACh is known to act. Further studies are required to clarify this possibility. Nevertheless, the observations reported here offer some implications for studies of synaptic mechanisms.

In this regard, the concept of "conditional" neurotransmitter interactions may be useful in explaining such interactions of peptides on neuronal activity. If the effects of iontophoretically applied SS-14 accurately reflect those of synaptically released SS-14, the peptide could be conceived to have at least two types of effects on hippocampal and cortical neurons. Its "primary" effect, in the absence of ACh, would be to inhibit spontaneous discharge. In the presence of ACh, the functional consequences of a conditional effect could vary the outcome, depending on the concentration and temporal context of the release of the two substances. An SS-14 release becomes pronounced, ACh excitations would be enhanced, while Glu excitations are depressed, selectively improving cholinergic transmission. As more of the chemical and electrophysiological variables that interact during the normal process of synaptic communication are defined, synaptic processes may emerge as even more complex. For example, it was recently found that systemic ethanol selectively enhances responses of hippocampal pyramidal cells to ACh and SS-14 [30]. However, given the interactions between these two substances, the increased responsiveness to ACh could be an indirect effect of ethanol, resulting from a primary enhancement of the actions of endogenous SS-14. Since SS-14 coexists in synaptic terminals with γ-aminobutyric acid, the interactive effects of these two substances with and without ACh should also be explored.

6. CONCLUSION

It is becoming increasingly evident that the vocabulary of neuronal communication is much larger and more complex than previously conceived. The results presented here suggest that deciphering the grammar of neuronal communication will require careful evaluation of the interactions of neuropeptides, regardless of how the cell we presume will secrete that peptide has transcribed and translated the gene that encodes it. However, in contrast with the rather rigorous proofs of synaptic transmitter status for the amino acids and monoamines (see Ref. 29), there are as yet no data for peptide-containing systems where a clustered group of neurons can be activated and their "peptidergic" effects recorded under conditions that would establish the possible temporal and spatial properties of the alleged peptidergic responses by the likely target cells. In fact, there are no known instances in which the effects of a peptide-containing system in the mammalian CNS have yet been identified as being peptidergic. Moreover, given the existing anatomic data, there are few places other than the hypothalamic paraventricular nucleus [32] where such stimulation paradigms might be effectively attempted.

Perhaps one of the many possible future lessons close to completion is the view that peptides play important regulatory roles in many organ and cell systems and are the mainstays of regulatory biological signaling. Their value so far has been chiefly one of expanding the lists of known regulators and possible sources of pathologic regulation. That value has the general utility of expanding our knowledge about the ways less complex molecules signal their cellular targets. Clearly, there is much more to be known about these signaling systems in both health and disease.

ACKNOWLEDGMENTS

I thank my colleagues, Drs. Siggins, Milner, Morrison, Mancillas, and Ferron, for allowing me to quote from their recent studies and Mrs. Nancy Callahan for preparing this manuscript. Supported by grants from the Whittier Foundation, the MacArthur Foundation, and McNeil Laboratories, and USPAS Grant NS-22347.

REFERENCES

1. Bloom, F.E. (1986). Whither Neuropeptides? In *Neuropeptides in Neurologic and Psychiatric Disease*, Martin, J.B. and Barchas, J.D., eds., Raven Press, New York, pp. 335–349.
2. Lewis, D.A. and Bloom, F.E. (1987). Clinical perspectives on neuropeptides. Ann. Rev. Med. 38, 143–148.
3. Hokfelt, T., Johansson, O., Ljungdahl, A., Lundberg, J.M. and Schultzberg, M. (1980). Peptidergic neurones. Nature (London) 284, 515–521.
4. Bloom, F.E. (1984). The functional significance of neurotransmitter diversity. Am. J. Physiol. 246, C184–C194.
5. Bloom, F.E. (1984). Chemical integrative processes in the central nervous system. In *Handbook of Chemical Neuroanatomy*, Bjorklund, A. and Hokfelt, T. eds., Elsevier Science Publishers, The Netherlands, pp. 51–58.
6. Vale, W., Spiess, J., Rivier, C. and Rivier, J. (1981). Characterization of a 41 residue ovine hypothalamic peptide that stimulates secretion of corticotropin and β-endorphin. Science 213, 1394–1397.
7. Guillemin, R., Brazeau, P., Bohlen, P., Esch, F., Ling, N., and Wehrenberg, W.B. (1982). Growth hormone-releasing factor from a human pancreatic tumor that caused acromegaly. Science 218, 585–587.
8. Tatemoto, K. and Mutt, V. (1980). Isolation of two novel candidate hormones using a chemical method for finding naturally occurring polypeptides. Nature 285, 417–418.
9. Tatemoto, K. and Mutt, V. (1981). Isolation and characterization of the intestinal peptide porcine PHI (PHI-27), a new member of the glucagon-secretin family. Proc. Natl. Acad. Sci. USA 78, 6603–6607.
10. Nakanishi, S., Inoue, A., Kita, T., Nakamura, M., Chang, A.C., Cohen, S.N. and Numa, S. (1979). Nucleotide sequence of cloned cDNA for bovine corticotropin-β-lipoprotein precursor. Nature 278, 423–427.
11. Bloom, F.E. (1987). Future directions, goals in basic psychopharmacology and neurobiology. In *Psychopharmacology — Generation of Progress*. H.Y. Meltcer, ed. Raven Press, N.Y., pp. 1685–1689.
12. Itoh, N., Obata, K., Yanaihara, N. and Okamoto, H. (1983). Human preprovasoactive intestinal polypeptide contains a novel PHI-27-like peptide PHM-27. Nature 304, 547–9.
13. Nawa, H., Hirose, T., Takashima, H., Inayama, S. and Nakanishi, S. (1983). Nucleotide sequences of cloned cDNAs for two types of bovine brain substance P precursor. Nature 306, 32–6.
14. Rosenfeld, M.G., Mermod, J.-J., Amara, S.G., Swanson, L.W., Sawchenko, P.E., Rivier, J., Vale, W. and Evans, R.M. (1983). Production of a novel neuropeptide encoded by the calcitonin gene via tissue-specific RNA processing. Nature 304, 129–135.
15. Sutcliffe, J.G., Milner, R.J. and Bloom, F.E. (1983). Cellular localization and function of the proteins encoded by brain-specific mRNAs. Cold Spring Harbor Symp. 48, 477–484.
16. Bloom, F.E., Battenberg, E.L., Milner, R.J. and Sutcliffe, J.G. (1985). Immunocytochemical mapping of 1B236, a brain specific neuronal polypeptide deduced from the sequence of a cloned mRNA. J. Neurosci. 5, 1781–1802.
17. Sutcliffe, J.G., Milner, R.J., Shinnick, T.M. and Bloom, F.E. (1983). Identifying the protein products of brain-specific genes with antibodies to chemically synthesized peptides. Cell 33, 671–682.
18. Malfroy, B., Bakhit, C., Bloom, F.E., Sutcliffe, J.G. and Milner, R.J. (1985). Brain-specific polypeptide 1B236 exists in multiple molecular forms. Proc. Natl. Acad. Sci. USA 82, 2009–2013.
19. Williams, A. (1985). Immunoglobulin-related domains for cell surface recognition. Nature 314, 579–580.
20. Morrison, J.H. and Magistretti, P.J. (1983). Monoamines and peptides in cerebral cortex: Contrasting principles of cortical organization. Trends in Neurosciences 6, 146–151.

21. Magistretti, P.J. and Morrison, J.H. (1985). VIP neurons in the neocortex. Trends in Neuroscience 8, 7–8.
22. Magistretti, P.J. and Schorderet, M. (1985). Norepinephine and histamine potentiate the increases in cyclic adenosine 3':5'-monophosphate elicited by vasoactive intestinal polypeptide in mouse cerebral cortical slices: Mediation by a_1-adrenergic and H_1-histaminergic receptors. J. Neurosci. 5, 363–368.
23. Morrison, J.H., Magistretti, P.J., Benoit, R. and Bloom, F.E. (1984). The distribution and morphological characteristics of the intracortical VIP-positive cell: An immunohistochemical analysis. Brain Res. 292, 269–282.
24. Foote, S.L., Bloom, F.E. and Aston-Jones, G. (1983). Nucleus locus ceruleus: New evidence of anatomical and physiological specificity. Physiological Reviews 63, 844–914.
25. Ferron, A., Siggins, G.R. and Bloom, F.E. (1985). Vasoactive intestinal polypeptide acts synergistically with noradrenaline to depress spontaneous discharge rates in cerebral cortical neurons. Proc. Natl. Acad. Sci. USA 82, 8810–8812.
26. Klein, D.C., Sugden, D. and Weller, J.L. (1983). Postsynaptic β-adrenergic receptors potentiate the β-adrenergic stimulation of pineal serotonin N-acetyltransferase. Proc. Natl. Acad. Sci. USA 80, 599–603.
27. Sugden, D., Vamecek, J., Klein, D.C., Thomas, T.P. and Anderson, W.B. (1985). Activation of protein kinase C potentiates isoprenaline-induced cyclic AMP accumulation in rat pinealocytes. Nature 314, 359–361.
28. Morgan, N.G., Charest, R., Blackmore, P.F. and Exton, J.H. (1984). Potentiation of alpha 1 adrenergic responses in rat liver by a cAMP-dependent mechanism. Proc. Natl. Acad. Sci. USA 81, 4208–4212.
29. Siggins, G.R. and Gruol, D.L. (1986). Mechanisms of transmitter action in the vertebrate central nervous system. In *Handbook of Physiology, Intrinsic Regulatory Systems of the Brain*, Bloom, F.E., ed., The American Physiological Society, Bethesda, Maryland, pp. 1–114.
30. Mancillas, J.R., Siggins, G.R. and Bloom, F.E. (1986), Systemic ethanol: Selective enhancement of responses to acetylcholine and somatostatin in hippocampus. Science 231, 161–163.
31. Mancillas, J.R., Siggins, G.R. and Bloom, F.E. (1986). Somatostatin-selectively enhances acetylcholine-induced excitations in rat hippocampus and cortex. Proc. Natl. Acad. Sci. USA 83, 7518–7521.
32. Buijs, R.M. and Van Heerikhuize, J.J. (1982). Vasopressin and oxytocin release in the brain — A synaptic event. Brain Res. 252, 71–76.

11. ROLE OF ATRIOPEPTIN IN CENTRAL CARDIOVASCULAR CONTROL*

CLIFFORD B. SAPER AND DAVID G. STANDAERT

Atriopeptin (AP), the atrial natriuretic peptide, is a 28 amino acid hormone that is synthesized in the atria of mammalian hearts [1]. During atrial stretch, AP is released into the circulation, where it binds to receptors in the renal glomeruli and papilla, resulting in profound natriuresis and diuresis (for review see Refs. 2–6). AP also binds to the adrenal glomerulosa, inhibiting the secretion of aldosterone, and to vascular smooth muscle, causing vasodilatation. AP, therefore, acts as a counterregulatory hormone to reduce blood volume and blood pressure, particularly during right atrial volume overload.

The rat AP gene contains three exons, which are spliced in atrial cells to yield an mRNA that codes for a 152 amino acid protein, including a 24 amino acid N-terminal signal sequence, two C-terminal arginines, and a 126 amino acid prohormone, atriopeptigen [7] (see Figure 11-1). The 28 carboxy-terminal amino acids of the prohormone constitute the circulating hormone, although other portions of the prohormone are secreted and may have as yet undiscovered effects [8].

Recent studies by Gardner and associates [9] and in our own laboratory [Standaert et al., in preparation] have demonstrated that the hypothalamus contains an mRNA that is similar, if not identical, to that coding for the AP

* The work described in this communication was supported by NINCDS grant NS22835, NIGMS grants GM07200 and GM07895, American Heart Association grant-in-aid 850894, the Washington University-Monsanto Grant, and a grant from the Brain Research Foundation.

Ferrendelli, J.A., Collins, R.C. and Johnson, E.M. (eds), Neurobiology of Amino Acids, Peptides, and Trophic Factors.

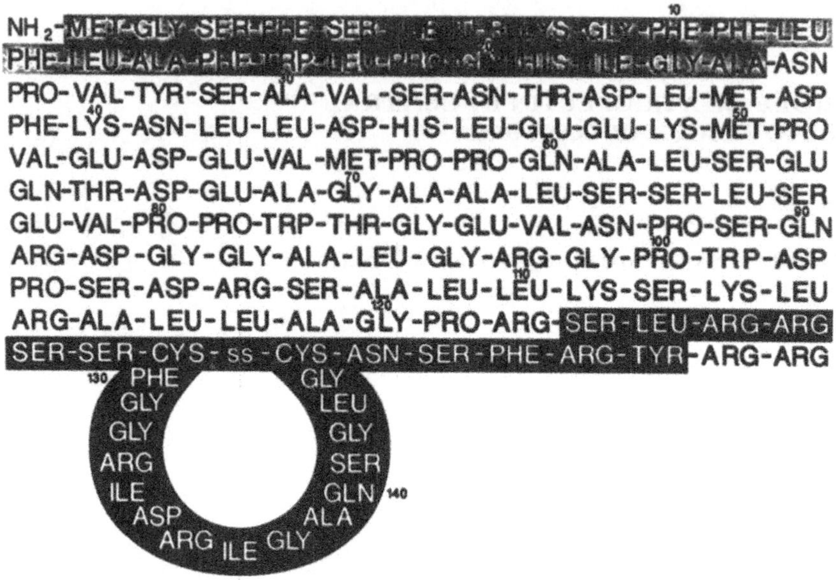

Figure 11-1. The complete amino acid sequence of the rat atriopeptin (atrial natriuretic peptide) preprohormone, as deduced from the nucleic acid sequence of its gene. The 26 N-terminal amino acids (shading) represent a signal sequence. The sequence shown in white lettering against a black background is the circulating hormone. This peptide forms a 17 amino acid ring structure that is necessary for the bioactivity of the hormone. (From Standaert et al. [31] with permission.)

prohormone in the heart. Both the prohormone and smaller immunoreactive peptides have also been identified in HPLC of brain extracts [10–14]. Immunoreactive AP can be released from brain by a calcium-dependent process during depolarization of hypothalamic explants [15].

1. IMMUNOHISTOCHEMICAL LOCALIZATION OF AP NEURONS AND PATHWAYS

The distribution of AP immunoreactive neurons in the brain has also been examined immunohistochemically in our own laboratory and by others [16–20] (see Figure 11-2). For most of our studies we have used an antiserum against a 93 amino acid C-terminal cyanogen bromide fragment of the AP prohormone. Staining with this antiserum is completely extinguished by pre-adsorption with the purified peptide, and partly adsorbed by incubation with the 24 C-terminal amino acid peptide, AP III [16]. (For a detailed description of the staining of the rat brain using this antiserum, see reference 19.)

Most of the AP immunoreactive (AP-ir) neurons in the brain were found in a limited number of cell groups in the brainstem and basal forebrain that have been implicated in cardiovascular regulation. The largest single collection of AP-ir cell bodies was found in the anterventral periventricular nucleus

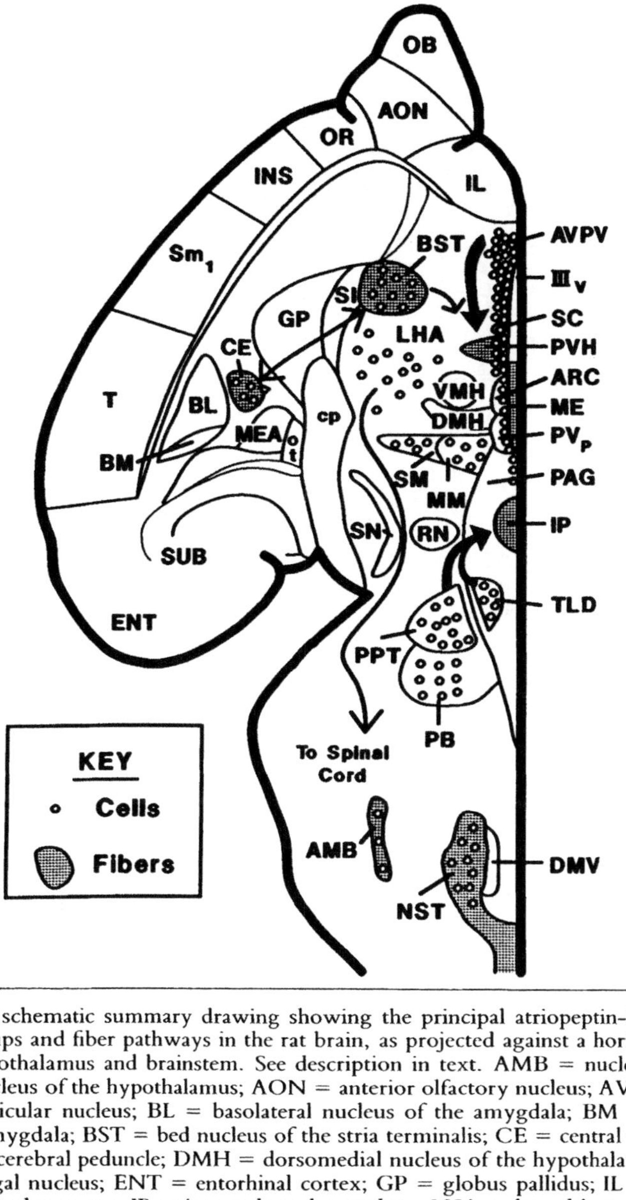

Figure 11-2. A schematic summary drawing showing the principal atriopeptin-like immunoreactive cell groups and fiber pathways in the rat brain, as projected against a horizontal section through the hypothalamus and brainstem. See description in text. AMB = nucleus ambiguus; ARC arcuate nucleus of the hypothalamus; AON = anterior olfactory nucleus; AVPV = anteroventral periventricular nucleus; BL = basolateral nucleus of the amygdala; BM = basomedial nucleus of the amygdala; BST = bed nucleus of the stria terminalis; CE = central nucleus of the amygdala; cp = cerebral peduncle; DMH = dorsomedial nucleus of the hypothalamus; DMV = dorsal motor vagal nucleus; ENT = entorhinal cortex; GP = globus pallidus; IL = infralimbic cortex; INS = insular cortex; IP = interpeduncular nucleus; LHA = lateral hypothalamic area; ME = median eminence; MEA = medial nucleus of the amygdala; MM = medial mammillary nucleus; NST = nucleus of the solitary tract; OB = olfactory bulb; OR = orbitofrontal cortex; ot = optic tract; PAG = periaqueductal gray matter; PB = parabrachial nucleus; PPT = pedunculopontine tegmental nucleus; PVH = paraventricular nucleus of the hypothalamus; PVp = posterior periventricular nucleus of the hypothalamus; RN = red nucleus; SC = suprachiasmatic nucleus; SI = substantia innominata; SM = supramammillary nucleus; SM1 = primary somatic sensory cortex; SN = substantia nigra; SUB = subiculum; T = temporal cortex; TLD = laterodorsal tegmental nucleus; VMH = ventromedial nucleus of the hypothalamus; III v = third ventricle. (From Standaert et al. [31] with permission.)

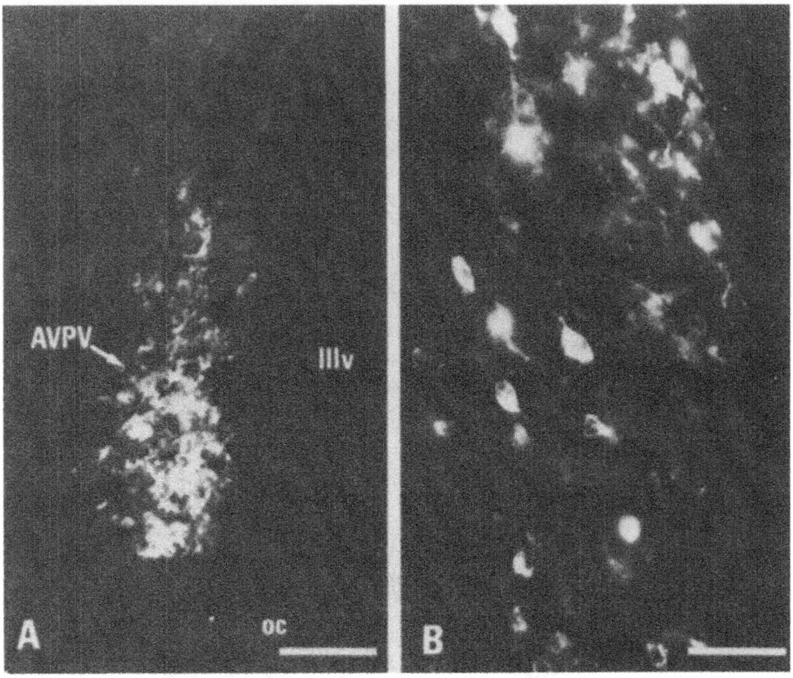

Figure 11-3. Immunofluorescence photomicrographs of the anteroventral periventricular (AVPV) nucleus, illustrating the clustering of AP-immunoreactive neurons in this cell group. At low magnification (panel A), the dense aggregation of the immunoreactive neurons can be seen in the wall of the anterior tip of the third ventricle. Scale = 100 μm. At higher magnification (panel B) the morphology of the cell bodies and dendrites can be appreciated. Scale = 50 μm. (From Standaert et al. [19] with permission.)

(AVPV), a small cell groups in the preoptic area, adjacent to the walls of the anteroventral tip of the third ventricle (see Figure 11-3). AP-ir cell bodies were found scattered caudally from the AVPV, throughout the periventricular zone along the wall of the third ventricle. These neurons invaded the arcuate and dorsomedial nuclei, and particularly the parvocellular part of the paraventricular nucleus (PVH). A separate collection of larger AP-ir cell bodies was found in the lateral hypothalamic area, and numerous AP-ir perikarya were also observed in the ventral and lateral parts of the bed nucleus of the stria terminalis. Smaller numbers of AP-ir cell bodies were found in the central nucleus of the amygdala, the parabrachial nucleus, Barrington's nucleus, and the nucleus of the solitary tract. The densest terminal fields related to these AP-ir neurons were in the PVH, involving primarily the parvocellular, but also the magnocellular, parts of the nucleus; the remainder of the periventricular hypothalamus and thalamus; the external lamina of the median eminence (see Figure 11-4); and the bed nucleus of the stria terminalis. AP-ir fibers were also prom-

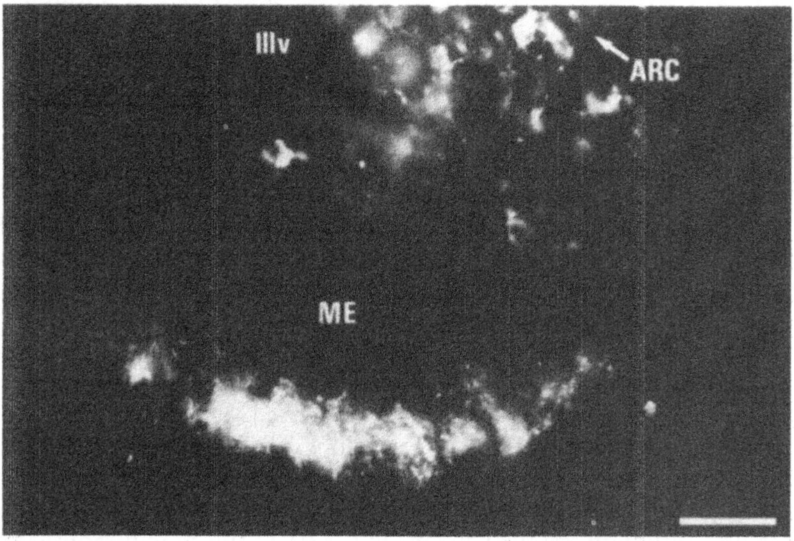

Figure 11-4. Immunofluorescence photomicrographs of the AP-immunoreactive arcuate nucleus (ARC) and median eminence (ME) in the rat. Note that there are numerous immunoreactive perikarya in the arcuate nucleus, with morphology similar to those in the AVPV (Figure 11-3). Fluorescent axons can be traced from the ARC and other immunoreactive neurons in the periventricular region into the median eminence, where they give rise to a dense terminal field in the external lamina, in proximity to the hypophysial portal vessels. Scale = 50 μm. (From Standaert et al. [19] with permission.)

inent in the parabrachial nucleus, Barrington's nucleus, and the nucleus of the solitary tract.

The remainder of the AP-ir cell groups and pathways can be loosely grouped, for want of a better term, with the limbic system. These include AP-ir cell bodies in the mammillary and habenular nuclei, and the laterodorsal and pedunculopontine tegmental nuclei. The latter cell groups, which also stain for choline acetyltransferase, give rise to a dense AP-ir fiber bundle that runs ventromedially into the interpeduncular nucleus, where they contribute to the most intensely innervated AP-ir terminal field found in the rat brain.

In another series of experiments, the origin of the AP-ir fibers was examined in the PVH [21]. Following injections of fluorescent dyes into the PVH, the largest number of retrogradely labeled, AP-ir cell bodies was found in the AVPV. Smaller numbers of double-labeled neurons were identified in the bed nucleus of the stria terminalis, the laterodorsal and pedunculopontine tegmental nuclei, and the nucleus of the solitary tract. Injections of PHA-L, an anterograde lectin tracer, into AVPV demonstrated that these neurons innervate all parts of the PVH, including both the parvocellular endocrine and autonomic areas, and the magnocellular neurons that secrete oxytocin and vasopressin from their axon terminals in the posterior pituitary gland [Saper et al., in preparation]. This was of considerable interest, as the AVPV is located in the heart of the anteroventral third ventricular (AV3V) area, in which lesions have been shown to cause hypodipsia and to impair the development of hypertension in a variety of renin-dependent and non-renin-dependent models [40].

2. ROLE OF AP-ir CELL GROUPS IN CARDIOVASCULAR REGULATION

The presence of AP immunoreactivity in so many of the cell groups that are thought to be involved in central cardiovascular control has naturally led to the speculation that AP in the CNS may act on many of the same functions that it regulates as a systemic hormone. One line of evidence supporting this hypothesis has come from studies of the effects of AP injected directly into the brain. Intraventricular AP inhibits both dehydration-induced drinking and the drinking elicited by intraventricular or intravenous administration of angiotensin II [22–24] and suppresses salt appetite [25, 26]. In addition, intraventricular AP suppresses basal VP secretion and VP release elicited by dehydration, hemorrhage, or angiotensin II infusion [27–30].

Such studies do not, however, provide information about the mechanism of action of AP. Although the VP neurons in the PVH and the supraoptic nucleus are directly innervated by AP-ir fibers, it is possible that the intraventricular AP may act at a distant site, affecting VP secretion by a polysynaptic mechanism. Therefore, an examination of the effect of AP applied directly to VP neurons in the PVH was attempted.

In these experiments, multibarrel micropipettes were used for simultaneous recording of extracellular potentials and injection of peptides [31]. Two of the injection barrels were filled with 10 or 100 μg/ml synthetic APIII in physio-

Figure 11-5. A firing rate histogram to illustrate the effect of application of AP to a vasopressin neuron. This neuron showed the phasic pattern of firing that is characteristic of vasopressin neurons. During phasic bursts, it would fire 10–20 action potentials per second (the bars on the histogram represent the number of action potentials fired during sequential 4-second periods). Application of the control peptide (des [17, 18] atriopeptin III) at a dosage of 150 pg (approx. 50 fm) produced no effect. Subsequent application of 75 pg (23 fm) of atriopeptin III (AP III, the 24 C-terminal amino acid peptide) caused a shortening of the duration of the bursting phases, with little change in the interburst interval. A second application of AP III at the same dosage again decreased the duration of the bursts, but also increased the interburst interval. A third application of 150 pg (45 fm) had the additional effect of initially decreasing the firing rate during the phasic bursts, with gradual recovery over the next 3 minutes. An additional application of 450 pg of AP III (136 fm) completely abolished firing of the neuron for about 1 minute. During recovery, the firing rate during the phasic bursts was initially reduced, gradually returning to the baseline firing rate over 2–3 minutes, at about the same pace as the recovery from the smaller dosage.

Note that the dosages indicated were calculated by multiplying the injection volume by the concentration of peptide loaded into the pipette. However, in this experiment, pipette barrels were employed that contained microfilaments to improve the ease of loading the peptide solutions. We later found that these pipettes were "wicking" up extracellular fluid by capillary action, so that the solution at the tips may have been considerably more dilute than that loaded into the pipettes. In later experiments, using plain micropipettes that did not "wick," we found thresholds for similar responses at dosages at least an order of magnitude lower. Thus, the dosages indicated in this figure may represent a considerable overestimate of the actual amount of peptide applied.

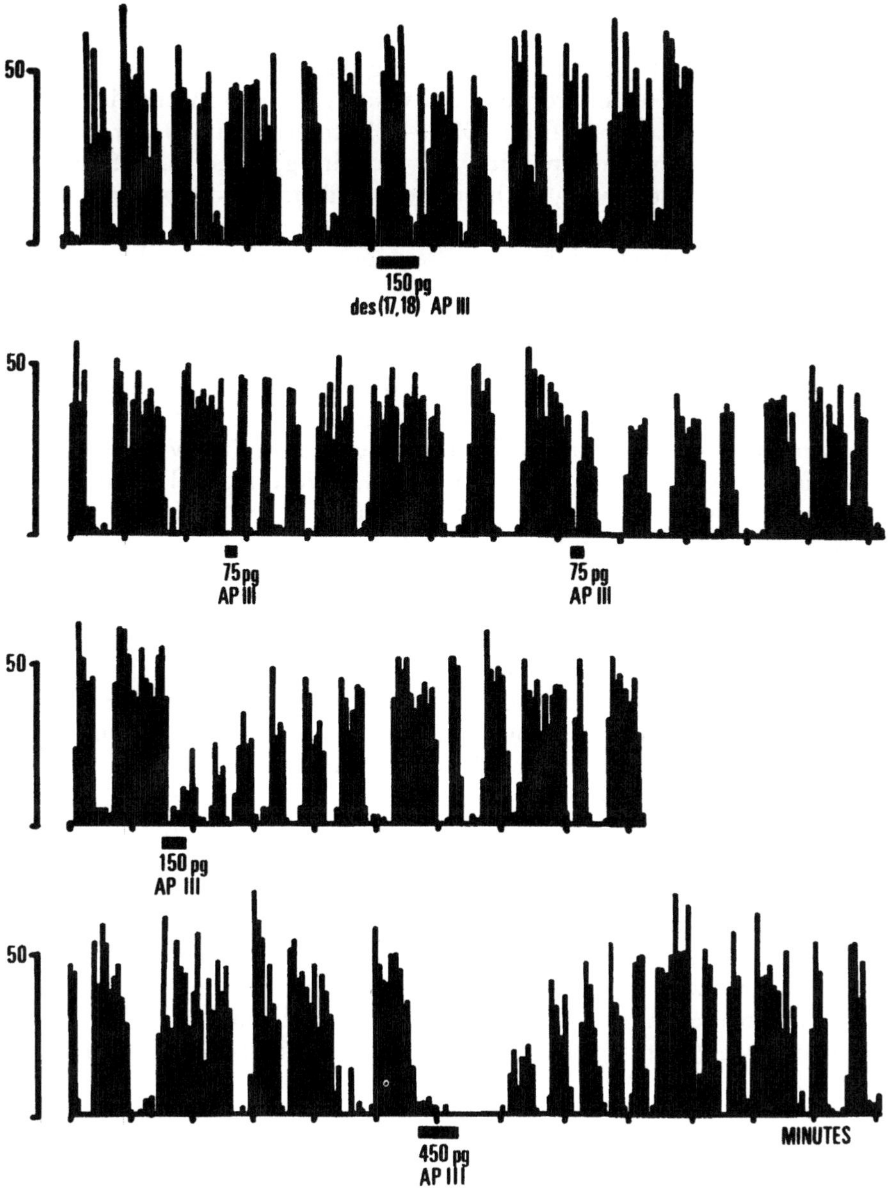
50
150 pg
des (17,18) AP III
50
75 pg
AP III
75 pg
AP III
50
150 pg
AP III
50
450 pg
AP III
MINUTES

logical saline, and an equivalent concentration of a peptide analog (des-[gly-18, leu-17] APIII-NH_2) that has no AP activity in bioassay. A third barrel was filled with 3 M NaCl and used for recording purposes. Single neurons in the vicinity of the PVH were recorded, and vasopressin units were identified by their characteristic pattern of firing [32–34]. Specifically, units were identified as VP neurons if they had a phasic pattern of firing, consisting of periods of 10–20 Hz activity alternating with periods of silence. Most of these neurons were also tested for responses to elevation of blood pressure, and all of the phasically active units were inhibited. Previous studies have established that in the rostral hypothalamus this activity profile is associated exclusively with VP neurons [33, 34].

AP and inactive peptide solutions were injected by applying multiple small puffs of air pressure, each of which ejected from 30–300 picoliters from the pipette tips. Injecting from 1.5 to 840 femtomoles (fm) of the inactive peptide was without effect. All 13 phasically active neurons in the PVH responded to application of AP. Four units, tested with 1.3–78 fm of AP, demonstrated either shortening of burst duration or prolongation of the interval between bursts, with little change in mean bursting firing rate (see Figure 11-5). This effect was gradual in onset, occurring over a period of one or more minutes, and lasting 240–3200 seconds. The remaining nine phasic neurons responded to the application of AP with a prolonged silent period (lasting 160–1680 seconds), following which their activity rapidly returned to baseline. None of these neurons responded to application of the control peptide, and none of the ten nonphasic neurons in the vicinity of the PVH that were tested showed any response to application of either AP or the inactive peptide.

In seven instances, graded responses to AP were obtained during application to phasic neurons in progressively increasing amounts. The mean threshold for response was 5.7 + 1.8 fm, but the range was 0.07–15 fm. The variability of time of onset of effect, and threshold dose was probably due to the differences in the geometric relationships of the injection pipette, the recording pipette, and the neuron being recorded. However, our results are most consistent with the AP solutions having their effect on neurons located no more than a few hundred microns from the injection site. As all of the injection sites were histologically verified within the vasopressin subnucleus of the PVH (see Figure 11-6), we are confident that the AP acted either directly on the VP neurons or on nearby interneurons. In any case, these findings demonstrate that the AP innervation of the PVH may act directly to regulate the secretion of VP.

3. AP AS A SYSTEMIC HORMONE AND CENTRAL NEUROTRANSMITTER IN CARDIOVASCULAR CONTROL

Our findings support the hypothesis that AP acts as a central neurotransmitter in regulating the same functions that it controls as a systemic peptide. This relationship may, in fact, be more the rule than the exception for neuropep-

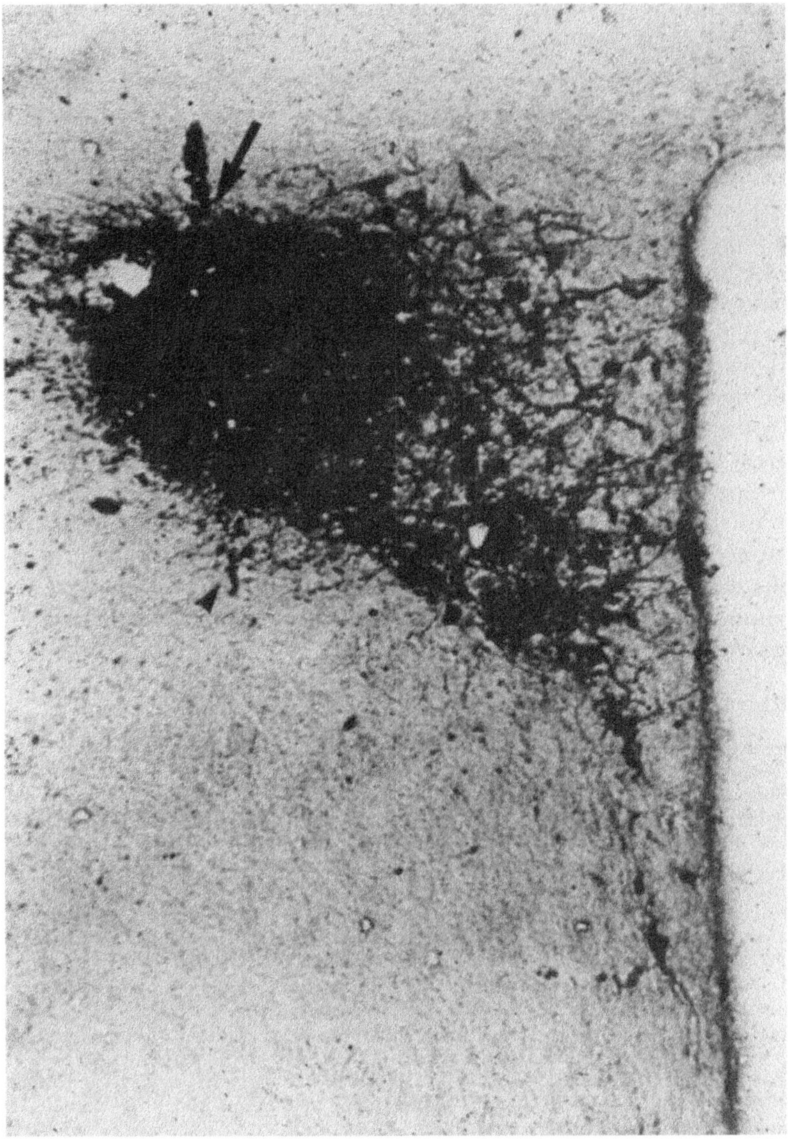

Figure 11-6. A photomicrograph of a section through the recording site of the neuron in Figure 11-5, stained by an immunoperoxidase method for vasopressin. A trail of peroxidase-positive red blood cells can be seen along the tract of the recording electrode, up to the recording site (arrow), amid the dense cluster of vasopressin neurons in the paraventricular nucleus of the hypothalamus. A second trail of red blood cells can be seen below the nucleus (arrowhead), marking the position of a more anterior electrode track.

tides. Similar suggestions have been made for angiotensin in cardiovascular regulation [35], corticotropin-releasing factor in stress [36, 37], and cholecystokinin in feeding [38]. The reason for this concordance of function remains to be elucidated, although it is interesting that, for each of these peptides, a major cluster of immunoreactive neurons is found in close association with a circumventricular organ. As circulating peptide may enter the central nervous system at these sites of attenuated blood-brain barrier [39], it is possible that the brain evolved sensitivity to these modulators as systemic hormones. The neurons that received this signal could then have coordinated the central response with the systemic hormonal signal. Neuronal systems employing the same peptide may have evolved to take advantage of this arrangement in regulating the same principal functions. Local neurons containing the peptide might function in part as interneurons whose peptidergic transmission would compete with or complement the systemic hormonal signal to the neurons in or near the circumventricular organs.

A great deal remains to be learned about the role of AP in central control of the cardiovascular system. For example, it will be necessary to determine the effects of the peptide on a variety of neurons involved in cardiovascular and other functions. In addition, the cellular mechanisms for the effects of AP on neurons will have to be determined. The elucidation of these and related problems should yield rich rewards in our continuing efforts to understand central control of the circulation.

REFERENCES

1. Schwartz, D., Geller, D.M., Manning, P.T., Seigel, N.R., Fok, K.F., Smith, C.E. and Needleman, P. (1985). Ser-Leu-Arg-Arg-atriopeptin III: The major circulating form of atrial peptide. Science 229, 397–400.
2. Needleman, P., Adams, S.P., Cole, B.R., Currie, M.G., Geller, D.M., Michener, M.L., Saper, C.B., Schwartz, D. and Standaert, D.G. (1985). Atriopeptins as cardiac hormones. Brief review. Hypertension 7, 469–482.
3. Needleman, P. and Greenwald, J.E. (1986). Atriopeptin: A cardiac hormone intimately involved in fluid, electrolyte and blood-pressure homeostasis. N. Engl. J. Med. 314, 828–834.
4. Cantin, M. and Genest, J. (1985). The heart and the atrial natriuretic factor. Endocrinol. Rev. 6, 107–127.
5. Atlas, S.A. and Laragh, J.H. (1986). Atrial natriuretic peptide: A new factor in hormonal control of blood pressure and electrolyte homeostasis. Ann. Rev. Med. 37, 397–414.
6. Laragh, J.H. (1985). Atrial natriuretic hormone, the renin-aldosterone axis, and blood pressure-electrolyte homeostasis. N. Engl. J. Med. 313, 1330–1340.
7. Geller, D.M., Currie, M.G., Sigel, N.R., Fok, K.F., Adams, S.P. and Needleman, P. (1984). The sequence of an atriopeptidogen: A precursor of the bioactive atrial peptide. Biochem. Biophys. Res. Commun. 121, 802–807.
8. Michener, M.L., Gierse, J.K., Seetharam, R., Fok, K.F., Olins, P.O., Mai, M.S. and Needleman, P. (1986). Proteolytic processing of atriopeptin prohormone. Mol. Pharmacol. 30, 552–557.
9. Gardner, D.G., Vlasuk, G., Fiddes, J., Baxter, J.D. and Lewicki, J. (1986). ANF genetic expression in the central nervous system. Hypertension 8, 826.
10. Tanaka, I., Misono, K.S. and Inagami, T. (1984). Atrial natriuretic factor in rat hypothalamus, atria, and plasma: Determination by specific radioimmunoassay. Biochem. Biophys. Res. Commun. 124, 663–668.
11. Glembotski, C.C., Wildey, G.M. and Gibson, T.R. (1985). Molecular forms of immunoreac-

tive atrial natriuretic peptide in the rat hypothalamus and atrium. Biochem. Biophys. Res. Commun. 129, 671–78.
12. Morii, N., Nakao, K., Sugawara, A., Sakamoto, M., Suda, M., Shimokura, M., Kiso, Y., Kihara, M., Yamori, Y. and Imura, H. (1985). Occurrence of atrial natriuretic polypeptide in bain. Biochem. Biophys. Res. Commun. 127, 413–419.
13. Shiono, S., Nakao, K., Morri, N., Yamada, T., Itoh, H., Sakamoto, M., Sugawara, A., Saito, Y., Katsuura, G. and Imura, H. (1986). Nature of atrial natriuretic polypeptide in rat brain. Biochem. Biophys. Res. Commun. 135, 728–734.
14. Zamir, N., Skofitsch, G., Eskay, R.L. and Jacobowitz, D.M. (1986). Distribution of immunoreactive atrial natriuretic peptides in the central nervous system of the rat. Brain Res. 365, 105–111.
15. Shibasaki, T., Naruse, M., Naruse, K., Masuda, A., Kim, Y.S., Imaki, T., Yamauchi, N., Demura, H., Inagami, T. and Shizume, K. (1986). Atrial natriuretic factor is released from rat hypothalamus in vitro. Biochem. Biophys. Res. Commun. 136, 590–595.
16. Saper, C.B., Standaert, D.G., Currie, M.G., Geller, D.M. and Needleman, P. (1985). Atriopeptin immunoreactive neurons in the brain: Presence in cardiovascular regulatory areas. Science 227, 1047–1049.
17. Jacobowitz, D.M., Skofitsch, G., Eskay, R.L. and Zamir, N. (1985). Distribution of atrial natriuretic factor-like immunoreactive neurons in the rat brain. Neuroscience 16, 917–948.
18. Kawata, M., Nakao, K., Morii, N., Kiso, Y., Yamashita, H., Imura, H. and Sano, Y. (1985). Atrial natriuretic polypeptide: Topographical distribution in the rat brain by radioimmunoassay and immunohistochemistry. Neuroscience 16, 521–546.
19. Standaert, D.G., Needleman, P. and Saper, C.B. (1986). Organization of atriopeptin-like immunoreactive neurons in the central nervous system of the rat. J. Comp. Neurol. 253, 315–341.
20. Standaert, D.G., Saper, C.B., Rye, D. and Wainer, B.H. (1986). Colocalization of atriopeptin- with choline acetyltransferase- and substance P-like immunoreactivity in the pedunculopontine and laterodorsal tegmental nuclei. Brain Res. 382, 163–168.
21. Standaert, D.G. and Saper, C.B. (1987). Origin of the atriopeptin-like immunoreactive innervation of the paraventricular nucleus of the hypothalamus. J. Neurosci. in press.
22. Antunes-Rodrigues, J., McCann, J.M., Rogers, L.C. and Samson, W.K. (1985). Atrial natriuretic factor inhibits dehydration- and angiotensin II-induced water intake in the conscious, unrestrained rat. Proc. Natl. Acad. Sci. USA 82, 8720–8723.
23. Lappe, R.W., Dinish, J.L., Bex, F., Michalak, K. and Wendt, R.L. (1986). Effects of atrial natriuretic factor on drinking responses to central angiotensin II. Pharmacol. Biochem. Behav. 24, 1573–1576.
24. Masotto, C. and Negro-Vilar, A. (1985). Inhibition of spontaneous or angiotensin II-stimulated water intake by atrial natriuretic factor. Brain Res. Bull. 15, 523–526.
25. Fitts, D.A., Thunhorst, R.L. and Simpson, J.B. (1985). Diuresis and reduction of salt appetite by lateral ventricular infusions of atriopeptin II. Brain Res. 348, 118–124.
26. Atunes-Rodrigues, J., McCann, S.M. and Samson, W.K. (1986). Central administration of atrial natriuretic factor inhibits saline preference in the rat. Endocrinology 118, 1726–1728.
27. Samson, W.K. (1985). Atrial natriuretic factor inhibits dehydration and hemorrhage-induced vasopressin release. Neuroendocrinology 40, 277–279.
28. Iitake, K., Share, L., Crofton, J.T., Brooks, D.P., Ouchi, Y. and Blaine, E.H. (1986). Central atrial natriuretic factor reduces vasopressin secretion in the rat. Endocrinology 119, 438–440.
29. Yamada, T., Nakao, K., Morri, N., Itoh, H., Shiono, S., Sakamoto, M., Sugawara, A., Saito, Y., Ohno, H., Kanai, A., Katsuura, G., Eigyo, M., Matsushita, A. and Imura, H. (1986). Central effect of atrial natriuretic polypeptide on angiotensin II-stimulated vasopressin secretion in conscious rats. Eur. J. Pharmacol. 125, 453–456.
30. Samson, W.K., Aguila, M.C., Martinovic, J., Antunes-Rodrigues, J. and Norris, M. (1987). Hypothalamic action of atrial natriuretic factor to inhibit vasopressin release. Peptides 453–456.
31. Standaert, D.G., Cechetto, D.F., Needleman, P. and Saper, C.B. (1987). Inhibition of the firing of vasopressin neurons by atriopeptin. Nature, 329, 151–153.
32. Wakerley, J.B., Poulain, D.A., Dyball, R.E. and Cross, B.A. (1975). Activity of phasic neurosecretory cells during haemorrhage. Nature 258, 82–84.

33. Poulain, D.A. and Wakerley, J.B. (1982). Electrophysiology of hypothalamic magnocellular neurones secreting oxytocin and vasopressin. Neuroscience 7, 773–808.
34. Renaud, L.P., Bourque, C.W., Day, T.A., Ferguson, A.V. and Randle, J.C. (1985). Electrophysiology of mammalian hypothalamic supraoptic and paraventricular neurosecretory cells. In *The Electrophysiology of the Secretory Cell*, Poisner, A.M. and Trifaro, J.M., eds., Elsevier, Amsterdam, pp. 165–194.
35. Lind, R.W., Swanson, L.W. and Ganten, D. (1985). Organization of angiotensin II immunoreactive cells and fibers in the rats CNS. An immunohistochemical study. Neuroendocrinology 40, 2–24.
36. Swanson, L.W., Sawchenko, P.E., Rivier, J. and Vale, W.W. (1983). Organization of ovine corticotropin-releasing factor immunoreactive cells and fibers in the rat brain: An immunohistochemical study. Neuroendocrinology 36, 165–186.
37. Brown, M.R., Fisher, L.A., Spiess, J., Rivier, C., Rivier, J. and Vale, W. (1982). Corticotropin-releasing factor: Actions on the sympathetic nervous system and metabolism. Endocrinology 111, 928–931.
38. Fulwiler, C.E. and Saper, C.B. (1985). Cholecystokinin-immunoreactive innervation of the ventromedial hypothalamus in the rat: Possible substrate for autonomic regulation of feeding. Neurosci. Lett. 53, 289–296.
39. Broadwell, R.D. and Brightman, M.W. (1976). Entry of peroxidase into neurons of the central and peripheral nervous systems from extracerebral and cerebral blood. J. Comp. Neurol. 166, 257–284.
40. Brody, M.J. and Johnson, A.K. (1981). Role of forebrain structures in models of experimental hypertension. In *Disturbances in Neurogenic Control of Circulation*, Abboud, F.M., Fozzard, H.A., Gilmore, J.P. and Reis, D.J., eds., American Physiological Society, Bethesda, pp. 105–117.

12. OPIOID PEPTIDES: POSSIBLE PHYSIOLOGICAL ROLE AS ENDOGENOUS ANTICONVULSANTS

FRANK C. TORTELLA

Among the most poorly understood and possibly least appreciated pharmacological actions of opioids (morphine, its congeners, and the enkephalins, endorphins, and dynorphins) is their effect on central nervous system (CNS) excitability relative to seizure states. Clinical reports dating back to the turn of the century describe proconvulsant and anticonvulsant actions of morphine in man [1]. Experimentally, a similar paradox exists wherein the convulsant properties of opioids in numerous species were recognized as early as 1824, while their anticonvulsant actions have also been repeatedly documented since the nineteenth century [1].

With the discovery of the endogenous opioid peptides over ten years ago, a new era began to unfold regarding opioids and seizures. However, after nearly a decade, the pro- and/or anticonvulsant effects of opioid systems are still being debated. Experimental evidence supporting both specific (opioid receptor-mediated) and nonspecific proconvulsant actions of opioids has been reported [2, 3], while other pharmacological studies have described anticonvulsant actions of opioids [4; and see Section 3]. This latter finding, and the demonstration of a postictal activation of endogenous opioid systems [5], formulated the basis of the working hypothesis that endogenous CNS opioids may act as one of the brain's natural anticonvulsants [4, 5], possibly playing a critical physiological role in the inhibitory mechanisms of seizure arrest and refractoriness [6–11]. More recently, the existence of an endogenous anticonvulsant substance in rat cerebrospinal fluid (CSF) following generalized seizures has been

Ferrendelli, J.A., Collins, R.C. and Johnson, E.M. (eds), Neurobiology of Amino Acids, Peptides, and Trophic Factors.

demonstrated, and this substance appears to be an endogenous opioid peptide [12, 13].

For the past several years, our research efforts have focused on the pharmacological issue of opioids and seizures and their physiological role as possible modulators of seizure states, directly addressing the proconvulsant versus anticonvulsant paradox. The effects of i.c.v. injections of numerous peptide and nonpeptide opioids have been examined using chemical and electrical models of seizure activity in rodents, as well as the spontaneous cortical and subcortical EEG of the rat. In addition, the experimental strategy of administering opioid antagonists has been employed to study the effects of exogenously administered and endogenously activated opioids on ictal and postictal phenomena, and to identify the specific receptor subtypes through which these effects are mediated. Using the latter approach, one can infer that the resulting changes in measured endpoints reflect the "functional" consequences of an altered endogenous opioid system.

This review will focus on the anticonvulsant properties of opioid peptides. Data will be presented to support their functional involvement in the inhibitory mechanisms responsible for the self-limitation of seizures, and their possible physiological role as endogenous anticonvulsants will be discussed. The primary experimental models of seizure activity used in these studies have been the rat flurothyl and maximal electroshock (MES) tests and threshold and spreading models of seizure activity.

1. ANTICONVULSANT ACTIONS OF OPIOID PEPTIDES

Anticonvulsant effects of opium were first reported in animals over 100 years ago, when Rodolfi in 1855 [14] and Beatty in 1871 [15] described morphine as an antidote to strychnine poisoning in the dog. During the ensuing 100 years, the references to opioids as anticonvulsant agents in both man and animal were numerous [1]. However, present-day interpretation of the results of these pioneering studies has been greatly hampered, not only due to the absence of proper control groups, particularly in the early clinical reports, but also to the unavailability of pharmacological antagonists with which to verify the opioid specificity of the pro- and/or anticonvulsant responses.

Since the initial reports by Tortella and coworkers [4] demonstrating that, like morphine and etorphine, the centrally administrated opioid peptides such as D-ala^2-D-met^5-enkephalin (DAME), D-ala^2-D-leu^5-enkephalin (DADLE), and beta-endorphin increased the threshold to flurothyl-induced seizures in rats, several studies have shown opioid peptides to be potent anticonvulsant agents against a variety of experimentally-induced seizures. For example, the anticonvulsant actions of various opioid peptides has been demonstrated against MES and flurothyl seizures in rats [7, 16–21], focal penicillin seizures in rabbits [22], audiogenic seizures in mice [22, 23], photic-induced seizures in baboons [24, 25], and against spontaneous seizures elicited in the epilepsy-prone gerbil [26]. Interestingly, while several nonpeptide opioids exhibit an anticonvulsant profile against kindled seizures in rats [27, 28], few studies have evaluated the effects of opioid peptides in this seizure model. Using the enkephalin analog ENK 146104, a decrease in seizure severity, but not in after discharge duration, has been reported [28]. In addition, microinjections of dynorphin A (1–13) into the substantia nigra of kindled rats was shown to suppress both motor and limbic seizures [29].

From the reports cited in the preceding paragraph, it is obvious that the opioid peptides may represent a novel class of anticonvulsant agents. However, defining these anticonvulsant actions as specific opioid responses based upon the pharmacological administration of agonists alone is tenuous, at best. Characterization of opioid activity requires that the action of the agonist be blocked or reversed by the administration of a specific opioid antagonist. In all of the studies cited above, the anticonvulsant effects observed as a result of opioid peptide injection were antagonized by low to moderate doses of naloxone. Therefore, unlike many of the reported seizureogenic or proconvulsant actions of opioid peptides that are either insensitive to naloxone antagonism or require high doses of naloxone to show partial attenuation [3], the anticonvulsant actions of opioid peptides are sensitive to naloxone antagonism. As such, the protective effects of various opioid peptides in a variety of experimental seizure models apparently represent specific opioid receptor-mediated actions.

Evidence accumulated over the past few years has demonstrated that the opioid receptor population is not homogenous. Based on in vivo [30–32], in vitro, and binding evidence [33–37], the existence of at least four opioid receptor subtypes — the mu, delta, kappa, and epsilon receptors — upon which opioid peptides may interact to produce pharmacological responses, have been firmly established. Using agonist and antagonist ligands selective for these opioid receptor subtypes, the role of mu, delta, and kappa receptors in the anticonvulsant action of opioid peptides has been extensively studied in the rat flurothyl and MES seizure models.

Table 12-1 summarizes the in vivo receptor profile for various opioid peptides to raise seizure thresholds in rats exposed to flurothyl. To date, all of the opioids listed in Table 12-1 have demonstrated anticonvulsant activity in this seizure model. For example, it has been shown [19] that one of the most selective agonist for mu opioid binding sites, D-Ala^{2}-N-methyl-Phe^{4}-Gly^{5}-ol-enkephalin (DAGO) [31, 37–39], produces dose-related increases in seizure threshold that are selectively antagonized by very low doses of naloxone or the irreversible mu selective antagonist beta-funaltrexamine (beta-FNA) [40], but not by the selective delta opioid receptor antagonist ICI 154, 129 [41, 42]. The mixed mu-delta directed opioid ligand, DADLE [37, 43, 44], is also a potent anticonvulsant against flurothyl seizures. However, complete dose-response antagonist studies with this ligand demonstrate that DADLE increases seizure threshold predominantly through delta opioid receptors [7]. Consistent with

Table 12-1. In vivo receptor profile of various opioid ligands as defined in the rat flurothyl seizure model.

Ligand	Seizure threshold	Antagonized By[a] NLX	BFNA	ICI154	Putative receptor
Morphine	↑	++			μ
Etorphine	↑	+++	+++	−	μ
DAGO (Glyol)	↑	+++	+++	−	μ
Beta-endorphin	↑	+			μ, δ, ε(?)
Metkephamid	↑	+		+	μ, δ
DADL	↑	+	−	+++	δ
DPDPE	↑			+++[b]	δ
U50, 488	no effect				ϰ
Dynorphin (1–13)	↑	−			non-opioid
Dynorphin (3–13)	↑				non-opioid

[a] Sensitivity to the respective antagonists: +++ (high), + (low), − (absent).
[b] ICI174,864.

this, it has recently been discovered [L. Robles, unpublished observation] that D-Pen^2-D-Pen^5-enkephalin (DPDPE), the highly selective, conformationally constrained delta opioid agonist [31, 37, 45] increases the seizure threshold to flurothyl. Moreover, the DPDPE-induced increase in seizure threshold is blocked by ICI 174,864, the recently developed delta selective opioid receptor antagonist [46]. While nonpeptide kappa opioid ligands, including the highly selective kappa agonist U50,488 [47], demonstrate no effect against flurothyl seizures in rats [48, 49], one of the putative endogenous peptides for the kappa opioid site, dynorphin A (1–13) [50, 51], is anticonvulsant. However, the results of experiments using naloxone and the inactive fragment of dynorphin (1–13), dynorphin (3–13), suggest that its anticonvulsant profile is at least, in part, due to a non-opioid action of this dynorphin fragment [21, 52].

Using representative ligands from Table 12-1, the anticonvulsant effects of selective mu (DAGO) and delta (DPDPE) opioid peptides were shown to exhibit an identical profile of responses in the rat MES seizure model. Namely, the ability of DAGO [19] and DPDPE [L. Robles, unpublished observation] to block tonic hindlimb extension and to decrease the duration of tonic forelimb extension can be selectively antagonized by beta-FNA and ICI 174,864, respectively. Interestingly, in contrast to flurothyl seizures, the nonpeptide kappa agonist U50,488 is a potent, long-acting anticonvulsant agent against MES seizures [49]. This effect is mediated by non-mu (possibly kappa) opioid receptors. The findings of these studies, as summarized in Table 12-2, indicate that each ligand is working through its own respective receptor system to elicit anticonvulsant activity.

Based upon the results of these many pharmacological studies, one can conclude that opioid peptides possess specific opioid receptor-mediated anticonvulsant properties. This conclusion is supported by two electrophysiological

Table 12-2. In vivo receptor profile of highly selective mu, delta, and kappa opioid ligands as defined in the rat MES seizure test.

Ligand	Blockade of THE[a]	Antagonized By[b] NLX	BFNA	ICI154	Putative receptor
DAGO (Glyol)	High[c]	+++	+++	−	μ
DPDPE	Moderate		−	+++[d]	δ
U50, 488	High	+			κ

[a] Tonic hindlimb extension
[b] Sensitivity to the respective antagonists: +++ (high), + (low), − (absent)
[c] Anticonvulsant efficacy
[d] ICI174,864

observations. Firstly, similar to anticonvulsant agents in general, a common characteristic of opioid peptides is their ability to hyperpolarize neurons [53]. Secondly, EEG studies uniformly reveal a general depressant action of opioid peptides on CNS activity. For example, central injections of enkephalins and beta-endorphin produce a profound slowing of spontaneous EEG activity characterized by high-amplitude slow waves and depressed behavior [54–59]. Critically, there appears to be a close temporal association between the opioid peptide-induced EEG slowing, behavioral stupor, and their anticonvulsant actions.

In light of the anticonvulsant properties associated with pharmacologically administered doses of opioids, in particular the enkephalins and endorphins, how can one reconcile the other body of literature that deals with the putative epileptogenic effects of the opioid peptides? Indeed, our own recent studies utilizing a complete dose-response analysis of the most selective agonists and antagonists for the mu and delta opioid binding site have revealed an exclusive role for the mu opioid receptor in the mediation of enkephalin-induced non-convulsive EEG seizures [32]. However, this excitatory response occurs as a result of the disinhibition of inhibitory interneurons [53], an action which appears to be unique to hippocampal loci [53], the major site of action for opioid peptide epileptiform activity [3, 57]. On the basis of this electrophysiological mechanism, it might be suggested that the EEG seizures produced by exogenously administered opioid peptides reflect an isolated pharmacological or toxicological artifact, rather than a physiologically relevant cellular mechanism of epileptogenesis. Indeed, clinical data using naloxone in a variety of seizure disorders, thereby implicating a causative role for opioid peptides in epilepsy, have been inconclusive [60–62].

2. SEIZURE ACTIVATION OF ENDOGENOUS OPIOID SYSTEMS

The fact that endogenous opioid peptides had been implicated in the etiology or pathophysiology of a variety of mental disorders [63–65] prompted the idea that the therapeutic effects of electroconvulsive therapy may in part be mediated by the activation of endogenous opioid systems [66]. Although it remains to be determined whether or not opioid peptides play a mechanistic or even a functional role in mental illness, a great deal of evidence has accumulated over the past several years demonstrating that endogenous opioid systems are activated as a consequence of seizures, such as those produced by electroconvulsive shock.

It was originally reported that immediately following an electroconvulsive shock (ECS) seizure in rats, a spectrum of measurable effects ensued not unlike those often associated with an acute opioid injection. An opioid form of catalepsy was reported [67], as well as increased nociceptive latencies, hyperthermia, respiratory depression, and cardiovascular changes, including post-ECS bradycardia. Many of the postictal opioid-like effects of ECS were antagonized by naloxone [68]. Using electroencephalographic (EEG) and electromyographic (EMG) activity in rats, it has been shown [5] that a single ECS seizure produced a similar pattern of EEG and behavioral responses to those previously reported by centrally administered opioid peptides [54–59], including polyspike discharges and a postictal isoelectric state, a prolonged period of high-voltage EEG slowing, EMG quieting, and an associated behavioral stupor. These postictal effects of ECS were antagonized by naloxone [5] and reduced by hypophysectomy [69], implicating an activation of endogenous opioids, possibly pituitary in origin, by a generalized tonic-clonic seizure.

Other studies further clarified the relation between postictal phenomena and endogenous opioid systems. It was demonstrated that the EEG and behavioral activating properties of the dihydrocodeinone RX 336-M, which were attenuated by beta-endorphin or enkephalin injection [70], were also attenuated by ECS [71]. Naloxone pretreatment significantly reversed this effect of ECS on the RX 336-M responses. Cross-tolerance [6, 72, 73] and cross-sensitization [74] between repeated ECS and morphine treatment have also been reported. Furthermore, there is extensive evidence showing that seizures increase the endogenous levels of CNS opioid peptides [75–80] and that ECS increases the number of opioid binding sites in rat brain [81].

From the results summarized above, there is little doubt that endogenous opioid systems are activated as a consequence of seizures. The supporting evidence includes information gained from behavioral, EEG, EMG, autonomic, biochemical, and binding studies. There is also extensive evidence indicating that other neurotransmitter and hormonal systems are similarly activated as a consequence of seizures [82–83]. Consequently, it can be concluded that endogenous opioids activated by seizures, and working in concert along with these other systems, may play an important modulatory role in postictal states.

3. ROLE OF ENDOGENOUS OPIOIDS IN THE SELF-LIMITATION OF SEIZURES

A unique pathophysiological consequence of a seizure is its capacity to spontaneously arrest and self-limit the recurrence of subsequent seizures. Although postseizure inhibition has been demonstrated experimentally [6, 84–89] and its

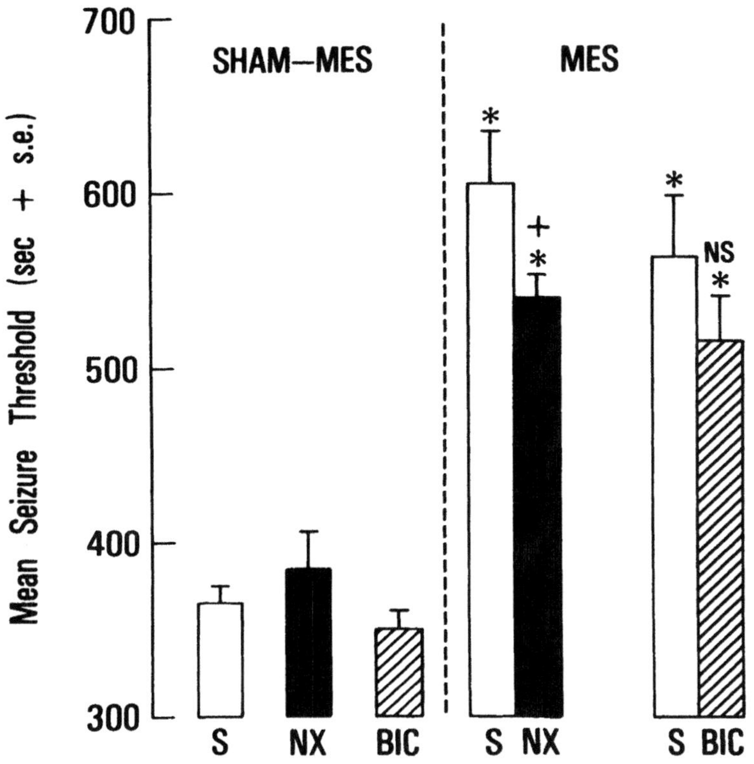

Figure 12-1. Effect of naloxone or bicuculline on flurothyl seizure thresholds after MES in rats. ★ = significantly different from corresponding sham-MES, $p < 0.05$; $^+$ = significantly different from corresponding saline group, $p < 0.05$; NS = not significantly different from corresponding saline group. (Modified from Reference 8.)

physiological importance recognized clinically [90, 91], the mechanism(s) underlying this state remain obscure.

As reviewed above, several studies have demonstrated that opioid peptides are anticonvulsants and that seizures activate endogenous opioid systems. Based upon such evidence, it was proposed that the postictally active endogenous opioids may participate in inhibitory mechanisms underlying the postictal refractory period [4, 5]. In our initial studies [8], the effect of a single maximal electroshock (MES) seizure on seizure thresholds in rats subsequently exposed to the volatile convulsant, flurothyl was evaluated. A prior MES seizure resulted in significantly increased convulsive thresholds when the same rats were subsequently exposed to flurothyl. Moreover, this postictal MES-induced increase in flurothyl seizure thresholds was selectively antagonized by naloxone, but not by subconvulsive doses of the GABA antagonist bicuculline, which themselves did not affect baseline threshold measures (Figure 12-1).

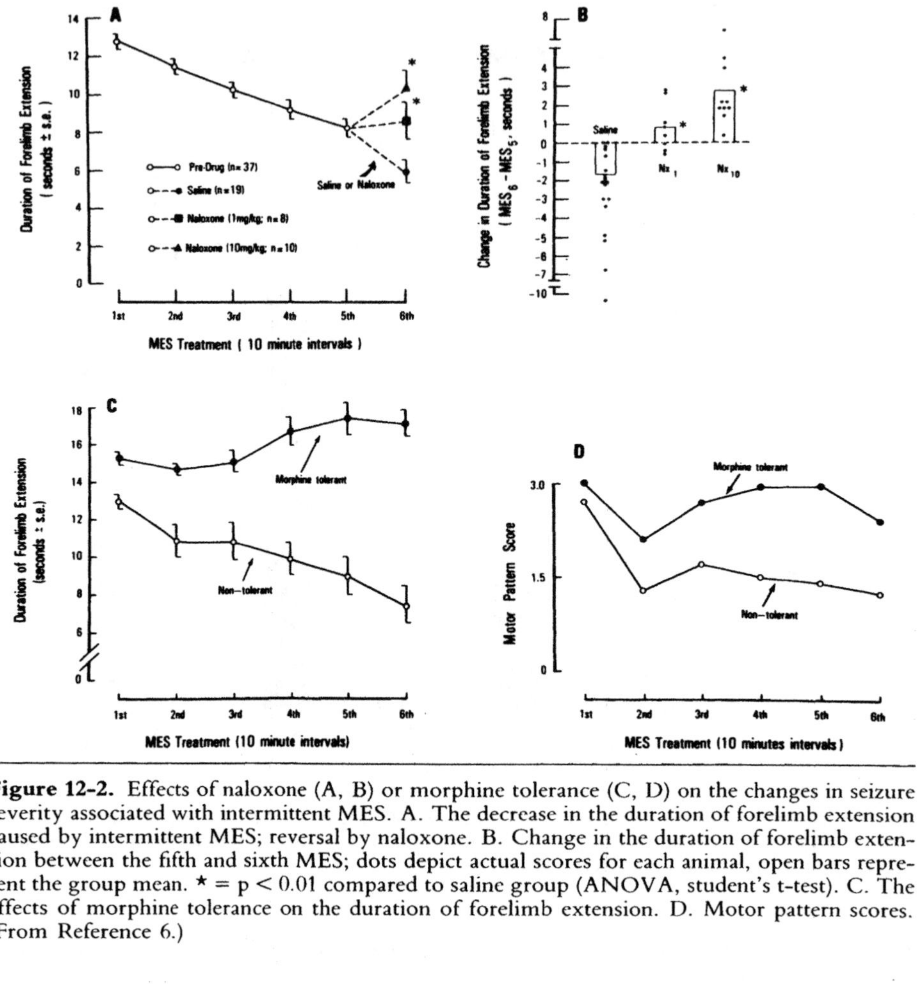

Figure 12-2. Effects of naloxone (A, B) or morphine tolerance (C, D) on the changes in seizure severity associated with intermittent MES. A. The decrease in the duration of forelimb extension caused by intermittent MES; reversal by naloxone. B. Change in the duration of forelimb extension between the fifth and sixth MES; dots depict actual scores for each animal, open bars represent the group mean. * = $p < 0.01$ compared to saline group (ANOVA, student's t-test). C. The effects of morphine tolerance on the duration of forelimb extension. D. Motor pattern scores. (From Reference 6.)

Thus, these events do not appear to involve inhibitory GABA systems.

These findings were recently reinforced by studies examining the effects of intermittent MES on seizure severity in rats [6]. Seizures produced by a single 2 second MES in naive rats were characterized by tonic forelimb extension (persisting for approximately 13 seconds) and complete hindlimb extension. Associated with a series of six intermittent MES seizures given at 10 minute intervals, there was a progressive decrease in seizure severity (Figure 12-2A, 12-2B, and 12-2D), which could be significantly reversed by naloxone (Figure 12-2A, 12-2B) and prevented by morphine tolerance (Figure 12-2C, 12-2D). Moreover, naloxone stereospecifically reversed the anticonvulsant actions of repeated seizures [6]. More recently, it has been demonstrated [92] that hypophysectomy, but not adrenalectomy, attenuated the normal anticonvulsant

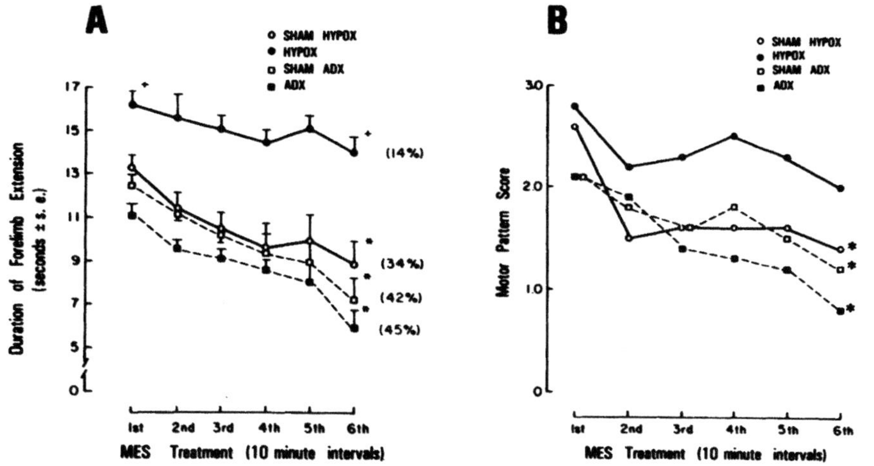

Figure 12-3. The effect of adrenalectomy (ADX) and hypophysectomy (HYPOX) on the durations of forelimb extension (A) and motor seizure patterns (B) associated with six consecutive MES seizures. Percentages (A) refer to the reduction in duration of forelimb extension following the sixth MES relative to those recorded following the first MES. $^{+}$ = $p < 0.05$ compared to sham-HYPOX rats; ★ = $p < 0.05$ compared to the first MES-induced seizure in this treatment group (Mann-Whitney U-test). (From Reference 92.)

effect of intermittent MES (Figure 12-3), suggesting that pituitary (but not adrenal) derived opioid peptides may play a prominent role in the inhibitory mechanisms responsible for the self-limitation of seizures.

Several other studies have demonstrated an involvement of endogenous opioid systems in the postictal inhibition of seizures. Naloxone has been reported to significantly reduce the anticonvulsant effect of electroconvulsive shock against kindled seizures [11], as well as reverse the postictal inhibition of seizures associated with massed kindling trials [9]. In addition, the opioid antagonist naltrexone was reported to attenuate the postictal anticonvulsant effect of spontaneous seizures on pentylenetetrazol-induced seizures in the genetically epilepsy-prone mongolian gerbil [10].

4. IDENTIFICATION OF AN ENDOGENOUS ANTICONVULSANT SUBSTANCE WITH OPIOID PEPTIDE-LIKE CHARACTERISTICS

Recent studies suggest that seizure arrest and refractoriness may occur as a result of the activation of the brain's own endogenous anticonvulsant substances or systems. For example, it has been proposed that the inhibitory modulator adenosine acts as the brain's own endogenous anticonvulsant, regulating postictal seizure arrest and refractoriness [83]. Other potential candidates for endogenous anticonvulsant substances include inosine [93], cyclic AMP [94], inhibitory amino acids [95], biogenic amines [96], prostaglandins [97], and various neuropeptides [98].

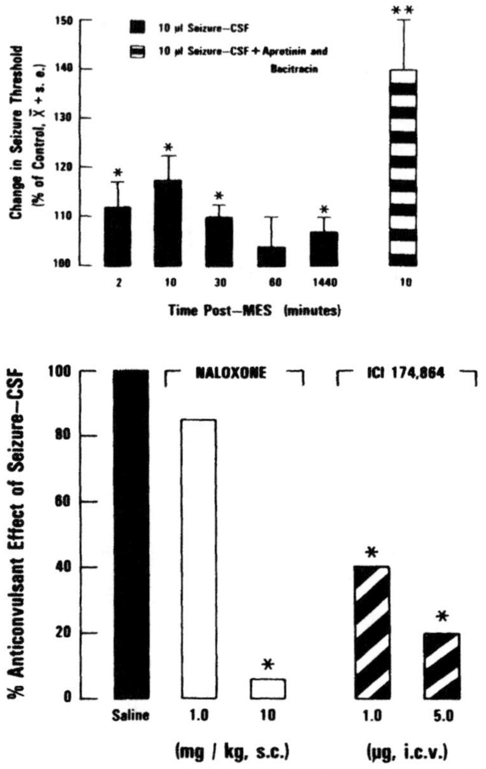

Figure 12-4. Top — effect of seizure CSF collected at various times after MES on the seizure thresholds of recipient rats challenged with the convulsant, flurothyl. Solid bars represent the response to seizure CSF not protected by protease inhibitors; the banded bar represents the response to seizure CSF protected by aprotinin and bacitracin. ⋆ = significantly different from control CSF ($p < 0.05$, student's t-test); ⋆⋆ = significantly different from seizure CSF without aprotinin and bacitracin ($p < 0.01$). Bottom — antagonist effect of naloxone or ICI 174,864 on the anticonvulsant bioactivity of the seizure CSF taken 10 minutes after MES. Anticonvulsant bioactivity of seizure CSF in drug-treated animals is expressed as the percentage of the total anticonvulsant effect of seizure CSF on saline-treated rats (normalized to 100%). ⋆ = significantly different from the respective control groups (p. < 0.05, student's t-test). (From Reference 12.)

Studies directly aimed at determining the existence of endogenous opioids in the CNS acting as endogenous anticonvulsant substances. It was hypothesised that if a seizure results in the activation of an endogenous anticonvulsant, it may be possible to detect the bioactive material from the cerebrospinal fluid (CSF) of donor rats following the seizure. It follows that re-administration of the donor CSF to recipient animals should offer protection against subsequent convulsive agents. Using transauricular MES as the priming seizure, and flurothyl as the second convulsive agent, it was observed (Figure 12-4, top) that CSF collected from the cisternal space of donor rats at various times post-MES and injected i.c.v. to recipient rats resulted in an increased seizure

Table 12-3. Potency comparison of the opioid antagonists ICI 174,864 and naloxone to antagonize the anticonvulsant action of seizure CSF (S-CSF).

Treatment	Dose range	AD50 (95% CL) (nmol, i.c.v.)
S-CSF + ICI 174,864	0.28 – 7.0	1.09 (0.85 – 1.39)
S-CSF + naloxone	29.0 – 290	91.2 (81.2 – 100.7)

Table 12-4. Effect of seizure CSF on the thresholds of recipient rats to flurothyl convulsions.

Seizure CSF	Maximal change in ST* (% of control)
No peptidase inhibitors	+18%
Thiorphin + Bestatin	+12%
Aprotinin + Bacitracin	+40%
Trypsin	−2%

* Seizure threshold

threshold to flurothyl convulsions in the recipients [12]. It was determined that the anticonvulsant bioactivity of the seizure CSF was enhanced by the peptidase inhibitors aprotinin and bacitracin (Figure 12-4, top), and was antagonized by prior treatment of recipient rats with high doses of peripherally administered naloxone or the centrally administered delta receptor selective opioid antagonist ICI 174,864 (Figure 12-4, bottom). These initial results suggested the existence of an endogenous anticonvulsant substance (EAS) in rat CSF following generalized seizures that appeared to be opioid peptide in nature.

A more thorough assessment of the antagonism by naloxone and ICI 174,864 of the EAS has revealed that when both antagonists were administered i.c.v. and compared on an equimolar basis, the bioactivity of the EAS was approximately 100 times more sensitive to antagonism by ICI 174,864 than by naloxone (Table 12-3). Thus, similar to the delta receptor mediation of the anticonvulsant effects of other delta-directed opioid peptides such as metkephamid [20], DADLE [7] and the highly selective delta opioid peptide DPDPE [L. Robles, unpublished observation], the anticonvulsant activity of the EAS in seizure CSF appears to be mediated through a delta opioid receptor.

The peptide nature of the EAS has been confirmed by a series of experiments using trypsin and specific peptidase inhibitors (Table 12-4). The bioactivity of the EAS can be inactivated by trypsin and selectively enhanced by aprotinin and bacitracin (see above), but not by thiorphan and bestatin, specific inhibitors of enzymes principally involved in the degradation of the small molecular weight enkephalins (approximately 600 daltons) and dynorphin A (approximately 2000 daltons). These results indicate that the EAS may represent a larger molecular weight opioid peptide.

Radioimmunoassays have been conducted on the seizure-CSF using anti-

Table 12-5. Changes in levels of opioid peptide-like immunoreactivity in seizure CSF.

Opioid peptide	% change in IR
Dynorphin A	no change
Leu-enkephalin	no change
Beta-endorphin	+427%
Met-enkephalin	
nondigested	no change
digested	+60%

bodies specific for met- and leu-enkephalin, dynorphin A and beta-endorphin. The results of these studies have been summarized in Table 12-5. Seizure CSF levels of dynorphin A, leu-enkephalin, or met-enkephalin-like immunoreactivity remained unchanged compared to control baseline CSF levels [99]. In contrast, beta-endorphin-like immunoreactivity was significantly increased in the seizure-CSF [12, 99]. In addition, it has recently been shown that following exposure of the seizure-CSF with trypsin and carboxypeptidase B, met-enkephalin-like immunoreactivity was increased 60% [13], indicating that the seizure-CSF may contain increased levels of a larger molecular weight form of met-enkephalin not recognized immunologically prior to digestion. The results of these radioimmunoassay studies support the possible large molecular weight nature of the seizure-CSF. Furthermore, preliminary molecular weight sizing experiments using gel exclusion chromatography (Sephadex G-75) reveal a molecular weight of 8700 daltons for the major species yielding met-enkephalin-like immunoreactivity [13].

Ultrafiltration of the EAS using membranes of varying molecular weight size have revealed the following: The bioactivity of the EAS was retained in the filtrate of seizure CSF passed through 10 K molecular weight membranes, but not 1 K or 5 K molecular weight membranes. Critically, while the retentate of the 10 K molecular weight ultrafiltration was devoid of bioactivity, complete recovery of bioactive material was measured in the retentate of the 5 K molecular weight ultrafiltration. Consequently, the bioactivity of the EAS resides in the 5 K to 10 K molecular weight range, a finding highly consistent with the observations described in the preceding paragraphs.

Based on the evidence presented, the existence of an EAS with affinity for, and bioactivity at, delta opioid receptor binding sites has been confirmed. Our present research efforts are focused on the purification and molecular identification of this factor.

5. CONCLUSION

Evidence gleaned from numerous experimental approaches has revealed the importance of endogenous opioid systems in seizure arrest and postictal refractoriness. Indeed, while there is little evidence supporting a tonic involvement of these systems in the cellular mechanisms of epileptogenesis, once activated by a seizure, there is ample evidence to support their potential physiological importance as endogenous anticonvulsants.

In order for any neuromodulator to be considered a viable candidate for an EAS, it is suggested that several criteria must be fulfilled. None of the least being: 1) the neuromodulator should be anticonvulsant when exogenously administered, 2) this would represent a pharmacological (receptor-mediated) action of the compound, identified by specific receptor antagonists, 3) it should be possible to measure seizure-related changes in endogenous levels of the putative EAS, 4) the administration of specific antagonists should attenuate postictal increases in seizure threshold or decreases in seizure severity, and 5) the endogenous anticonvulsant candidate should hyperpolarize, rather than depolarize, central neurons.

Among the potential neuromodulator candidates for an EAS [83], opioid peptides appear to most fully satisfy these criteria. It has been shown that they possess marked anticonvulsant activity against a variety of experimentally induced seizures, effects specifically antagonized by the various receptor selective opioid antagnoists. Their regional brain levels and CSF content are increased following seizures. Several important studies have demonstrated efficacy of opioid antagonists to decrease the postictal rise in seizure threshold and behavioral depression, or attenuate the anticonvulsant effect of a prior seizure. Importantly, common to all anticonvulsant agents, opioids also hyperpolarize neurons throughout the CNS.

Thus, while it would be premature to attribute the phenomena of seizure arrest and refractoriness to a single inhibitory modulator system or substance, the data reviewed herein indicate the potential importance of opioid physiology and pharmacology in developing novel strategies of epilepsy research. Despite the preliminary nature of these convincing data, it is interesting to speculate that in addition to their putative role as the brain's endogenous pain relieving system, endogenous opioids may also subserve an important function to quiet the "seizing" brain.

ACKNOWLEDGMENTS

The author acknowledges with gratitude a number of outstanding scientists and associates to the studies described in this review. Singular mention should be made of Drs. Joseph B. Long and John W. Holaday for their scientific collaborations and contributions to this manuscript and Ms. Lydia E. Robles and Mr. Clifton E. Johnson for their excellent technical assistance over the years.

REFERENCES

1. Krueger, H., Eddy, N.B. and Sumwalt, M. (eds.) (1941). *The Pharmacology of the Opium Alkaloids*, Supplement No. 165 to the Public Health Reports, U.S. Government Printing Office, Washington, DC.
2. Urca, G., Frenk, H., Liebeskind, J.C. and Taylor, A.N. (1977). Morphine and enkephalin: Analgesic and epileptic properties. Science 197, 83–86.

3. Frenk, H. (1983). Pro- and anticonvulsant actions of morphine and the endogenous opioids: Involvement and interactions of multiple opiate and non-opiate systems. Brain Res. Rev. 6, 197–210.
4. Tortella, F.C., Cowan, A. and Adler, M.W. (1981). Comparison of the anticonvulsant effects of opioid peptides and etorphine in rats. Life Sci. 29, 1039–1045.
5. Tortella, F.C., Cowan, A., Belenky, G.L. and Holaday, J.W. (1981). Opiate-like electroencephalographic and behavioral effects of electroconvulsive shock in rats. Eur. J. Pharmacol. 76, 121–128.
6. Tortella, F.C., Long, J.B. and Holaday, J.W. (1985). Endogenous opioid systems: Physiological role in the self-limitation of seizures. Brain Res. 332, 174–178.
7. Tortella, F.C., Robles, L. and Holaday, J.W. (1985). The anticonvulsant effects of DADL are primarily mediated by activation of delta opioid receptors: Interactions between delta and mu receptor antagonists. Life Sci. 37, 497–503.
8. Tortella, F.C. and Cowan, A. (1982). Studies on the role of opioid peptides as endogenous anticonvulsants. Life Sci. 31, 2225–2228.
9. Kelsey, J.E. and Belluzi, J.D. (1982). Endorphin mediation of postictal effects of kindled seizures in rats. Brain Res. 253, 337–340.
10. Lee, R.J. and Lomax, P. (1985). The effect of spontaneous seizures on pentylenetetrazole and maximal electroshock induced seizures in the mongolian gerbil. Eur. J. Pharmacol. 106, 91–96.
11. Shavit, Y., Caldecott-Hazard, S. and Liebeskind, J.C. (1984). Activating endogenous opioid systems by electroconvulsive shock or footshock stress inhibits recurrent kindled seizures in rats. Brain Res. 305, 203–207.
12. Tortella, F.C. and Long, J.B. (1985). Endogenous anticonvulsant substance in rat cerebrospinal fluid after a generalized seizure. Science 228, 1106–1108.
13. Tortella, F.C., Long, J.B. and Liston, D. (1986). Endogenous opioid peptide-like substance: Physiological and molecular characterization of its properties. Soc. Neurosci. Abstr. 12, 776.
14. Rodolfi, R. (1855). Nuove osservazioni su l' azione della stricnina. Gazz. Med. Ital. Lomb. 6, 61–63.
15. Beatty, T.C. (1871). Morphia as antidote to strychine (correspondence). Lancet 2, 907.
16. Berman, E.F. and Adler, M.W. (1984). The anticonvulsant effect of opioids and opioid peptides against maximal electroshock seizures in rats. Neuropharmacol. 23, 367–371.
17. Puglisi-Allegr, S., Castellano, C., Csanyl, V., Doka, A. and Oliverio, A. (1984). Opioid antagonism of electroshock-induced seizures. Pharmacol. Biochem. Behav. 20, 767–769.
18. Garant, D.S. and Gale, K. (1985). Infusion of opiates into substantia nigra protects against maximal electroshock seizures in rats. J. Pharmacol. Exp. Ther. 234, 45–48.
19. Robles, L., Tortella, F.C. and Holaday, J.W. (1986). Anticonvulsant effects of the mu selective ligand DAGO in rats. Pharmacologist 28, 170.
20. Tortella, F.C., Robles, L., Holaday, J.W. and Cowan, A. (1983). A selective role for delta receptors in the regulation of opioid-induced changes in seizure threshold. Life Sci. 33, 603–606.
21. Tortella, F.C. and Holaday, J.W. (1987). Dynorphin (1–13): In vivo antagonist actions and non-opioid anticonvulsant effects in the rat flurothyl test. Natl. Inst. Drug Abuse Monograph, in press.
22. Baccelliere, L., Ferrillo, F., Montano, V.F., Rodriguez, G. and Rosadini, G. (1980). Inhibitory effects of met^5-enkephaline on different models of experimental epilepsy. Acta. Neurol. Scand. 62 (Suppl. 79).
23. Plotnikoff, N.P., Kastin, A.J., Coy, D.H., Christensen, C.W., Schally, A.V. and Spirtes, M.A. (1976). Neuropharmacological actions of enkephalin after systemic administration. Life Sci. 19, 1283–1288.
24. Meldrum, B.S., Menini, C., Stutzmann, J.M. and Naquet, R. (1979). Effects of opiate-like peptides, morphine, and naloxone in the photosensitive baboon, *Papio Papio*. Brain Res. 170, 333–348.
25. Meldrum, B.S. and Menini, C. (1981). Effect of morphine, enkephalins, beta-endorphin, and related compounds on seizure thresholds. In *Neurotransmitters, Seizures, and Epilepsy*, Morselli, P.L. et al, eds., Raven Press, New York, pp. 185–194.
26. Bajorek, J.G. and Lomax, P. (1982). Modulation of spontaneous seizures in the mongolian gerbil: Effects of beta-endorphin. Peptides 3, 83–86.
27. Albertson, T.E., Joy, R.M. and Stark, L.G. (1984). Modification of kindled amygdaloid

seizures by opiate agonists and antagonists. J. Pharmacol. Exp. Ther. 228, 620–627.

28. Caldecott-Hazard, S., Shavit, Y., Ackermann, R.F., Engel, J., Frederickson, R.C. and Liebeskind, J.C. (1982). Behavioral and electrographic effects of opioids on kindled seizures in rats. Brain Res. 251, 327–333.
29. McNamara, J.O., Rigsbee, L.C., Legg, S. and Galloway, M.T. (1983). Microinjection of dynorphin 1–13 into substantia nigra suppresses kindled seizures. Soc. Neurosci. Abst. 9, 485.
30. Holaday, J.W. and Tortella, F.C. (1984). Multiple opiate receptors: Possible physiological functions of mu and delta binding sites in vivo. In *Central and Peripheral Endorphins: Basic and Clinical Aspects*, Muller, E.E. and Genazzani, R. eds., Raven Press, New York, pp. 237–250.
31. Porreca, F., Mosberg, H.I., Hurst, R., Hruby, V.J. and Burks, T.F. (1984). Roles of mu, delta and kappa opioid receptors in spinal and supraspinal mediation of gastrointestinal transit effects and hot-plate analgesia in the mouse. J. Pharmacol. Exp. Ther. 230, 341–348.
32. Tortella, F.C., Robles, L. and Mosberg, H.I. (1987). Evidence for mu-opioid receptor mediation of enkephalin-induced EEG seizures. J. Pharmacol. Exp. Ther., in press.
33. Lord, J.A., Waterfield, A.A., Hughes, J. and Kosterlitz, H.W. (1977). Endogenous opioid peptides: Multiple agonists and receptors. Nature 267, 495–499.
34. Chang, K.J. and Cuatrecasas, P. (1979). Multiple opiate receptors: Enkephalins and morphine bind to receptors of different specificity. J. Biol. Chem. 254, 2610–2618.
35. Wuster, M., Schultz, R. and Herz, A. (1981). Multiple opiate receptors in peripheral tissue preparations. Biochem. Pharmacol. 30, 1883–1887.
36. James, I.F. and Goldstein, A. (1984). Site-directed alkylation of multiple opioid receptors. I. Binding selectivity. Mol. Pharmacol. 25, 337–342.
37. Goldstein, A. and James, I.F. (1984). Site-directed alkylation of multiple opioid receptors. II. Pharmacological selectivity. Mol. Pharmacol. 30, 343–348.
38. Handa, B.K., Lane, A.C., Lord, J.A., Morgan, B.A., Rance, M.J. and Smith, C.F. (1981). Analogs of beta-LPH_{61-64} possessing selective agonists at mu-opiate receptors. Br. J. Pharmacol. 70, 531–540.
39. Kosterlitz, H.W. and Paterson, S.J. (1981). TYR-D-ALA^2-GLY-MePHE-$NH(CH_2)_2$ is a selective ligand for the mu opiate binding site. Br. J. Pharmacol. 73, 299P.
40. Takemori, A.E., Larson, D.L. and Portoghese, P.S. (1981). The irreversible narcotic antagonist and reversible agonist properties of the fumaramate ester methyl derivative of naltrexone. Eur. J. Pharmacol. 70, 445–451.
41. Shaw, J.S., Miller, L., Turnbull, M.J., Gormley, J.J. and Morley, J.S. (1982). Selective antagonists at the opiate delta-receptor. Life Sci. 31, 1259–1262.
42. Tortella, F.C., Robles, L., Holaday, J.W. and Cowan, A. (1984). ICI 154,129, a delta-opioid receptor antagonist raises seizure threshold in rats. Eur. J. Pharmacol. 97, 141–144.
43. Zajac, J.M., Gacel, G. Petit, F., Dodey, P. and Roques, B.P. (1983). Deltakephalin, TYR-D-THR-GLY-PHE-LEU-THR: A new highly potent and fully specific agonist for opiate delta receptors. Biochem. Biophys. Res. Commun. 111, 390–397.
44. Galligan, J.J., Mosberg, H.I., Hurst, R., Hruby, V.J. and Burks, T.F. (1984). Cerebral delta opioid receptors mediate analgesia but not the intestinal motility effects of intracerebroventricularly administered opioids. J. Pharmacol. Exp. Ther. 229, 641–648.
45. Mosberg, H.I., Hurst, R., Hruby, V.J., Galligan, J.J., Burks, T.F., Gee, K. and Yamamura, H.I. (1983). Bis-penicillamine enkephalins show pronounced delta opioid receptor selectivity. Proc. Natl. Acad. Sci. USA 80, 6871–6874.
46. Cotton, R., Giles, M.G., Miller, L., Shaw, J.S. and Timms, D. (1984). ICI 174,864: A highly selective antagonist for the opioid delta receptor. Eur. J. Pharmacol. 97, 331–332.
47. VonVoigtlander, P.F., Lahti, R.A. and Ludens, J.H. (1983). U-50,488: A selective and structurally novel non-mu (kappa) opioid agonist. J. Pharmacol. Exp. Ther. 224, 7–12.
48. Cowan, A., Geller, E.B. and Adler, M.W. (1979). Classification of opioids on the basis of change in seizure threshold in rats. Science 206, 465–467.
49. Tortella, F.C., Robles, L. and Holaday, J.W. (1985). U50,488, a highly selective kappa opioid: Anticonvulsant profile in rats. J. Pharmacol. Exp. Ther. 237, 49–53.
50. Chavkin, C., James, I.F. and Goldstein, A. (1982). Dynorphin is a specific endogenous ligand of the kappa opioid receptor. Science 215, 413–415.
51. Lee, N.M. and Smith, A.P. (1984). Possible regulatory function of dynorphin and its clinical implications. TIPS 5, 108–110.
52. Tortella, F.C., Robles, L. and Holaday, J.W. (1985). Seizure threshold studies with dynor-

phin (1–13) in rats: Possible interactions among kappa, mu and delta opioid binding sites. Pharmacologist 27, 179.
53. Duggan, A.W. and North, R.A. (1984). Electrophysiology of opioids. Pharmacol. Rev. 35, 219–281.
54. Tortella, F.C., Moreton, J.E. and Khazan, N. (1978). Electroencephalographic and behavioral effects of D-ala^2-methionine-enkephalinamide and morphine in the rat. J. Pharmacol. Exp. Ther. 206, 636–643.
55. Tortella, F.C., Moreton, J.E. and Khazan, N. (1979). Electroencephalographic and behavioral tolerance to and cross-tolerance between D-ala^2-methionine-enkephalinamide and morphine in the rat. J. Pharmacol. Exp. Ther. 210, 174–179.
56. Moreton, J.E., Tortella, F.C. and Khazan, N. (1978). EEG and behavioral effects of acute and chronic administration of opiate-like peptides in the rat. Dev. Neurosci. 4, 435–436.
57. Henriksen, S.J., Bloom, F.E., McCoy, F., Ling, N. and Guillemin, R. (1978). Beta-endorphin induces nonconvulsive limbic seizures. Proc. Natl. Acad. Sci. USA 75, 5221–5225.
58. Tortella, F.C., Robles, L., Mosberg, H.I. and Holaday, J.W. (1984). Electroencephalographic assessment of the role of delta receptors in opioid peptide-induced seizures. Neuropeptides 5, 213–216.
59. Tortella, F.C., Robles, L., Mosberg, H.I. and Holaday, J.W. (1985). Electroencephalographic characterization of mu and delta opioid receptor activity in rats. Soc. Neurosci. Abst. 11, 308.
60. Montplaisir, J., Saint-Hilaire, J.M., Walsh, J.T., Laverdiere, M. and Bouvier, G. (1981). Naloxone and focal epilepsy: A study with depth electrodes. Neurology 31. 350–352.
61. Engel, J., Ackermann, R.F., Caldecott-Hazard, S. and Chugani, H.T. (1984). Do altered opioid mechanisms play a role in human epilepsy? In *Neurotransmitters, seizures, and epilepsy II*. Fariello, R.G., Morselli, P.L., Lloyd, K.G., eds., Raven Press, New York, pp. 263–272.
62. Snead, O.C. (1986). Neuropeptides and seizures. Neurologic Clin. 4, 863–875.
63. Emrich, H.M., Hollt, H., Laspe, M., Fischler, M., Heinemann, H., Kissling, W. Zersen, D.V. and Herz, A. (1979). Studies on possible pathological significance of endorphins in psychiatric disorders. In *Neuropsychopharmacology*, Saletu, B., Berner, P. and Hollister, L., eds., Pergamon Press, New York, pp. 527–534.
64. Costa, E. and Trabucchi, M. (1980). Neural peptides and neural communication. Adv. Biochem. Psychopharmacol. 22, 435–563.
65. Holaday, J.W. and Loh, H.H. (1981). Neurobiology of beta-endorphin and related peptides. In *Hormonal Proteins and Peptides: Beta-endorphin*, Li, C.H., ed., Academic Press, New York, pp. 202–291.
66. Belenky, G.L. and Holaday, J.W. (1979). The opiate antagonist naloxone modifies the effects of electroconvulsive shock (ECS) on respiration, blood pressure and heart rate. Brain Res. 177, 414–417.
67. Holaday, J.W. and Belenky, G.L. (1980). Opiate-like effects of electroconvulsive shock in rats: A differential effect of naloxone on nociceptive measures. Life Sci. 27, 1929–1938.
68. Belenky, G.L., Tortella, F.C., Hitzemann, R.J. and Holaday, J.W. (1984). The role of endorphin systems in the effects of ECS. In *ECT: Basic Mechanisms*, Lerer, B., Weiner, R.D. and Belmaker, R.H., eds., John Libby & Co., Bondway, London, pp. 89–97.
69. Tortella, F.C., Cowan, A. and Holaday, J.W. (1984). Pituitary endorphin involvement in electroconvulsive shock-induced postictal electrogenesis and behavioral depression in rats. Peptides 5, 115–118.
70. Cowan, A. and Tortella, F.C. (1982). A quantitative analysis of the shaking behavior induced in rats by beta-endorphin and D-ala^2-met-enkephalinamide. Life Sci. 30, 171–176.
71. Tortella, F.C. and Cowan, A. (1982). EEG, EMG and behavioral evidence for the involvement of endorphin systems in postictal events after electroconvulsive shock in rats. Life Sci. 31, 881–888.
72. Katz, R.J. and Schmaltz, K. (1980). Reduction of opiate activation after chronic electroconvulsive shock: Possible role for endorphins in the behavioral effects of convulsive shock treatment. Neurosci. Lett. 19, 85–91.
73. Urca, G., Nof, A., Weissman, B.A. and Sarne, Y. (1983). Analgesia induced by electroconvulsive shock: Brain enkephalins may mediate tolerance but not the induction of analgesia. Brain Res. 260, 271–277.
74. Belenky, G.L. and Holaday, J.W. (1981). Repeated electroconvulsive shock (ECS) and morphine tolerance: Demonstration of cross-sensitivity in the rat. Life Sci. 29, 553–563.
75. Green, A.R., Peralta, E., Hong, J.S., Mao, C.C., Atterwill, C.K. and Costa, E. (1978).

Alterations in GABA metabolism and met-enkephalin content in rat brain following repeated electroconvulsive shocks. J. Neurochem. 31, 607–611.
76. Hong, J.S., Wood, P.L., Gillen, J.C., Yang, H.-Y.T. and Costa, E. (1980). Changes of hippocampal met-enkephalin content after recurrent motor seizures. Nature (Lond.) 285, 231–232.
77. Vindrola, O., Briones, R., Asai, M. and Fernandez-Guardiola, A. (1981). Amygdaloid kindling enhances the enkephalin content in the rat brain. Neurosci. Lett. 21, 39–43.
78. Sarne, Y., Weissman, G. and Urca, G. (1982). Differential effects of long-term electroconvulsive shock on brain levels of enkephalin and humoral-endorphin. J. Neurochem. 39, 1478–1480.
79. Przewlocki, R., Lason, W., Stach, R. and Kacz, D. (1983). Opioid peptides, particularly dynorphin, after amygdaloid-kindled seizures. Regul. Peptides 6, 385–392.
80. McGinty, J.F., Kanamatsu, T., Obie, J., Dyer, R.S., Mitchell, C.L. and Hong, J.S. (1986). A mygdaloid kindling increases enkephalin-like immunoreactivity but decreases dynorphin-A-like immunoreactivity in rat hippocampus. Neurosci. Lett. 71, 31–36.
81. Holaday, J.W., Tortella, F.C., Long, J.B., Belenky, G.L. and Hitzemann, R.J. (1986). Endogenous opioids and their receptors: Evidence for involvement in the postictal effects of electroconvulsive shock. In *Electroconvulsive Therapy: Clinical and Basic Research Issues*, Malitz, S. and Sackeim, H.A., eds., Ann. New York Acad. Sci. 462, 124–139.
82. Malitz, S. and Sackeim, H.A. (eds.) (1986). In *Electroconvulsive Therapy: Clinical and Basic Research Issues*, New York Acad. Sci. 462, 76–172.
83. Dragunow, M. (1986). Endogenous anticonvulsant substances. Neurosci. Biobehav. Rev. 10, 229–244.
84. Essig, C.F. and Flanary, H.G. (1966). The importance of the convulsion in occurrence and rate of development of electroconvulsive threshold elevation. Exp. Neurol. 14, 448–452.
85. Herberg, L.J., Trees, K.H. and Blundell, J.E. (1969). Raising the threshold in experimental epilepsy by hypothalamic and septal stimulation and by audiogenic seizures. Brain 92, 313–328.
86. Ramer, D. and Pinel, J.P. (1976). Progressive intensification of motor seizures produced by periodic electroconvulsive shock. Exp. Neurol. 51, 421–433.
87. Mucha, R.F. and Pinel, J.P. (1977). Postseizure inhibition of kindled seizures. Exp. Neurol. 54, 266–282.
88. Sainsbury, R.S., Bland, B.H. and Buchan, D.H. (1978). Electrically induced seizure activity in the hippocampus: Time course for postseizure inhibition of subsequent kindled seizures. Behav. Biol. 22, 479–488.
89. Handforth, A. (1982). Postseizure inhibition of kindled seizures by electroconvulsive shock. Exp. Neurol. 78, 483–491.
90. Kalinowsky, L.B. and Kennedy, F. (1943). Observations in electric shock therapy applied to problems of epilepsy. J. Nerv. Ment, Dis. 98, 56–67.
91. Holmberg, G. (1954). Effect on electrically induced convulsions of the number of previous treatments in a series. Arch. Neurol. Psychiat. 71, 619–623.
92. Long, J.B. and Tortella, F.C. (1987). Effects of adrenalectomy and hypophysectomy on postictal seizure protection. Brain Res., in press.
93. Lewin, E. and Bleck, V. (1985). Effect of inosine on seizures induced with metrazol, bicuculline, or picrotoxin. Epilepsia 26, 258–261.
94. Ferrendelli, J.A. (1980). Epilepsy and cyclic nucleotides. Adv. Cyclic Neucleotide Protein Phosphorylation Res. 12, 199–211.
95. Meldrum, B. (1984). Amino acid neurotransmitters and new approaches to anticonvulsant drug action. Epilepsia 25, S140–S149.
96. Ferrendelli, J.A. (1984). Roles of biogenic amines and cyclic nucleotides in seizure mechanisms. Ann. Neurol. 16, S98–S103.
97. Forstermann, U., Heldt, R., Knappen, F. and Hertting, G. (1982). Potential anticonvulsive properties of endogenous prostaglandins formed in mouse brain. Brain Res. 240, 303–310.
98. Bajorek, J.G., Lee, R.J. and Lomax, P. (1984). Neuropeptides: A role as endogenous mediators or modulators of epileptic phenomena. Ann. Neurol. 16, S31–S38.
99. Long, J.B., Molineaux, C.J. and Tortella, F.C. (1985). Further characterization of an endogenous opioid anticonvulsant: Measurement of opioid peptide immunoreactivity in rat cerebrospinal fluid following a generalized seizure. Soc. Neurosci. Abst. 11, 468.

13. ALPHA- AND BETA-ENDOPSYCHOSINS: PHYSIOLOGICAL ACTIONS AND INTERACTIONS WITH EXCITATORY AMINO ACIDS

THOMAS H. LANTHORN, DEBORA A. DIMAGGIO, PATRICIA C. CONTRERAS, JOSEPH B. MONAHAN, LINDA M. PULLAN, GAIL HANDELMANN, NANCY M. GRAY AND THOMAS L. O'DONOHUE

Phencyclidine (1-(1-cyclohexylphenyl)piperidine) was synthesized in 1957 by the Parke Davis company. Phencyclidine (PCP) is an excellent general anesthetic because it produces anesthesia with analgesia, while producing minimal cardiorespiratory depression. However, in clinical trials PCP was found to produce postanesthetic hallucinations, which could last more than 12 hours, in about 30% of patients [1]. Clinical use of PCP in humans was discontinued. Later, PCP was approved for use as a veterinary anesthetic and an analog, ketamine, was approved for use in humans. Although ketamine can produce psychotomimetic side effects, these are not as prolonged as with PCP.

In recent years there has been an increasing interest in the actions of PCP and the neuronal mechanisms that underlie them. This increased interest has been spurred by several diverse developments. Much of what is known about the effects of PCP in humans has been due to the nonmedical use of PCP. The nonmedical use of PCP first appeared in the 1960s, but PCP did not gain popularity until recently. The recent and rapid rise in the nonmedical use of PCP has provided a strong impetus to understand its mechanisms of action, not only for what they can tell us about the neural regulation of behavior, but also to find a selective antagonist of PCP for use in cases of PCP intoxication. The similarity between the symptoms of schizophrenia and PCP-induced psychosis [2–5] suggests that PCP intoxication may be a useful model for testing for antipsychotics and also that PCP may interact with an endogenous system that is involved in the pathogenesis of schizophrenia.

Ferrendelli, J.A., Collins, R.C. and Johnson, E.M. (eds), Neurobiology of Amino Acids, Peptides, and Trophic Factors.

This impetus to understand the mechanisms has been matched by scientific developments. The recognition and isolation of endogenous ligands for PCP receptors indicates that PCP-like compounds reveal fundamental processes of brain-behavior integration. In this context, the actions of PCP-like compounds probably represent the hypo- or hyperactivity of normal, ongoing psychological processes. The discovery of multiple radioligand binding sites has provided an important tool for investigating and separating the mechanisms of action. Finally, the discovery that certain PCP-like compounds potently and selectively block the actions of the N-methyl-D-aspartate (NMDA) type acidic amino acid receptor has provided a possible mechanism to unify and explain some of the diverse actions of PCP. This paper will discuss the current state of these developments in the field of PCP research and present some models to try to explicate the PCP/NMDA interaction.

1. EVIDENCE FOR MULTIPLE RECEPTORS

Specific binding sites for PCP have been shown to exhibit reversible, saturable, and high-affinity binding of [^{3}H]PCP [6, 7]. The binding of [^{3}H]PCP was rapidly inactivated by heat and by proteases, indicating that the binding was to a protein [8]. Furthermore, binding to the site labeled by [^{3}H]PCP was stereoselective [9] and had a unique distribution in the central nervous system [9, 10].

There is still some controversy concerning the number of receptors for phencyclidine and related compounds. Originally, it was believed that sigma opioids, which are opioids that produce psychotomimetic effects, and PCP exert their psychotomimetic effects through a common receptor. However, it is more likely that there are at least two different binding sites because of numerous reports indicating distinct PCP and sigma opioid receptors. There are differences in the structure-activity requirements for binding of PCP, N-allylnormetazocine (SKF-10,047), and dexoxadrol [11–14] and differences in the distribution of binding sites labeled by PCP and sigma opioids [10, 15, 16]. Also, it was shown that haloperidol and chlorpromazine only inhibit the binding the sigma opioids and not that of PCP [17, 18]. So far, there is only one selective ligand for the PCP receptor, MK-801, which like PCP produced stereotyped behavior and ataxia [19]. It has been more difficult to demonstrate a separate physiological role for the sigma opioid receptor.

Part of the difficulty in determining whether there were separate sigma opioid and PCP receptors was due to the lack of selective ligands for sigma opioid receptors. Until recently, the only selective ligands for sigma opioid receptors consisted of haloperidol [13], (+)3-PPP [16, 20], and (−)butaclamol [13]. It was difficult to use haloperidol as a tool to study sigma opioid receptors in vivo because haloperidol is more potent at dopamine receptors than at sigma opioid receptors; its effects could be attributed to dopaminergic effects. (−)Butaclamol was also not the ideal compound to study in behavioral assays because of its poor solubility. (+)3-PPP, which is believed by many to also be a presynaptic dopaminergic receptor agonist, has been shown to generalize to a PCP stimulus [21]. More recently, 1,3-di-o-tolylguanidine (DTG) [22], BMY-14802-1 [23], cinuperone (HR-375) [24], and rimcazole (BW234U) [25] were found to selectively interact with sigma opioid receptors and not PCP receptors. DTG and (+)3-PPP behaviorally appeared to be sigma opioid agonists, because they produced stereotyped behavior and ataxia [19]. These results suggest that there are two receptors, a PCP and sigma opioid receptor, which can mediate similar behavioral effects in the rat. Thus, there may be a role for both the PCP receptor and the sigma opioid receptor in schizophrenia.

2. ENDOGENOUS LIGANDS FOR PCP AND SIGMA OPIOID RECEPTORS

2.1. Alpha- and beta-endopsychosin

The characterization of specific PCP and sigma opioid receptors raises the possibility that there might be an endogenous ligand for PCP and/or sigma opioid receptors. This is particularly interesting in light of the profound behavioral effects of PCP and the finding that PCP can produce a psychosis that is indistinguishable from schizophrenia. Thus, it could be that some type of disturbance in an endogenous PCP system in the CNS might be involved in the pathogenesis of schizophrenia. Characterization of endogenous ligands for the PCP and sigma opioid receptor will also help in the understanding of the physiological role of endogenous PCP and sigma opioid systems.

A factor was isolated from porcine brain, alpha-endopsychosin, that inhibited the binding of [^{3}H]PCP in a concentration-dependent manner [26–28]. This PCP-like factor did not inhibit the binding of [^{3}H]dihydromorphine, [^{3}H]-D-ala$_2$-D-leu$_5$-enkephalin, [^{3}H]ethylketocyclazocine, [^{3}H]diazepam or [^{3}H]neurotensin. These results indicate that the PCP-like material is specific and selective for PCP receptors. Similarly, no inhibition of [^{3}H]haloperidol was apparent with this same active material.

The distribution of the PCP-like activity was determined and found to roughly parallel the distribution of PCP receptors [26]. The highest concentration of alpha-endopsychosin was found in the hippocampus and cortex, while lesser amounts were found in the striatum and very little in the brainstem and cerebellum.

An aliquot of the PCP-like activity was tested to determine whether it could induce PCP-like electrophysiological effects [26]. On hippocampal and cortical cells, the alpha-endopsychosin mimicked the actions of PCP; PCP inhibited spontaneous cortical and hippocampal cell firing. Chromatographic fractions that did not possess PCP-like activity in the radioreceptor assay had no effect on spontaneous neuronal activity.

Similarly, using a behavioral paradigm where unilateral injection of PCP into the substantia nigra induces contralateral turning in rats, alpha-endopsychosin also mimicked the actions of PCP [26]. Once again, chromatographic fractions inactive in the radioreceptor assays elicited no response in this test.

To study the nature of the PCP-like factor, the effect of various enzymes on the PCP-like activity was examined [26]. The potency of the PCP-like activity was markedly reduced following incubation of sample with pronase, carboxypeptidase A, and trypsin. No significant change in activity was seen following incubation with alpha-chymotrypsin. Also, the ability of the PCP-like fractions to inhibit the binding of [^{3}H]PCP was not attenuated following incubation with boiled enzymes. These data indicate that the endogenous material is a protein or a peptide with few aromatic amino acid residues. Spectroscopic analysis confirmed this finding, because no absorbance bands were seen when the sample was scanned at 280 nm and 254 nm [14].

Studies using gel filtration and SDS gel electrophoresis were carried out to determine the relative size of the alpha-endopsychosin [26]. PCP-like fractions were chromatographed over columns of Sephadex G-10, G-25, and G-50. Aliquots of collected fractions were assessed for their ability to inhibit the binding of [^{3}H]PCP. The results indicated that the endogenous PCP-like material has a molecular weight of about 3000. In contrast, studies using SDS gel electrophoresis showed two distinct bands migrating with marker proteins at molecular weights of 3000 and 13,000 [John Bishop, personal communication].

When alpha-endopsychosin was purified, there were three peaks of absorbance at 214 nm [27]. An aliquot of the most active material was hydrolyzed in acid and the amino acid composition determined using OPA detection. It was apparent that the peptide contained approximately 26 amino acids, in close agreement with the molecular weight predicted by Sephadex gel filtration studies. N-terminal analysis revealed that the peptide was blocked at this site. The nature of this blockade is yet to be determined. Studies are under way to determine the amino acid sequence of the peptide.

Another peptide, beta-endopsychosin, was also isolated from porcine brain. It selectively inhibited the binding of [^{3}H]-(+)SKF-10,047 and not that of [^{3}H]PCP [28]. A partial sequence for this peptide was determined and synthesized. This partial sequence inhibited only the binding of [^{3}H]-(+)-SKF-10,047 in a concentration-dependent manner [29].

2.2. Other endogenous ligands for PCP and sigma opioid receptors

Other investigators have also found evidence for endogenous ligands for the PCP and sigma opioid receptors. Like alpha-endopsychosin, Zukin and coworkers have isolated an endogenous material that, like PCP, will inhibit NMDA-induced release of acetylcholine [30].

Two other groups have isolated endogenous ligands for the sigma opioid receptor. Su and coworkers [24] have isolated two endogenous peptides with molecular weights of about 10,000 and 4000. These two peptides inhibited binding of [^{3}H]-(+)SKF10,047 in a concentration-dependent manner, but did not inhibit binding of [^{3}H]PCP and did not inhibit the binding of [^{3}H]-ethylketocyclazocine, [^{3}H]naloxone, or [^{3}H]-D-ala-D-leu-enkephalin. A second group has isolated a compound that is not a peptide, which selectively binds to sigma opioid receptors [31].

3. INTERACTION WITH ACIDIC AMINO ACIDS

3.1. Electrophysiological evidence

PCP and other sigma opioid compounds have been reported to have many electrophysiological actions. For example, in the hippocampus alone, phencyclidine has been reported to increase and decrease spontaneous discharge rates of neurons [32, 33], to decrease the population spike [34–36], to decrease the population excitatory postsynaptic potential (EPSP) [35], to decrease inhibition [34, 36], to raise afterdischarge thresholds [37], to block induction of long-term potentiation (LTP) [38], and to reduce glutamate-induced excitation [35].

Lodge and Anis [39] were the first to show that PCP can block increases in neuronal discharge induced by acidic amino acids. Moreover, this blockade is selective for excitation induced by acidic amino acids that act at the N-methyl-D-aspartate (NMDA) receptor. PCP-like compounds do not block excitation induced by acidic amino acids acting at the kainate (KA) or quisqualate (QA) receptors. Given that PCP will block an action of NMDA, at least four questions arise: How widespread is this effect, how specific is it for a sigma receptor, what is the mechanism of this effect, and how many of the other actions of PCP-like compounds can be explained by antagonism of the actions of NMDA?

Lodge and coworkers have reported that PCP and related compounds block the discharge rate induced by NMDA in unidentified dorsal horn interneurons [39–46], on Renshaw cells in cat and rat in vivo [40–42, 45], and in frog motorneurons in vitro [43]. This effect is also observed in dissociated mouse spinal neurons [51]. The blockade of NMDA-induced excitation has also been shown in neurons in the rat medulla [47] and in rat cortical slices [48–50]. The blockade of NMDA-induced excitation occurs on several neuronal types in different regions of the CNS in several species. This suggests that the effect is generalized to most cells which have NMDA receptors.

The specificity for sigma receptors has been approached in a number of studies. The first question is whether an interaction with mu or kappa opioid receptors plays a role in antagonism of NMDA-induced excitation. Several compounds with potent actions at the mu opioid receptor, such as naloxone, morphine, and levorphanol do not selectively block NMA-induced excitation [43, 46, 52]. In contrast, dextrorphan, the inactive isomer of the analgesic levorphanol, selectively antagonized the electrophysiological effects of NMDA and was seven times more potent than levorphanol [46]. Opioids interacting with the kappa opioid receptor, such as ethylketocyclazocine, U-50,488, and tifluadom, do not antagonize the actions of NMDA is a selective manner [45, 53]. Only opioids that also interact with PCP and sigma opioid receptors, such as dextrorphan and cyclazocine, were able to selectively antagonize NMDA-induced excitation.

Another question is whether compounds structurally diverse from PCP but that share the ability to bind to PCP and sigma opioid receptors can antagonize NMDA-induced excitation. Some dioxolanes, such as etoxadrol and dexoxadrol, which potently bind to the PCP receptor and induce PCP-like stereotyped behavior and ataxia, selectively reduced NMA (N-methyl-D,L,-aspartate)-induced excitation. The (−)-isomer of dexoxadrol, levoxadrol, is much less potent in antagonizing NMA effects [44]. Another structurally dissimilar compound, 2-methyl-3,3-diphenyl-3-propanolamine (2-MDP), and, in particular, the (−)-isomer, is a selective antagonist of NMA-induced excitation [47]. In addition, some benz(f)isoquinolines, such as LY154045, have actions similar to PCP and other sigma opioid compounds. LY154045 selectively antagonized NMA-induced excitation, but the behaviorally inactive analogue, LY154005, was inactive [54]. The ability of structurally diverse compounds, which share the quality of being able to act at PCP receptors, to block the effects of NMDA strongly suggests that a PCP or sigma opioid receptor is mediating the antagonism of NMDA responses.

Support for a role of the PCP receptor in mediating the antagonism of NMDA is found in the similar stereoselectivity in binding to the PCP receptor and antagonizing NMDA-induced excitation. The (+)-isomer of ketamine, which is the behaviorally active isomer, is 2.5–3 times more potent than (−)-ketamine [40]. Cis-N-(1-phenyl-4-methylcyclohexyl) piperidine (GK5) was more potent than the trans-enantiomer (GK4) [41]. In addition, (+)-N-(1-phenylcyclohexyl)-3-methyl-piperidine (PCMP) is more potent than (−)-PCMP [41]. The (−) isomer of cyclazocine, a sigma opioid, was twice as potent as the (+) isomer [43]. Both isomers of SKF-10,047 selectively antagonize NMDA-induced excitation, but the (+)-isomer appeared to be slightly more potent [44]. In each case, the more potent isomer in antagonizing NMDA-induced excitation was also the more potent isomer in the PCP radioreceptor assay and in behavioral assays.

The next question is whether only PCP or both PCP and sigma opioid receptors mediate the antagonism of NMDA. MK-801, which selectively binds to PCP receptors versus sigma opioid receptors, is a potent NMDA antagonist [55]. It is clear, then, that PCP receptors can mediate the antagonism of NMDA-induced excitation, but the actions of sigma opioid receptor agonists are not yet defined.

As was mentioned earlier, PCP-like compounds have been reported to have many electrophysiological actions. Overall, competitive NMDA antagonists have been directly compared to PCP-like compounds for only a few of these actions. PCP has been reported to block the induction of long-term potentiation (LTP) in vivo and in vitro [38]. The induction of LTP is also blocked by the competitive NMDA antagonists 2-amino-5-phosphonopentanoate (AP5) and 2-amino-7-phosphonoheptanoate (AP7) in vivo and in vitro [56–58]. PCP, in vivo and in vitro, has been shown to strongly reduce the population spike in CA1 neurons evoked by stimulation of the Schaffer collateral/commissural fibers. The average dose, i.v., required to reduce the population spike by half is 1–2 mg/kg [34, 35]. In the in vitro hippocampal slice, only high doses of PCP 100 μM has been reported to reduce the amplitude of the population spike [36, 38] (by about 25%). Since the in vivo effect can be blocked by some manipulations that affect norepinephrine, the effect seen in vivo may be indirect [34, 35]. PCP can also reduce the slope of the rising phase of the population EPSP, but this was much less sensitive than the population spike. PCP, i.v., in doses from 1.9–7.5 mg/kg decreased the slope by only 8%–40% [36, 38]. In general, AP5 or AP7 do not affect the size of the population EPSP [56, 57], but exceptions have been noted [59]. No effect on the primary population spike has been reported. Ketamine has been observed to block polysynaptic excitation in the spinal cord to a greater extent than monosynaptic excitation [40]. AP5 and AP7 have also been reported to preferentially block polysynaptic excitation. In general, the effects of PCP-like compounds appear to be mimicked by competitive NMDA antagonists. However, the ability of competitive NMDA antagonists to mimic many of the effects of PCP-like compounds has not been examined. Studies of this kind will be important to determine the mechanisms of action of PCP-like compounds as well as the function of NMDA receptors in the CNS.

3.2. Neurochemical evidence

Ketamine [60] and PCP [61] have been shown to antagonize NMDA-stimulated release of ACh from cortical tissue. The NMDA subclass of acidic amino acid receptors appears to mediate the excitatory effects of glutamate on striatal cholinergic interneurons because the rank order of potency of agonists, the antagonism by magnesium, and the antagonism by 2-amino-5-phosphonopentano (AP5) [62] are all characteristic of the NMDA receptor. PCP-like drugs antagonize the stimulation of ACh release by NMDA in a stereospecific manner, and this inhibition does not appear to be competitive [61]. There is also a correlation between the ability of these drugs to interact with the PCP receptor and their ability to inhibit NMDA-induced release of ACh [63]. PCP does not antagonize the release of ACh stimulated by kainate or quisqualate [63]. The PCP-induced inhibition of NMDA-stimulated ACh release is not reversed by haloperidol [61], which indicates that antagonism of NMDA-induced release of ACh may not be mediated by the sigma opioid receptor and is likely to be mediated by the PCP receptor.

Glutamate stimulates dopamine release in the striatum in a calcium-dependent and TTX-sensitive manner [64]. This can be antagonized by PCP [61].

There is also a good correlation between the ability of these compounds to interact with the PCP receptor and their ability to inhibit NMDA-induced release of dopamine, but PCP and PCP-like drugs are less potent at blocking dopamine release than release of ACh [63].

Other interactions between PCP and NMDA have been found. PCP non-competitively antagonizes the efflux of sodium-22 [65]. PCP has been shown to antagonize NMDA-mediated excitotoxicity in the chick retina [66]. The protective effect of PCP-like compounds and competitive NMDA antagonists against neuronal damage in models of ischemia has also been documented [66]. Both MK-801 and CPP (3-(2-carboxypiperazin-4-yl)propyl-1-phosphonic acid), a competitive NMDA antagonist, have been shown to afford some cellular protection following bilateral carotid occlusion in the gerbil [67, 68], while AP7 has been shown to protect against ischemic damage in the rat [69].

3.3. Behavioral evidence

In addition to the electrophysiological and biochemical studies, there are behavioral studies indicating an interaction between PCP and acidic amino acids transmitters. PCP and AP7 have similar anticonvulsant properties: both antagonize chemically-induced [70, 71] and electroconvulsant shock-induced seizures [72, 73] in mice. AP7 and ketamine have also been shown to antagonize NMDA-induced seizures in mice [74, 75]. In addition, PCP and AP7 blocked the biting and scratching behavior in mice induced by intrathecal injection of NMDA, suggestive of antinociceptive activity [76].

If the behavioral actions of PCP are due to antagonism of NMDA receptor-mediated transmission, then competitive NMDA antagonists should induce PCP-like behaviors. PCP produces certain characteristic behaviors in animals, including catalepsy and stereotyped behavior in pigeons [77] and stereotyped behavior and ataxia in rats [10, 78]. The ability of PCP analogs to produce these behaviors correlates with their potency in inhibiting binding of [^{3}H]-PCP [10]. Recently, AP5 has been shown to induce PCP-like catalepsy and stereotyped behavior in pigeons in a time- and dose-dependent manner following either i.c.v. or i.m. administration [79, 80]. Two other NMDA-selective antagonists, AP7 and CPP, produce PCP-like stereotyped behavior and ataxia in rats [81, 82]. AP7 produced this behavioral response in a stereoselective manner and in a time-dependent manner consistent with concentrations in the cerebrospinal fluid [83]. These results indicate that competitive NMDA antagonists (i.e., AP5, AP7, CPP) produce similar behaviors to those produced by PCP-like compounds in rats and pigeons. This supports an NMDA receptor-mediated mechanism in the behavioral effects induced by PCP.

Competitive NMDA antagonists have been tested for their ability to produce a PCP-like cue in discriminitive stimulus paradigms in pigeons and rats. AP5 produced PCP-appropriate responding in pigeons at doses similar to that used to induce catalepsy [80]. Comparable results were obtained with AP7 in rats trained to discriminate PCP from saline [84]. In these experiments, AP7 administered i.c.v. shared some discriminative stimulus properties with systemically administered PCP. These results are, again, consistent with antagonism of the NMDA receptor as mediating many of the behaviors induced by PCP.

3.4. Possible mechanisms of the interaction with acidic amino acids

The behavioral comparisons, together with the biochemical and electrophysiological studies, provide convincing evidence that an important physiological action of PCP-like compounds is the specific and potent antagonism of NMDA receptor-mediated neurotransmission. The mechanism by which PCP-like compounds antagonize NMDA-induced excitation has been addressed in a number of studies. It seems likely that the interaction occurs at the NMDA receptor/channel complex, since the autoradiographic distribution of [^{3}H]TCP and NMDA-sensitive L-[^{3}H]glutamate binding sites are very similar [85, 86].

Initial attempts using ionophoretic application of compounds to determine whether the antagonism was competitive or noncompetitive suggested that a parallel (competitive) shift in the NMA dose-response curve occurred [42]. However, studies using more quantitative techniques have indicated that a non-competitive type of interaction occurs [49, 87]. Magnesium ions can also selectively block NMA-induced responses, but ketamine and magnesium ions appear to act at separate sites [49, 87]. However, the blockade induced by magnesium ions, and that produced by ketamine and PCP, are similar in that both types of blockade are highly voltage-sensitive and are relieved at membrane potentials positive to the normal resting state [51]. A voltage-dependent blockade is often presumed to imply a blockade of the ion channel [51]. Moreover, the gradual development of the blockade during repetitive stimulation has been suggested to indicate an open-channel blockade [51]. Open-channel blockade is defined by the occurrence of agonist-dependent (use-dependent) blockade. Use-dependent blockade has been shown with MK-801 in vitro [55; Lodge, personal communication], but not in vivo [Lodge, personal communication]. Use-dependent blockade was not seen with PCP or ketamine, in vivo or in cortical wedges in vitro. However, agonist-dependent blockade, and unblockade, have been shown for ketamine in dissociated mouse spinal neurons [88]. Evidence for open-channel blockade by PCP of the glutamate-activated currents in locust muscle has also been reported [89]. However, since the acidic amino acid receptors in locust muscle are not sensitive to NMDA, it is not clear what relevance these results have.

The actions of PCP-like compounds on NMDA responses are voltage-sensitive and agonist- (or use-) dependent. These results are often taken to imply that a compound is blocking the ion channel by being an intrachannel plug.

However, it is possible to imagine that voltage dependence could be due to an element of the receptor/channel complex, outside of the channel itself, that is influenced by voltage changes. This could, perhaps, be as simple as the polar head-group of phosphatidylserine, which might shift position depending on membrane potential and cover or uncover a part of the binding site. Agonist dependence may also be explained without recourse to intrachannel blockade. Agonist dependence could be a reflection of a change in the binding site conformation that increases the affinity of the receptor for PCP-like compounds. That is, the binding of an NMDA agonist increases the affinity for PCP-like compounds. In fact, binding experiments indicate that NMDA agonists change the Kd for PCP-like compounds without much change in the Bmax.

Although the data may be explained without postulating intrachannel blockade, an increase in affinity alone does not seem enough to explain the use-dependent unblockade reported by MacDonald and Miljkovic [88]. This fact seems to return us to a requirement for an occluded receptor. However, in place of a fully occluded receptor, as an intrachannel binding site implies, a partially occluded receptor may be postulated to explain both the physiological and binding data. In this model, NMDA agonists modify the conformation of the receptor channel complex to allow more of the points of attachment on the PCP-like molecule easy access to the binding site. When the NMDA agonist dissociates from its binding site, the PCP binding site is once again partially occluded, trapping part of the PCP molecule. Such a model also predicts that different PCP-like molecules would exhibit different degrees of use-dependency based on whether the occluded part of the binding site is necessary for their initial binding. This model of a partially occluded receptor can explain why MK-801 appears to be more use-dependent than PCP or ketamine.

Additional insight into the functional interaction may be gained by comparing the actions of PCP to those of noncompetitive modulators at other receptor/channel complexes. The effects of modulators at the GABA receptor/channel complex have been extensively studied. These modulators include the benzodiazepines, picrotoxin and cage convulsants, barbiturates, penicillin, and ethanol. Classically, benzodiazepines have been regarded as allosteric modulators of the GABA receptor, while picrotoxin has been regarded as a channel blocker. However, channel blockade as a mechanism of action of picrotoxin has become less tenable [90–92]. It has been suggested, in fact, that penicillin is more likely to act by blocking the channel than is picrotoxin [90]. The actions of barbiturates and ethanol are less defined. In radioligand binding studies, benzodiazepines have been shown to affect the binding of GABA and, in turn, GABA affects the binding of benzodiazepines [93]. With respect to picrotoxin, GABA has been reported to modulate picrotoxin-like binding, but picrotoxin has generally been reported not to affect GABA binding [94, 95, but see 96]. Barbiturates are known to enhance the binding of GABA [95]. As of yet, the only interaction known between NMDA and PCP is that NMDA compounds modulate PCP-like binding. Effects of PCP on NMDA-sensitive binding have not been reported. Thus, given the known data, PCP is most like picrotoxin. It is interesting, then, to note again that both picrotoxin and PCP have been characterized as channel blockers. However, while NMDA enhances PCP-like binding by an effect on the Kd, GABA decreases picrotoxin binding by reducing the Bmax [93]. It is clearly too early to say which modulators of GABA are most similar to PCP-like compounds, but the analogy with the GABA receptor/channel complex will be very useful in suggesting future experiments. The comparison with picrotoxin, however, predicts another fact of clinical importance. It is difficult to imagine an antagonist of an intrachannel plug, since the antagonist itself must bind within the channel and is likely to, at least partially, block it. However, it is known that alpha-substituted gammabutyrolactones act as picrotoxin antagonists and act at the picrotoxin-sensitive binding site [97]. This suggests that PCP antagonists can exist. PCP antagonists will be very important therapeutic agents.

4. CONCLUSION

In this paper we have reviewed evidence for multiple receptors for PCP and sigma opioid compounds, for the existence of endogenous ligands for PCP and sigma opioids, and for the interactions of PCP-like compounds with actions of the NMDA type acidic amino acid receptor. As a whole, this evidence leads to the conclusion that PCP compounds have selective actions in the CNS. The profusion of effects reported for PCP may now begin to be more simply categorized. The existence of two binding sites for PCP and sigma opioid compounds suggests that some of the actions of PCP and other compounds can be dissociated into actions at two sites. Selective agonists such as MK-801 can be utilized to start to determine the actions at the specific receptors. However, selective PCP and sigma opioid antagonists will be critical for a complete assessment of the role of the different receptors.

The finding that endogenous ligands exist confirms that PCP and sigma opioids are modulating some normal neural processes. However, it is not clear that all the effects of synthetic compounds are via these normal processes. The investigation of the electrophysiological, neurochemical, and behavioral actions of the endogenous compounds will determine which of the effects of PCP and sigma opioids are physiologically important.

The understanding that PCP-like compounds, but apparently not sigma opioids, block the actions of NMDA agonists helps to unify a large number of diverse actions of PCP. The similar distribution of PCP and NMDA-type binding sites in the CNS suggests that a single mechanism of action of PCP may account for a number of effects. However, although one mechanism may account for many effects, PCP-like compounds have been shown to have numerous actions, and future research must be directed toward determining how many of the actions of PCP can be mimicked by NMDA antagonists. In particular, there are three general effects of PCP-like compounds that are not obviously related to NMDA antagonism. 1) PCP has actions on peripheral organs [98–100]. The peripheral actions of acidic amino acids have not been extensively examined but are usually considered to be minimal. The interaction between PCP and NMDA in the CNS provides a strong impetus to look for interactions between PCP and NMDA on peripheral organs. 2) PCP also has effects at the nicotinic receptor/channel complex in several muscle preparations [101–103]. Whether this is indirectly mediated by NMDA receptors is not known. 3) A third effect of PCP in which a PCP/NMDA interaction is not obvious is the blockade of some potassium channels [104–106]. The ability of PCP to block potassium channels has been used to explain the transmitter releasing properties of PCP, as well as its psychotomimetic property. Data from two laboratories indicate that compounds which act at the NMDA recognition site do not affect PCP-sensitive potassium channels [107; D. Bartschat, unpublished observations].

Perhaps the most interesting direction for future research will be in determining the behavioral, neurochemical, and electrophysiological actions of the endogenous ligands themselves. It is certain that the knowledge gained will contribute to our understanding of the neural control of behavior and of the processes underlying schizophrenia.

REFERENCES

1. Greifenstein, F.E., Devault, M., Yoshitake, J. and Gajewski, J.E. (1985). A study of 1-arylcyclohexylamine for anesthesia. Anesthesia Anesth. Analg. 37, 283–294.
2. Luby, E.D., Cohen, R.C., Rosenbaum, G., Gottlieb, J.S. and Kelly, R. (1959). Study of a new schizophrenomimetic drug: Sernyl. Arch. Neurol. Psychiat. 81, 363–369.
3. Randrup, A. and Munkvad, I. (1967). Stereotypic activities produced by amphetamine in several species and man. Psychopharmacologica 11, 300.
4. Cohen, B.D., Luby, E.D., Rosenbaum, E.D. and Gottlieb (1960). Combined sernyl and sensory deprivation. Comp. Psychiatr. 1, 135.
5. Allen, R.M. and Young, S.J. (1978). Phencyclidine-induced psychosis. Am. J. Psychiatr. 135, 1081.
6. Vincent, J.P., Cavey, D., Kamenka, J.M., Geneste, P. and Lazdunski, M. (1979). Interaction of phencyclidine ("angle dust") with a specific receptor in rat brain membranes. Proc. Natl. Acad. Sci. USA 76, 4678–4682.
7. Zukin, S.R. and Zukin, R.S. (1978). Specific [^{3}H]-phencyclidine binding in rat central nervous system. Proc. Natl. Acad. Sci. USA 76, 5372–5376.
8. Vignon, J., Vincent, J.P., Bidard, J.N., Kamenka, J.M., Geneste, P., Monier, S. and Lazdunski, M. (1982). Biochemical properties of the brain phencyclidine receptor. Eur. J. Pharmacol. 81, 531–542.
9. Quirion, R., Hammer, R.P., Jr., Herkenham, M. and Pert, C.B. (1981). Phencyclidine (angle dust)/sigma "optiate" visualization by tritium-sensitive film. Proc. Natl. Acad. Sci. USA 78, 5881–5885.
10. Contreras, P.C., Quirion, R., O'Donohue, T.L. (1986). Autoradiographic distribution of phencyclidine receptors in the rat brain using [^{3}H]1-(1-(2-thienyl)cyclohexyl)piperidine (^{3}H)TCP). Neurosci. Lett. 67, 101–106.
11. Su, T.-P. (1982). Evidence for sigma opioid receptor: Binding of [^{3}H]SKF 10,047 to etorphine-inaccessible sites in guinea pig brain. J. Pharmacol. Exp. Ther. 223, 284–290.
12. Martin, B.R., Katzen, J.S., Woods, J.A., Tripathi, J.L., Harris, L.S. and May, E.L. (1984). Steroisomers of [^{3}H]-N-allylnormetazocine bind to different sites in mouse brain. J. Pharmocol. Exp. Ther. 231, 539–544.
13. Tam, S.W. (1985). (+)-[^{3}H]SKF 10,047, (+)[^{3}H]ethylketocyclazocine, mu, kappa delta and

phencyclidine binding sites in guinea pig brain membranes. Eur. J. Pharmacol. 109, 33–41.
14. Contreras, P.C., DiMaggio, D.A. and O'Donohue, T.L. (1987). An endogenous ligand for the sigma opioid binding site. Synapse 1, 57–61.
15. Pilapil, C., Contreras, P.C., O'Donohue, T.L. and Quirion, R. (1986). Autoradiographic distribution of [^{3}H]dexoxadrol, a phencyclidine-related ligand, binding sites in rat and human brain. Neurosci. Lett. 56, 1–6.
16. Gundlach, A.L., Largent, B.L., Snyder, S.H. (1985). Phencyclidine and sigma opiate receptors in the brain: Biochemical and autoradiographical differentiation. Eur. J. Pharmacol. 113, 465.
17. Tam, S.W. (1983). Naloxone-inaccessible sigma receptor in rat central nervous system. Pro. Natl. Acad. Sci. USA 80, 6703–6707.
18. Tam, S.W. and Cook, L. (1984). Sigma opiates and certain antipsychotic drugs mutually inhibit (+)-[^{3}H]SKF 10,047 and [^{3}H]haloperidol binding in guinea pig brain membranes. Proc. Natl. Acad. Sci. USA 81, 5618–5621.
19. Contreras, P.C., Lair, C.C., Compton, R.P., Monahan, J.B. and O'Donohue, T.L. (1987). Comparison of behavioral effects of selective PCP and sigma opioid ligands. ASPET Abst., in press.
20. Contreras, P.C., Quirion, R. and O'Donohue, T.L. (1985). Comparison of the binding and regional distribution of sigma opioid and phencyclidine receptors. Soc. Neurosci. Abst. 11, 583.
21. Steinfels, G.F., Tam, S.W. and Cook, L. (1987). (+)-3-(3 hydroxyphenyl)-N-(1-propyl)-piperidine [(+)-3-PPP] but not (−)-3-PPP produces (+)-N-allynormetazocine-like (SKF 10,047) discriminate stimuli. Life Sci., in press.
22. Weber, E., Sonders, M., Quarum, M., McLean, S., Pou, S. and Keana, J.F. (1986). 1,3-Di(2-^{3}H)tolyl)guanidine: A selective ligand that labels sigma-type receptors for psychotomimetic opiates and antipsychotic drugs. Proc. Nat. Acad. Sci. 83, 8784–8788.
23. Taylor, D.P. and Dekleva, J. (1987). The potential antipsychotic BMY14802 selectively binds to sigma sites. Fed. Proc. 46, 1304.
24. Su, T-P., Weissmanm A.D. and Yeh S.-Y. (1986). Endogenous ligands for sigma opioid receptors in brain ("Sigmaphin"): Evidence from binding assays. Life Sci. 38, 2199–2210.
25. Ferris, R.M., Tang, R.L., Chang, K.J. and Russell, A. (1986). Evidence that the potential antipsychotic agent rimcazole (BW 234U) is a specific, competitive antagonist of sigma sites in brain. Life Sci. 39, 2329–2337.
26. Quirion, R., DiMaggio, D.A., French, E.D., Contreras, P.C., Shiloach, J. Pert, C.B., Everist, J., Pert, A. and O'Donohue, T.L. (1984). Evidence for an endogenous peptide ligand for the phencyclidine receptor. Peptides 5, 967–973.
27. DiMaggio, D.A., Contreras, P.C., Quirion, R. and O'Donohue, T.L. (1986). Isolation and identification of an endogenous ligand for the phencyclidine receptor in phencyclidine: An update. Clouet D.H., ed., NIDA, MD, pp. 24–37.
28. Contreras, P.C., DiMaggio, D.A., Quirion, R., and O'Donohue, T.L. (1985). An endogenous peptide ligand for the PCP/sigma opioid receptor. In *Neural and endocrine peptides and receptors*, Moody T., ed., Plenum Press, New York, pp. 1–13.
29. DiMaggio, D.A., Contreras, P.C. and O'Donohue, T.L. (1987). Distinct endogenous ligands for PCP and sigma opioid receptors. Tenth Am. Peptide Symp., in press.
30. Sircar, R., Samaan, G.H., Nichtenhauser, R.G., Snell, L.D., Monson, K.C., Rivier, J., Vale, W., Zukin, R.S. and Zukin, S.R. (1986). The brain PCP/sigma receptor and its exogenous and endogenous ligands: Functional relationship to NMDA. Soc. Neurosci. Abst. 12, 59.
31. Sonders, M., Campbell, B. and Weber, E. (1986). Identification and partial characterization of an endogenous compound that competitively and reversibly inhibited [^{3}H]-DTG from binding to the haloperidol-sensitive sigma (opioid) receptor, Soc. Neurosci. Abst. 12, 172.
32. Rose, G., Pang, K., Palmer, M. and Freedman, R. (1984). Differential effects of phencyclidine upon hippocampal complex-spike and theta neurons. Neurosci. Lett. 45, 141–161.
33. Bickford, P.C., Palmer, M.R., Rice, K.C., Hoffer, B.J. and Freedman, R. (198). Electrophysiological effects of phencyclidine on rat hippocampal pyramidal neurons. Neuropharmacology, 20, 733–743.
34. Stringer, J.L. and Guyenet, P.C. (1982). Effect of phencyclidines on hippocampal pyramidal cells. Br. Res. 252, 343–352.

35. Raja, S.N. and Guyenet, P.G. (1982). Action of phencyclidine on synpatic transmission in the hippocampus. Brain Res. 236, 289–304.
36. Bourne, G.W., Theoret, Y., Esplin, B. and Capek, R. (1983). Naunyn-Schmiedeberg's Arch. Pharmacol. 323, 168–172.
37. Matsuzaki, M. and Dowling, K.C. (1984). Phencyclidine (PCP): Effects on limbic afterdischarges in the rhesus monkey. Br. Res. Bull. 13, 635–641.
38. Stringer, J.L., Greenfield, L.J., Hackett, J.T. and Guyenet, P.G. (1983). Blockade of long-term potentiation by phencyclidine and opiates in the hippocampus in vivo and in vitro. Br. Res. 280, 127–138.
39. Lodge, D. and Anis, N.A. (1982). Effects of phencyclidine on excitatory amino acid activation of spinal interneurones in the cat. Eur. J. Pharmacol. 77, 203–204.
40. Lodge, D., Anis, N.A. and Burton, N.R. (1982). Effects of optical isomers of ketamine on excitation of cat and rat spinal neurones by amino acids and acetylcholine. Neurosci. Lett. 29, 281–286.
41. Berry, S.C., Burton, N.R., Anis, N.A. and Lodge, D. (1983). Stereoselective effect of two phencyclidine derivatives on N-methylaspartate excitation of apical neurones in the cat and rat. Eur. J. Pharmacol. 96, 261–267.
42. Anis, N.A., Berry, S.C., Burton, N.R. and Loge, D. (1983). The dissociative anesthetics, ketamine and phencyclidine, selectively reduce excitation of central mammalian neurones by N-methyl-aspartate, Br. J. Pharmcol. 79, 565–576.
43. Lodge, D., Berry, S.C., Church, J., Martin, D., McGhee, A., Lai, H-M. and Thomson, A.M. (1984). Isomers of cyclazocine as excitatory amino acid antagonists. Neuropeptides 5, 245–248.
44. Berry, S.C., Anis, N.A. and Lodge, D. (1984). The effect of the dioxolanes on amino acid induced excitation in the mammalian spinal cord. Brain Res. 307, 85–90.
45. Berry, S.C., Dawkins, S.L. and Lodge, D. (1984). Comparison of O- and kopiate receptor ligands as excitatory amino acid antagonists. Br. J. Pharmacol. 83, 179–185.
46. Church, J., Lodge, D. and Berry, S.C. (1985). Differential effects of dextrorphan and levorphanol on the excitation of rat spinal neurons by amino acids. Eur. J. Pharmacol. 111, 185–190.
47. Black, J.C., Davies, S.N., Church, J., Martin, D. and Lodge, D. (1986). 2-methyl-3,3-diphenyl-3-propanolamine (2-MDP) selectively antagonizes N-methyl-aspartate (NMDA). Pharmacol. Biochem. Behav. 24, 23–25.
48. Thomson, A.M., West, D.C. and Lodge, D. (1985). An N-methylaspartate receptor-mediated synapse in rat cerebral cortex: A site of action of ketamine? Nature 313, 479–481.
49. Harrison, N.L. and Simmonds, M.A. (1985). Quantitative studies on some antagonists of N-methyl-D-aspartate in slices of rat cerebral cortex. Br. J. Pharmacol. 84, 381–391.
50. Thomson, A.M. and Lodge, D. (1985). Selective blockade of an excitatory synapse in rat cerebral cortex by the sigma opiate cyclazocine: An intracellular, in vitro study. Neurosci. Lett. 54, 21–26.
51. Honey, C.R., Miljkovic, Z. and MacDonald, J.F. (1985). Ketamine and phencyclidine couse a voltage-dependent block of responses to L-aspartic acid. Neurosci. Lett. 61, 135–139.
52. Anis, N.A., Berry, S.C., Burton, N.R. and Lodge, D. (1983). Cyclazocine, like ketamine, blocks N-methyl-aspartate actions on spinal neurones in cat and rat. J. Physiol. 338, 37–38P.
53. Parsons, C.G., Martin, D., Franklin, R.J., Wood, J.L. and Headley, P.M. (1986). Do kappa opioids mimic sigma agonists as amino acid antagonists? Neuropharmacology. 25, 217–220.
54. Berry, S.C. and Lodge, D. (1984). Benz (f) isoquinolines as excitatory amino acids antagonists: An indication of their mechanism of action? Biochem. Pharmacol. 33, 3829–3832.
55. Wong, E.H., Kemp, J.A., Priestley, T., Knight, A.R., Woodruff, G.A. and Iversen, L.L. (1986). The anticonvulsant MK-801 is a potent N-methyl-D-aspartate antagonist. Proc. Natl. Acad. Sci. USA 83, 7104–7109.
56. Collingridge, G.L., Kehl, S.J. and McLennan, H. (1983). Excitatory amino acids in synaptic transmission in the Schaffer collateral-commissural pathway of the rat hippocampus. J. Physiol. 334, 33–46.
57. Harris, E.W., Ganong, A.H. and Cotman, C.W. (1984). Long-term potentiation in the hippocampus involves activation of N-methyl-D-aspartate receptors. Brain Res. 323, 132–137.
58. Morris, R.G., Anderson, E., Lynch, G.S. and Baudry, M. (1986). Selective impairment of

learning and blockade of long-term potentiation by an N-methyl-D-aspartate receptor antagonist, A5. Nature 27, 774–776.
59. Hablitz, J.J. and Langmoen, I.A. (1986). N-methyl-D-aspartate receptor antagonists reduce synaptic excitation in the hippocampus. J. Neurosci. 6, 102–106.
60. Johnston, G.A. and Lodge, D. (1983). Ketamine and magnesium selectively block the N-methylaspartate-evoked release of acetylcholine from rat cortex slices in vitro. J. Physiol. (Lond.) 349, 15p.
61. Snell, L.D. and Johnson, K.M. (1985). Antagonism of N-methyl-D-aspartate-induced transmitter release in the rat striatum by phencyclidine-like drugs and its relationship to turning behavior. J. Pharmacol. Exp. Ther. 235, 50–57.
62. Lehmann, J. and Scatton, D. (1982). Characterization of the excitatory amino acid receptor-mediated release of [^{3}H]acetylcholine from rat striatal slices. Brain Res. 252, 77–89.
63. Snell, L.D. and Johnson, K.M. (1986). Characterization of the inhibition of excitatory amino acid-induced neurotransmitter release in the rat striatum by phencyclidine-like drugs. J. Pharmacol. Exp. Ther. 238, 938–946.
64. Roberts, P.J. and Anderson, S.D. (1979). Stimulatory effect of L-glutamate and related amino acids on [^{3}H]dopamine release from rat striatum: An in vitro model for glutamate actions. J. Neurochem. 32, 1539–1545.
65. Pullan, L.M. and Hood, W.F. (1987). Phencyclidine (PCP) inhibition of N-methyl-D-aspartate stimulated sodium flux. J. Neurochem. in press.
66. Olney, J.W., Price, M.T.,Fuller, T.A., Labruyere, J., Samson, L., Carpenter, M. and Mahan, K. (1986). The anti-excitotoxic effect of fertain anesthetics, analgesics and sedative-hypnotics. Neurosci. Lett. 68, 29–34.
67. Foster, A.C., Gill R., Iverson, L.L. and Woodruff, G.N. (1986). Systemic administration of MK-801 protects agsinst ischaemia-induced hippocampal neurodegeneration in the gerbil.
68. Gerhardt. S.C., Bernar, P.S., Pastor, G. and Boast, C.A. (1986). Effects of systemic administration of the NMDA antagonist, CPP, on ischemic brain damage in gerbils. Soc. Neurosci. Abst. 12, 59.
69. Simon, R.P., Swan, J.H., Griffiths, T. and Meldrum, B.S. (1984). Blockade of N-methyl-D-aspartate receptors may protect against ischemic damage in the brain. Science 226, 850–852.
70. Croucher, M.J., Collins, J.F. and Meldrum, B.S. (1982). Anticonvulsant action of excitatory amino acid antagonists. Science 216, 899–901.
71. Hayes, B.A. and Balstar, R.L. (1985). Anticonvulsant properties of phencyclidine-like drugs in mice. Eur. J. Pharmcol. 117, 121–125.
72. Leccese, A.P., Marquis, K.L., Mattis, A. and Moreton, J.E. (1986). The convulsant and anticonvulsant effect of phencyclidine (PCP) and PCP analogues in the rat. Behav. Brain Res. 19, 163–169.
73. DeSarro, G., Meldrum, B.s. and Reavill, G. (1985). Anticonvulsant action of 2-amino-7-phosphonoheptanoic acid in the rat substantia nigra. Eur. J. Pharmacol. 106, 175–179.
74. Czuczwar, S.J. and Meldrum, B.S. (1982). Protection against chemically induced seizures by 2-amino-7-phosphonoheptanoic acid. Eur. J. Pharmacol. 83, 335–338.
75. Amrick, C.L., Bernard, P.S. and Bennett, D.A. (1986), A comparison of PCP-like compounds in two in vivo models for NMDA antagonism. The Pharmacologist 28, 114.
76. Aaronsen, L.M. and Wilcox, G.L. (1987). Phencyclidine selectively blocks a spinal action of N-methyl-D-aspartate in mice. Neurosci. Lett. 67, 191–197.
77. Koek, W., Woods, J.H., Rice, K.C., Jacobson, A.E., Huguenin, P.N. and Burke, T.R., Jr. (1984). Phencyclidine-induced catalepsy in pigeons: Specificity and stereoselectivity. Eur. J. Pharmacol. 106, 635–638.
78. Koek, W., Kleer, E., Mudar, P.J. and Woods, J.H. (1986). Phencyclidine-like catalepsy induced by the excitatory amino acid antagonist DL-2-amino-5-phosphonovalerate. Behav. Brain Res. 19, 257–259.
79. Sturgeon, R.D., Fessler, R.G. and Meltzer, H.Y. (1979). Behavioral rating scales for assessing phencyclidine-induced locomotor activity, stereotyped behavior and ataxia in rats. Eur. J. Pharmacol. 59, 169–179.
80. Koek, W., Woods, J.H. and Ornstein, P. (1986). Phencyclidine-like behavioral effects in pigeons induced by systemic administration of the excitatory amino acid antagonist, 2-amino-5-phosphonovalerate. Life Sci. 39, 973–978.

81. Bernard, P.S. and Bennett, D.A. (1986). Similarity of behavioral effects produced by an N-methyl-D-aspartate antagonist and phencyclidine-type drugs. Soc. Neurosci. Abst. 12, 60.
82. Compton, R.P., Contreras, P.C., O'Donohue, T.L. and Monahan, J.B. (1987). The N-methyl-D-aspartate antagonist, 2-amino-7-phosphonoheptanoate, produces phencyclidine-like behavioral effects in rats. Eur. J. Pharmacol., in press.
83. Compton, R.P., Kreiter, P.A., Smith, R.G., Harken, R.D. and Monahan, J.B. (1987). Determination of the pharmacokinetics of 2-amino-7-phosphonoheptanoate in plasma and cerebrospinal fluid. *The Third International Symposium on the Neuronal Control of Bodily Functions*, in press.
84. Willetts, J., Chapman, M.Y. and Balstar, R.L. (1986). Discriminative stimulus effects of 2-amino-7-phosphonoheptanoic acid (APH) in phencyclidine trained rats. Soc. Neurosci. Abst. 12, 909.
85. Monaghan, D.T., Nguyen, L. and Cotman, C.W. (1986). Localization of NMDA, PCP and AmPA receptors: Comparison of their distributions and the effects of selective lesions. Soc. Neurosci. Abs. 12, 1385.
86. Penney, J.B., Maragos, W.F., Chu, D.C.M. and Young, A.B. (1986). Correlation between localization of [^{3}H]TCP and NMDA binding sites. Soc. Neurosci. Abs. 12, 1285.
87. Lodge, D. and Johnston, G.A. (1985). Effect of ketamine on amino acid-evoked release of acetylcholine from rat cerebral cortex in vitro. Neurosci Lett. 56, 371–375.
88. MacDonald, J.F. and Miljkovic, Z. (1986). The voltage- and agonist-dependent blockade of excitatory amino acid currents by the dissociative anesthetic ketamine. Soc. Neurosci. Abs. 12, 959.
89. Idriss, M. and Albuquerque, E.X. (1985). Phencyclidine (PCP) blocks glutamate-activated postsynaptic currents. FEBS Letts. 189, 150–156.
90. Simmonds, M.A. (198). Evidence that bicuculline and picrotoxin act at separate sites to antagonize γ-aminobutyroic acid in rat cuneate nucleus. Neuropharmacology., 19, 39–45.
91. Barker, J.L. and Owen, D.G. (1986). In *Benzodiazepine/GABA Receptors and Chloride Channels*, R.W. Olsen and J.C. Venter, eds., pp. 135–166.
92. Ticku, M.K. (1986). In *Benzodiazepine/GABA Receptors and Chloride Channels*, R.W. Olsen and J.C. Venter, eds., pp. 195–208.
93. Ticku, M.K. (1983). Benzodiazepine-GABA receptor-ionophore complex. Neuropharmacology., 22, 1459–1470.
94. Olsen, R.W. (1981). GABA-benzodiazepine-barbiturate receptor interactions. J. Neurochem. 37, 1–13.
95. Karobath, M., Drezley, G.P. and Supavilai, P. (1981). Modulation by picrotoxin and IPTBO of [^{3}H]flunitrazepam binding to the GABA-benzodiazepine receptor complex of rat cerebellum. Life Sci. 28, 307–317.
96. Supavilai, P., Mannonen, A., Collins, J.F. and Karobeth, M. (1982). Anion-dependent modulation of [^{3}H]muscimol binding and of GABA-stimulated [^{3}H]flunitrazepam binding by picrotoxin and related CNS convulsants. Eur. J. Pharmacol. 81, 687–691.
97. Klunk, W.E., Covey, D.F. and Ferrendelli, J.A. (1982). Structure-activity relationships of alkyl-substituted y-butyrolactones and succinimides.
98. Bayorh, M.A., Lozovsky D., Rice, K.C., Burke, T.R., Jr. and Kopin, I.J. (1983). Cardiovascular and plasma prolactin responses to stereoisomers of phencyclidine. Pharmacol. Biochem. Behav. 19, 365–367.
99. Altura, B.T., Quirion, R., Pert, C.B. and Altura, B.M. (1983). Phencyclidine ("angle dust") analogs and sigma opiates couse cerebral arterial spasms. Proc. Natl. Acad. Sci. USA 80, 865–869.
100. Gintzler, A.R., Zukin, R.S. and Zukin, S.R. (1982). Effects of phencyclidine and its derivatives on enteric neurones. Br. J. Pharmacol. 75, 261–267.
101. Haring, R., Kloog, Y. and Sokolovsky, M. (1984). Localization of phencyclidine binding sites on alpha and beta subunits of the nicotinic acetylcholine receptor from *Torpedo ocellata* electric organ using azido phencyclidine. J. Neurochem. 4, 627–637.
102. Oswald, R.E., Bamberger, J.J. and McLaughlin, J.T. (1984). Mechanisms of phencyclidine binding to the acetylcholine receptor from *Torpedo* electroplaque. Mol. Pharmacol. 25, 360–368.
103. Aguayo, L.G., Warnick, J.E., Maayani, S., Glick, S.D., Weinstein, H. and Alburquer-

que, E.X. (1982). Site of action of phencyclidine. IV. Interaction of phencyclidine and its analogues on ionic channels of the electrically excitable membrane and nicotinic receptor: Implications for behavioral effects. Mol. Pharmacol. 21, 637–647.
104. Albuquerque, E.X., Aguayo, L.G., Warnick, J.E., Weinstein, H., Glick, S.D., Maayani, S., Ickowicz, R.K. and Balustein, M.P. (1981). The behavioral effects of phencyclidines may be due to their blockade of potassium channels. Pro. Natl. Acad. Sci. USA 78, 7792–7796.
105. Bartschat, D.K. and Blaustein, M.P. (1986). Phencyclidine in low doses selectively blocks a presynaptic voltage regulated potassium channel in rat brain. Pro. Natl. Acad. Sci. USA 83, 189–192.
106. Sorensen, R.G. and Blaustein, M.P. (1986). m-Azido-phencyclidine covalently labels the rat brain PCP receptor, a putative K^+ channel. J. Neurosci. 6, 3676–3681.
107. Rothman, S.M. (1987). Non-competitive N-methyl-D-aspartate antagonists affect multiple ion channels. Soc. Neurosci. Abs. 13, in press.

14. NEUROPEPTIDE ABNORMALITIES IN ALZHEIMER'S AND HUNTINGTON'S DISEASES

JOSEPH B. MARTIN AND M. FLINT BEAL

Neuropeptides are widely distributed in the central nervous system where they serve as neuroregulators. Recent interest has focused on their role in degenerative neurologic diseases. In this review is described the anatomy of neuropeptides in cerebral cortex and basal ganglia as a framework for interpreting neuropeptide alterations in Alzheimer's disease (AD) and Huntington's disease (HD).

1. NEUROPEPTIDES IN DISEASES OF CEREBRAL CORTEX

1.1. Normal anatomy of neuropeptides in cerebral cortex

A knowledge of normal neuropeptidergic anatomy is essential to understand the relevance of neuropeptide abnormalities to neurological illnesses. It is also important to understand the relationship of neuropeptides to conventional neurotransmitters. One can then speculate whether alterations in neuropeptides reflect changes in intrinsic neurons, afferent terminals, altered turnover or degradation, or interactions with other neurotransmitters.

Neurons of the cerebral cortex can be divided into two general categories: intrinsic (or local circuit) neurons, and projection neurons. Intrinsic neurons are characterized by their multipolar, bipolar, or stellate shape and have axons that arborize within a local region of cortex. It has been suggested that up to 40% of intrinsic cortical neurons use GABA as a transmitter [1], while others use a variety of neuropeptides. Cortical projection neurons (pyramidal neurons) in layers II–III are involved in cortico-cortical connections, while those in

Ferrendelli, J.A., Collins, R.C. and Johnson, E.M. (eds), Neurobiology of Amino Acids, Peptides, and Trophic Factors.

deeper layers (V) project to the striatum, thalamus, brainstem, and spinal cord [2, 3]. On the basis of both lesion and uptake experiments, it has been proposed that pyramidal neurons utilize glutamate or aspartate as their principal neurotransmitters [2]. Many neuropeptides are found in neurons of the cerebral cortex in higher primates and humans [4–8]. Vasoactive intestinal polypeptide (VIP), somatostatin, cholecystokinin (CCK), neuropeptide Y (NPY), corticotropin-releasing factor (CRF), substance P, and dynorphin have each been demonstrated in intrinsic cortical neurons and fiber plexuses [9–13]. The work of Jones, Hendry and collaborators in the macaque monkey has provided detailed anatomical analysis of neuropeptide localization in cerebral cortex [13]. Our own work in the human brain, although less extensive, shows nearly identical observations. Several generalizations can now be made from these observations.

All peptide-containing cortical neurons are essentially similar. Neuronal perikarya immunoreactive for each neuropeptide are particularly concentrated in two striata: layer II and the upper part of layer III, and in layer VI and the underlying white matter [13]. The neurons are small, 8–10 microns in diameter, and those containing VIP, CCK, somatostatin, and NPY each account for 2%–3% of the total population in most areas of cortex examined [13]. Cells staining for substance P, dynorphin, and CRF are found in smaller numbers. The concentration of peptidergic neurons is greatest in the entorhinal and piriform cortex, followed by motor, premotor, and parietal cortex.

The processes of all types of peptidergic cells project in a vertical orientation, interconnecting various layers in a columnar fashion [12]. The neuronal processes of peptidergic cells tend to be beaded, and multiple axonal processes often arise from a single individual cell. All form plexuses, arising from the vertical orientation of fibers, which are concentrated in layers I, II, and VI and in the subjacent white.matter. The density of plexuses is greatest for NPY and somatostatin.

There is a striking paucity of peptidergic fibers entering the cortex from other parts of the CNS. No peptidergic fibers have been found in deeper white matter of the centrum semiovale or in the corpus callosum. These observations, taken together with the morphology of the cortical peptidergic somata, suggest that peptide-containing cells of the cerebral cortex are local, intrinsic neurons without efferent projections.

Studies in monkey and human cerebral cortex indicate that over 90% of somatostatin positive cells colocalize with NPY [4, 5, 8, 12]. In extensive double labeling experiments in the monkey cortex, Hendry and coworkers found that at least 95% of cells containing somatostatin, NPY and/or CCK are also immunoreactive for glutamic acid decarboxylase (GAD) or GABA [7, 11, 14]. Some substance P neurons also contain GABA [15]. In rats, Eckenstein and Baughman showed that VIP and choline acetyl-transferase are colocalized in a small number of peptidergic intrinsic neurons [16].

Evidence suggests that although there are eight or nine morphological subtypes of cortical intrinsic neurons which are GABAergic, only the one class described above contains neuropeptides [17–19]. The GABA-containing basket cells, which are much larger than the peptidergic neurons, have not, to date, shown any immunoreactivity to the known neuropeptides found in cortex [18, 19]. Some peptidergic cells also contain acetylcholine [16]. In conclusion, the data obtained to date suggest that all neuropeptides in primate cortex colocalize with either GABA or acetylcholine. On the other hand, morphologic evidence suggests that neuropeptides do not colocalize with the excitatory neurotransmitters glutamate and aspartate in pyramidal neurons of layers II, III, V, and VI [2].

1.2. Postmortem studies of cerebral cortex

1.2.1. Alzheimer's disease

Neurochemical analysis of postmortem brain and cortical biopsy tissue in AD samples reveal that the best characterized neurochemical deficiency is that of cortical acetylcholine, attributed to neuronal loss in the basal nucleus of Meynert from which cortical cholinergic projections arise [20–22]. Loss of choline acetyltransferase activity correlates both with the degree of dementia and the density of senile plaques [23]. In addition, less prominent deficits in cortical noradrenaline and serotonin are caused by neuronal degeneration in the locus coeruleus and raphe nuclei, respectively [1, 24–28]. Pathologic studies document that there is also neuronal loss in AD cerebral cortex [29–31]. Since both neuropeptides and amino acid neurotransmitters are localized to intrinsic cortical neurons, they are attractive candidates to reflect the neuronal loss.

The most consistent peptidergic abnormality in cerebral cortex in AD is a loss of somatostatin [32]. Several laboratories have confirmed the early reports of Davies and colleagues [32], although the extent and degree of somatostatin depletion has varied [33–36]. We have found a widespread reduction of somatostatin in virtually all cortical regions examined [37]. The most profound changes are in the temporal lobe, but there were also major reductions in both frontal and occipital cortex and hippocampus. In contrast to some previous studies, we have found no changes in somatostatin in subcortical regions, including the amygdala and substantia innominata.

As is the case with all neuropeptide changes, several possibilities may account for altered concentrations. The possibilities include altered degradation or processing, increased release with insufficient synthesis, a transynaptic effect as a consequence of alteration of another neurotransmitter, or selective neuronal degeneration. The finding of reduced levels of CSF somatostatin argues against increased release, since CSF somatostatin is remarkably stable [38, 39]. The reductions in somatostatin do not appear to be a consequence of altered degradation or processing since chromatographic profiles in AD and control frontal cortex are identical [37, 40].

These considerations raise the possibility that decreased somatostatin may reflect degeneration of somatostatin-containing neurons or terminals. Because somatostatin and neuropeptide Y are at least 80% colocalized in both monkey and human cortical neurons, one would expect parallel losses of both peptides in AD if these neurons or their terminals are indeed degenerating in AD. Concentrations of neuropeptide Y in AD cerebral cortex have recently been measured and widespread reductions which correlate with reductions of somatostatin were found [41], however they are of lesser magnitude than those of somatostatin.

It was found that somatostatin receptors are also reduced in AD cerebral cortex [42]. The loss of receptors correlates with reductions of somatostatin. The localization of these receptors is unknown, but it is possible that the loss of receptors could result in transneuronal degenerative changes of somatostatin neurons or terminals.

Substance P was reported to be reduced in AD cerebral cortex in an initial study [43], however in subsequent studies the result was not replicated [34, 44]. The discrepant reports may be due to patient age, since more severe neurochemical pathology is found in younger patients. We have recently studied a relatively young group of AD cases (mean age 72) and found widespread reductions in substance P-like immunoreactivity in cerebral cortex [45]. The decreases are not as profound as those of somatostatin and neuropeptide Y and typically range from 30% to 40%. Substance P coexists with acetylcholine in the caudal ascending cholinergic projection from the brainstem (lateral tegmental nucleus) [46]. It is possible, therefore, that reduced cortical substance P might reflect degeneration of this pathway. More recent evidence in both monkeys and humans has shown that substance P is localized to a small number of intrinsic cortical neurons [15, 47]. In the monkey, substance P is colocalized in deeper cortical layers, with some neurons containing both somatostain and neuropeptide Y [13]. Reduced cortical substance P may, therefore, reflect degeneration of these neurons.

Corticotropin-releasing factor (CRF) is also localized in a small number of cortical neurons, and concentrations of this neuropeptide have recently been found to be reduced in AD cerebral cortex [48, 49]. In contrast to somatostatin, however, CRF receptors are increased in regions where CRF concentrations are decreased [49]. Neither VIP nor CCK concentrations are altered in AD cerebral cortex [23, 34, 50, 51], although in one study aqueous extracted CCK was decreased in severe cases [34]. CCK receptors are normal in AD cortex [52]. Since VIP and CCK are contained in cortical neurons showing similar morphologic features to those of somatostatin and neuropeptide Y, their preservation indicates selectivity of the degenerative process. Met-enkephalin and neurotensin concentrations are also unaltered in AD cerebral cortex [34, 53–55].

Hypothalamic neuropeptides are, for the most part, localized within neuronal perikarya confined to the hypothalamus with terminals projecting to other regions. Concentrations of both thyrotropin-releasing hormone [44, 53] and luteinizing hormone releasing hormone [44] are unaltered in AD. Vasopressin is of particular interest in AD because of its putative role in memory functions [56]. We have found reduced concentrations of vasopressin in AD in globus pallidus, nucleus accumbens, and hippocampus [57]. Interestingly, concentrations were increased in cerebral cortex, presumably reflecting tissue atrophy with preserved vasopressin terminals. Oxytocin concentrations are increased in hippocampus [58].

Because gamma-aminobutyric acid (GABA) accounts for as many as 40% of all cortical synapses [59], and GABA is colocalized with somatostatin, neuropeptide Y, and cholecystokinin in cortical neurons [7, 11, 14], its levels in AD are of interest. GABA content was found to be reduced in AD cerebral cortex by Rossor and associates, and we have confirmed this finding, documenting a widespread reduction in cortical GABA content of 30%–40%, with the most marked reductions found in temporal cortex [60]. It is possible that reduced somatostatin and neuropeptide Y and AD reflect loss of a subpopulation of GABAergic neurons, whereas cholecystokinin neurons, colocalized with GABA in another subpopulation of neurons, are preserved.

1.2.2. Relationship of neuropeptide deficits to pathologic findings

The utilization of both histochemical and immunohistochemical techniques has allowed studies to be made of morphologic alterations of neuropeptide neurons in AD and their relationship to senile plaques and neurofibrillary tangles. In 1907, Alois Alzheimer identified senile plaques and neurofibrillary tangles as the neuropathologic hallmarks of AD [61]. Neurofibrillary tangles consist of pained helical filaments containing microtubule antigenic components. Senile plaques consist of disordered nerve terminals or neurites, microglia, and a central amyloid core [62].

Several immunocytochemical studies have shown abnormalities in somatostatin neurons in AD. One study showed somatostatin-staining neurons to be shrunken and irregularly shaped in AD cortex as compared with age-matched controls [63]. In another, cortical somatostatin perikarya exhibited morphologic changes, which were interpreted as being consistent with neuronal degeneration, and some were shown to contain tangles [64]. In a third study, swollen bulbous profiles and beaded processes were interpreted as representing degenerating somatostatin neurons [65].

Nakamura and Vincent [66] recently compared the density of somatostatin neurons in five cortical regions in AD as compared with aged controls. No decrease in density was found. These authors, however, did note that many somatostatin-positive fibers were abnormally swollen and bulbous in shape. They therefore suggested that the primary degenerative process may be begin at the fiber terminals of somatostatin neurons.

Neuropeptide Y neurons show similar morphologic changes in AD cerebral cortex. Chan-Palay and colleagues [67, 68] have also found marked morphologic changes in neuropeptide Y neurons in AD cortex and hippocampus.

They noted that neuropeptide Y neurons became distorted, with large misshapen cell somata and reduced, thickened, and gnarled dendrites. It was noted that there appeared to be a reduction in the extensiveness of the axonal plexus and fewer neuronal cell bodies.

Both somatostatin and neuropeptide Y have been localized to senile plaques [65, 67–70]. Neuropeptide Y has been estimated to be present in 10%–20% of plaques, and somatostatin has been found in 20%–50% of plaques. In our own studies, it has been shown that somatostatin and neuropeptide Y are colocalized in plaques [71]. We have used histochemical staining for NADPH-diaphorase and immunocytochemical staining for both somatostatin and neuropeptide Y to show similar morphologic alterations in somatostatin and neuropeptide Y neurons, as reported by other authors [65–68]. We found markedly distorted swollen and bulbous neuronal processes and apparent reductions in axonal plexuses. In agreement with Nakamura and Vincent, we found alterations in cell density in a small number of cases [5]. In contrast to the report of Roberts and coworkers [64], however, we have not been able to localize neurofibrillary tangles to somatostatin neurons [5]. We have found somatostatin and neuropeptide Y in 10% of plaques [71]. Our findings therefore confirm the findings of markedly altered somatostatin and neuropeptide Y neuronal processes in AD with relatively preserved numbers of neurons.

Much less is known about the relationship of other neuropeptides to the pathologic stigmata of AD. Substance P has been localized to approximately 5% of plaques [72]. Substance P fibers have also been shown to show abnormalities consisting of distentions and abnormal curvatures [72, 73]. Similar findings have been observed with CRF fibers, and CRF has been found in a few senile plaques, although appreciably fewer than those staining with either somatostatin or substance [73]. In addition CCK, VIP, bombesin, leu-enkephalin, and neurotensin have been localized to plaques [74].

2. NEUROPEPTIDES IN DISEASES OF THE BASAL GANGLIA

2.1. Normal anatomy of neuropeptides in basal ganglia

The complexity of striatal organization has recently become apparent. Nissl-stained sections of striatum show two neuronal populations based on size and dendritic morphology [75, 76]. Medium-sized (10–20 micron) neurons account for 90% of the total, and a larger-sized group makes up the remainder. These neuronal groups based on size can be further subdivided by Golgi studies into subsets of neurons. The majority (70%–80%) of neurons are medium-sized *spiny* neurons. A second spiny type is medium to large, with sparse spiny dendrites (10%). *Aspiny* neurons (10%–20%) are comprised of medium and large types. The neurons can be identified by their indented nuclei. They have locally arborizing axons and do not project outside the striatum. The final category consists of small neurons with variable dendritic morphology (1%–2%). Retrograde transport experiments have shown that the medium-sized spiny neurons account for most of the projecting neurons in the striatum, while aspiny neurons are involved exclusively in local intrinsic striatal circuits [76].

Several neurotransmitters have been localized to *spiny* type neurons. Spiny neurons contain the GABA synthetic enzyme, glutamic acid decarboxylase, as well as GABA itself [77]. These neurons project to both segments of the pallidum and the substantia nigra reticulata. Enkephalin is contained in about half of the GABA neurons [78, 79]. These neurons project preferentially to the external pallidum and substantia nigra. Both substance P and dynorphin are also localized to striatal spiny neurons, which project preferentially to the internal pallidum and substantia nigra reticulata [80–82].

Aspiny neurons contain a variety of neurotransmitters. Some neurons are GABAergic [83]. The best characterized are medium-sized aspiny neurons that contain both somatostatin and neuropeptide [21, 84–86]. The somatostatin-neuropeptide Y neurons account for 3%–4% of the total striatal neuronal population [85]. Of interest, these neurons also contain the histochemical marker NADPH-diaphorase [85, 87, 88]. VIP and CCK are also found in small populations of striatal aspiny neurons [89, 90]. Large aspiny neurons contain both choline acetyltransferase and the enzyme acetylcholinesterase [91].

Afferents to the striatum include substantia nigra dopaminergic projections, raphe nuclei serotonergic projections, and locus coeruleus noradrenergic projections [76]. Other neuropeptide afferents, including VIP, CRF, TRH, vasopressin, and oxytocin, are thought to originate in hypothalamic or brainstem neurons. CCK striatal projections originate in the amygdala and entorhinal cortex [92]. Cortical-striatal inputs contain the excitatory amino acids glutamate and aspartate [76].

Golgi studies show marked alterations in the morphology of dendrites of medium-sized *spiny* neurons in HD [33]. These abnormalities include changes in the size and shape of spines with recurved endings and collateralization. Pathological changes are rarely observed in *aspiny* neurons. Consistent with these observations, there is a depletion of neurotransmitter markers associated with spiny neurons (GABA, substance P, dynorphin, and enkephalin), while increased concentrations of some, but not all, neurotransmitter markers (somatostatin-neuropeptide Y) associated with aspiny neurons are found. Neurotransmitter markers in striatal afferents, including dopamine, TRH, neurotensin, CCK, and VIP, are either unchanged in concentration or modestly increased as a consequence of tissue shrinkage.

Substance P was the first neuropeptide to be measured in HD brain. Its concentration is markedly reduced in the striatopallidal (medial pallidum) and striatonigral (pars reticulata) pathways [93–98]. Less marked reductions are found in caudate, putamen, substantia nigra, pars compacta, and lateral pallidum. Consistent with the neurochemical measurements, immunocytochemical studies have shown a marked decrease in substance P fiber density in both the substantia nigra and globus pallidus, and a reduction in the number of positive-staining striatal neurons [99].

We have recently measured substance P concentrations in a series of pathologically graded cases of HD. Significant reductions of substance P were found in the caudate, putamen, globus pallidus, and both segments of the globus pallidus. The reductions in substance P content were highly correlated with estimates of neuronal depletion in the striatum in the various grades. This provides strong corroborative evidence that the substance P striatal spiny neurons are preferentially affected by the HD pathologic process. We also found significant reductions in substance P in both the bed nucleus of the stria terminalis and the subthalamic nucleus, two regions that had not been previously examined in HD. We have also found reductions in GABA-concentrations that are correlated with worsening pathologic grade [60].

Dynorphin concentrations have been reported to be depleted in the striatum as well as its projection sites in two recent studies, consistent with its localization in striatal spiny neurons, which are preferentially affected by the disease process [100, 101]. A possible exception to the rule that spiny neurons are preferentially affected in HD is neurotensin, since this neuropeptide has recently been localized to striatal spiny neurons, and concentrations have been reported to be increased in HD striatum [102].

Somatostatin concentrations in HD are increased approximately threefold in the caudate, putamen, nucleus accumbens, and external pallidum [93, 102, 103]. Neuropeptide Y concentrations have been reported to be increased a similar magnitude in the same regions [103], consistent with colocalization of the two peptides in striatal aspiny neurons. We have recently measured both somatostatin and neuropeptide Y in a large number of brain regions in HD cases that were graded pathologically [104]. Increases of both somatostatin and neuropeptide Y of a comparable degree were found in both mild and severe grade cases. Since striatal atrophy is much more severe in the advanced grade cases, this suggests there is relative, but not absolute, sparing of somatostatin-neuropeptide Y neurons in these cases. Our more recent findings have shown that there are significant increases of both somatostatin and neuropeptide Y in a number of other subcortical nuclei, consistent with a widespread disease process. Of particular interest we have found significant increases of both somatostatin and neuropeptide Y in frontal cortex [104].

Several studies have sought the source of increased striatal somatostatin in HD. It is possible that some striatal somatostatin is present in fibers that originate outside the striatum [105, 106]. On the basis of lesion studies, we estimate that about 50% of basal ganglia somatostatin is contained within intrinsic striatal neurons. Initial immunocytochemical studies showed increased somatostatin fibers and some preserved neuronal perikarya in advanced Huntington's disease. We have recently used NADPH-diaphorase staining to show that these neurons are indeed preserved in HD striatum [107]. Due to tissue atrophy, the density of NADPH-d neurons is markedly increased. This finding has been confirmed in the study of Dawbarn and associates in which the density of neuropeptide Y-stained neurons was demonstrated to be increased in HD striatum [103].

Our recent work has shown that the large acetylcholinesterase positive aspiny neurons in HD are also relatively spared [108]. This occurs despite concomitant reductions in choline acetyltransferase activity, which may reflect a loss of axonal terminals due to a loss of synaptic contacts. At least two populations of aspiny neurons are therefore relatively preserved in HD striatum. The nature of their resistance is unknown, however, an intriguing possibility is that it may be a consequence of their paucity of dendritic spines. It is known that glutamatergic cortico-striatal afferents terminate preferentially on dendritic spines. If glutamate interacts with an endogenous excitotoxin, this could explain a preferential vulnerability of spiny neurons.

The possibility of an endogenous excitotoxin being involved in the pathogenesis of HD was raised after it was shown that kainic acid lesions reproduce many of the neurochemical and neuropathologic features of HD [109]. We, however, found that they were an imperfect model of HD, since they do not spare somatostatin-neuropeptide Y neurons [106, 110]. More recently, Schwarcz and colleagues found that quinolinic acid, an endogenous metabolite of tryptophan present in human brain, can produce axon-sparing lesions similar to those observed in HD [111]. The lesions result in a depletion in neurotransmitters contained within striatal spiny neurons, such as GABA, while dopamine, which is contained in striatal afferents, is unaffected. We have recently found that quinolinic acid lesions are similar to HD is producing a depletion of both GABA and substance P, while there is relative sparing of both somatostatin and neuropeptide Y [110]. In addition, histologic studies showed that NADPH-diaphorase neurons were spared relative to other neuronal populations in a transition zone away from the core of the lesion. Quinolinic acid lesions, therefore, provide the best animal model of the neurochemistry of HD, and it is possible that quinolinic acid or a similar compound could be responsible for neuronal degeneration in HD. If an excitotoxin is involved in the pathogenesis of HD, then it is possible that early diagnosis using molecular genetics could be followed by therapeutic intervention with excitatory amino acid antagonists in an attempt to retard the degenerative process.

REFERENCES

1. Tomlinson, B.E., Irving, D. and Blessed, G. (1981). Cell loss in the locus coeruleus in senile dementia of Alzheimer type. J. Neurol. Sci. 49, 419–428.
2. Donoghue J.P., Wenthold, R.J., and Altschuler, R.A. (1985). Localization of glutaminase-like and aspartate aminotransferase-like immunoreactivity in neurons of cerebral cortex. J. Neurosci. 5, 2597–2608.
3. Fonnum, F. (1984). Glutamate: A neurotransmitter in mammalian brain. J. Neurochem. 42, 1–11.
4. Chronwall, B.M., Chase, T.N. and O'Donohue, T.L. (1984). Coexistence of neuropeptide Y and somatostatin in rat and human cortical and rat hypothalamic neurons. Neurosci. Lett. 52, 213–217.

5. Kowall, N.W., Beal, M.F. and Martin, J.B. (1986). Somatostatin, neuropeptide Y, NADPH diaphorase neurons do not contain neurofibrillary tangles in Alzheimer's disease cortex. Ann. Neurol. 20, 124.
6. Nakamura, S. and Vincent, S.R. (1985). Acetylcholinesterase and somatostatin-immunoreactivity coexist in human neocortex. Neurosci. Lett. 61, 183–187.
7. Somogyi, P., Hodgson, A.J., Smith, A.D., et al. (1984). Differential populations of GABAergic neurons in the visual cortex and hippocampus of the cat contain somatostatin or cholecystokinin immunoreactive material. J. Neurosci. 4, 2590–2603.
8. Vincent, S.R., Johansson, O., Hokfelt, T. et al. (1982). Neuropeptide coexistence in human cortical neurons. Nature 298, 65–67.
9. Emson, P.C. and Hunt, S.P. (1981). Anatomical chemistry of the cerebral cortex. In *The Organization of the Cerebral Cortex*, Schmitt, F.O., Worden, F.G., Adelman, G., Dennis, S.G., eds., MIT Press, Cambridge, MA, pp. 325–345.
10. Hendry, S.H., Jones, E.G. and Beinfeld, M.C. (1983). CCK immunoreactive neurons in rat and monkey cerebral cortex make symmetric synapses and have intimate associations with blood vessels. Proc. Natl. Acad. Sci. USA 80, 2400–2404.
11. Hendry, S.H., Jones, E.G., DeFelipe, J., et al. (1984). Neuropeptide-containing neurons of the cerebral cortex are also GABAergic. Proc. Natl. Acad. Sci. USA 81, 6526–6530.
12. Hendry, S.H., Jones, E.G. and Emson, P.C. (1984). Morphology, distribution, and synaptic relations of somatostatin- and neuropeptide Y-immunoreactive neurons in rat and monkey neocortex. J. Neurosci. 4, 2497–2517.
13. Jones, E.G. and Hendry, S.H. (1986). The peptide containing neurons of the primate cerebral cortex. In *Implications of Neuropeptides in Neurological and Psychiatric Diseases*, Martin, J.B., Barchus, J., eds., Raven, New York, pp. 163–178.
14. Schmechel, D.E., Vickrey, B.G., Fitzpatric, D. and Elde, R.P. (1984). GABAergic neurons of mammalian cerebral cortex: Widespread subclass defined by somatostatin content. Neurosci. Lett. 47, 227–232.
15. Jones, E.G. and Hendry, S.H. (1985). GABAergic, substance P-immunoreactive neurons in monkey cerebral cortex. Neurosci. Abst. 11, 145.
16. Eckenstein, F. and Baughman, R. (1984). Two types of cholinergic innervation in cortex, one co-localized with vasoactive intestinal polypeptide. Nature 309, 153–155.
17. Hendry, S.H., Houser, C.R., Jones, E.G. and Vaughn, J.E. (1983). Synaptic organization of immunocytochemically identified GABA neurons in the monkey sensory-motor cortex. J. Neurocytol. 12, 639–660.
18. Hendry, S.H. and Jones, E.G. (1981). Sizes and distributions of intrinsic neurons incorporating tritiated GABA in monkey sensory-motor cortex. J. Neurosci. 1, 390–408.
19. Houser, C.R., Hendry, S.H., Jones, E.G. and Vaughn, J.E. (1983). Morphological diversity of immunocytochemically identified GABA neurons in monkey sensory-motor cortex. J. Neurocytol. 12, 617–638.
20. Candy, J.M., Perry, R.H., Perry, E.K., et al. (1983). Pathological changes in the nucleus of Meynert in Alzheimer's and Parkinson's disease. J. Neurol. Sci. 54, 277–289.
21. Coyle, J.T., Price, D.L. and DeLong, M.R. (1983). Alzheimer's disease: A disorder of cortical cholinergic innervation. Science 219, 1184–1190.
22. Rossor, M.N., Garrett, N.J. and Johnson, A.I. (1982). A postmortem study of the cholinergic and GABA systems in senile dementia. Brain 105, 313–330.
23. Perry, E.K., Tomlinson, B.E., Blessed, G., et al. (1978). Correlation of cholinergic abnormalities with senile plaques and mental test scores in senile dementia. Br. Med. J. (Clin. Res.) 2, 1457–1459.
24. Bondareff, W., Mountjoy, C.Q. and Roth, M. (1981). Loss of neurons of origin of the adrenergic projection to cerebral cortex (nucleus locus coeruleus) in senile dementia. Lancet 1, 783–784.
25. Crow, T.J., Cross, A.J., Cooper, S.J., et al. (1984). Neurotransmitter receptors and monoamine metabolites in the brains of patients with Alzheimer-type dementia and depression, and suicides. Neuropharmacology 23, 1561–1569.
26. Curcio, C.A. and Kemper, T. (1984). Nucleus raphe dorsalis in dementia of the Alzheimer type: Neurofibrillary changes and neuronal packing density. J. Neuropath. Exp. Neurol. 143, 359–368.
27. Hardy, J., Adolfsson, R., Alafuzoff, I., et al. (1985). Transmitter deficits in Alzheimer's disease. Neurochem. Int. 7, 545–563.

28. Mann, D.M., Lincoln, J., Yates, P.O., et al. (1980). Changes in the monoamine containing neurons of the human central nervous system in senile dementia. Br. J. Psychiatry 136, 533–541.
29. Mann, D.M., Yates, P.O. and Marcyniuk, B. (1985). Correlation between senile plaque and neurofibrillary tangle counts in cerebral cortex and neuronal counts in cortex and subcortical structures in Alzheimer's disease. Neurosci. Lett. 56, 51–55.
30. Mountjoy, C.Q., Roth, M., Evans, N.J. and Evans, H.M. (1983). Cortical neuronal counts in normal elderly controls and demented patients. Neurobiol. Aging 4, 1–11.
31. Terry, R.D., Peck, A., DeTeresa, R., et al. (1981). Some morphometric aspects of the brain in senile dementia of the Alzheimer type. Ann. Neurol. 10, 184–192.
32. Davies, P., Katzman, R. and Terry, R.D. (1980). Reduced somatostatin-like immunoreactivity in cerebral cortex from cases of Alzheimer disease and Alzheimer senile dementia. Nature 288, 279–280.
33. Graveland, G.A., Williams, R.S. and Difiglia M. (1985). Evidence for degenerative and regenerative changes in neostriatal spiny neurons in Huntington's disease. Science 277, 770–773.
34. Ferrier, I.N., Cross, A.J., Johnson, J.A., et al. (1983). Neuropeptides in Alzheimer type dementia. J. Neurol. Sci. 62, 159–170.
35. Rossor, M.N., Emson, P.C., Mountjoy, C.Q., et al. (1980). Reduced amounts of immunoreactive somatostatin in the temporal cortex in senile dementia of Alzheimer type. Neurosci. Lett. 20, 373–377.
36. Rossor, M.N. Iversen, L.L., Reynolds, G.P., et al. (1984). Neurochemical characteristics of early and late onset types of Alzheimer's disease. Br. Med. J. (Clin. Res.) 288, 961–964.
37. Beal, M.F., Mazurek, M.F., Svendsen, C.N., et al. (1986). Widespread reduction of somatostatin-like immunoreactivity in the cerebral cortex in Alzheimer's disease. Ann. Neurol. 20, 489–495.
38. Beal, M.F., Growdon, J.H., Mazurek, M.F. and Martin, J.B. (1986). CSF somatostatin-like immunoreactivity in dementia. Neurology 36, 294–297.
39. Beal, M.F., Mazurek, M.F., Black, P.B. and Martin, J.B. (1985). CSF somatostatin in neurological diseases. J. Neurol. Sci. 71, 91–104.
40. Candy, J.M., Gascoigne, A.D., Biggins, J.A., et al. (1985). Somatostatin immunoreactivity in cortical and some subcortical regions in Alzheimer's disease. J. Neurol. Sci. 71, 315–323.
41. Beal, M.F., Mazurek, M.F., Chattha, G.K., et al. (1986). Neuropeptide Y immunoreactivity is reduced in cerebral cortex in Alzheimer's disease. Ann. Neurol. 20, 282–288.
42. Beal, M.F., Mazurek, M.F., Tran, V.T., et al. (1985). Somatostatin receptors are reduced in cerebral cortex in Alzheimer's disease. Science 229, 289–291.
43. Crystal, H.A. and Davies P. (1982). Cortical substance P-like immunoreactivity in cases of Alzheimer's disease and senile dementia of the Alzheimer type. J. Neurochem. 38, 1781–1784.
44. Yates, C.M., Harmar, A.J., Rosie, R., et al. (1983). Thyrotropin-releasing hormone, luteinizing hormone-releasing hormone and substance P immunoreactivity in post-mortem from cases of Alzheimer-type dementia and Down's syndrome. Brain Res. 258, 45–52.
45. Beal, M.F. and Mazurek, M.F. Substance P-like immunoreactivity is reduced in Alzheimer's disease cerebral cortex. Neurology, in press.
46. Vincent, S.R., Satoh, K., Armstrong, D.M. and Fibiger, H.C. (1983). Substance P in the ascending cholinergic reticular system. Nature 306, 688–691.
47. Sakamoto, N., Takatsuji, K., Shiosaka, S. and Tohyama, M. (1985). Evidence for the existence of substance P-like immunoreactive neurons in the human cerebral cortex: An immunohistochemical analysis. Brain Res. 325, 322–324.
48. Bissette, G., Reynolds, G.P., Kilts, C.D., et al. (1985). Corticotropin-releasing factor-like immunoreactivity in senile dementia of the Alzheimer type. JAMA 265, 3067–3069.
49. Desouza, E.B., Whitehouse, P.J., Kuhar, M.J., et al. (1986). Reciprocal changes in corticotropin-releasing factor (CRF)-like immunoreactivity and CRF receptors in cerebral cortex of Alzheimer's disease. Nature 319, 593–595.
50. Rossor, M.N., Fahrenkrug, J., Emson, P.C., et al. (1980). Reduced cortical choline acetyltransferase activity in senile dementia of Alzheimer type is not accompanied by changes in vasoactive intestinal polypeptide. Brain Res. 201, 249–253.
51. Rossor, M.N., Rehfeld, J.F., Emson, P.C., et al. (1981). Normal cortical concentrations of cholecystokinin-like immunoreactivity with reduced choline acetyltransferase activity in

senile dementia of Alzheimer type. Life Sci. 29, 405–410.
52. Hays, S.E. and Paul, S.M. (1982). CCK receptors and human neurological disease. Life Sci. 31, 319–322.
53. Nemeroff, C.B., Bissette, G., Busby, W.H., et al. (1983). Regional brain concentrations of neurotensin, thyrotropin releasing hormone and somatostatin in Alzheimer's disease. Neurosci. Abst. 9, 1052.
54. Rossor, M.N., Emson, P.C. and Mountjoy, C.A. (1982). Neurotransmitters of the cerebral cortex in senile dementia of Alzheimer's type. Exp. Brain Res. 5 (Suppl), 33–157.
55. Yates, C.M., Fink, G., Bennie, J.G., et al. (1985). Neurotensin immunoreactivity in postmortem brain is increased in Down's syndrome but not in Alzheimer-type dementia. J. Neurol. Sci. 67, 327–335.
56. Dewied, D. (1976). Behavioral effects of intraventricularly administered vasopressin and vasopressin fragments. Life Sci. 19, 685–690.
57. Mazurek, M.F., Beal, M.F. and Martin, J.B. (1985). Vasopressin in postmortem Alzheimer brain. Ann. Neurol. 18, 143–144.
58. Mazurek, M.F., Beal, M.F., Bird, E.D. and Martin, J.B. Oxytocin concentration is increased in the hippocampus in Alzheimer's disease. Neurology, in press.
59. Iversen, L.L. and Bloom, F.E. (1979). Studies of the uptake of ^{3}H-GABA and ^{3}H-glycine in slices and homogenates of rat brain and spinal cord by electron microscopic autoradiography. Brain Res. 41, 131–143.
60. Ellison, D.W., Beal, M.F., Mazurek, M.F., Malloy, J.R., Bird, E.D. and Martin J.B. Amino acid neurotransmitter abnormalities in Huntington's disease and the quinolinic acid animal model of Huntington's disease. Brain, in press.
61. Alzheimer, A. (1907). Uber ein eigenartige erkrankung der hinnrinde. Allg. Z. Psychiatr. 64, 146–148.
62. Probst, A., Basler, V., Brow, B. and Ulrich J. (1983). Neuritic plaques in senile dementia of Alzheimer type: A golgi analysis in the hippocampal region. Brain Res. 268, 249–254.
63. Joynt, R.J. and McNeill, T.H. (1984). Neuropeptides in aging and dementia. Peptides (Fayetteville) 5 (Suppl. 1), 269–274.
64. Roberts, G.W., Crow, T.J. and Rolak, J.M. (1985). Location of neuronal tangles in somatostatin neurons in Alzheimer's disease. Nature 314, 92–94.
65. Morrison, J.H., Rogers, J., Scherr, S., et al. (1985). Somatostatin immunoreactivity in neuritic plaques of Alzheimer's patients. Nature 31, 490–492.
66. Nakamura, S. and Vincent, S.R. (1986). Somatostatin and neuropeptide Y-immunoreactive neurons in the neocortex in senile dementia of Alzheimer's type. Brain Res. 370, 11–20.
67. Chan-Palay, V., Lang, W., Allen, Y.S., et al. (1985). Cortical neurons immunoreactive with antisera against neuropeptide Y are altered in Alzheimer's-type dementia. J. Comp. Neurol. 238, 390–400.
68. Chan-Palay, V., Lang, W., Haesler, U., Kohler, C. and Yasargil G. (1986). Distribution of altered hippocampal neurons and axons immunoreactive with antisera against neuropeptide Y in Alzheimer's-type dementia. J. Comp. Neurol. 248, 376–394.
69. Armstrong, D.M., Leroy, S., Shields, D., and Terry, R.D. (1985). Somatostatin-like immunoreactivity within neuritic plauqes. Brain Res. 338, 71–79.
70. Struble, R.G., Kitt, C.A., Walker, L.C., Cork, L.C. and Price D.L. (1984). Somatostatinergic neurities in senile plaques of aged non-human primates. Brain Res. 324, 394–396.
71. Kowall, N.W., Beal, M.F. and Martin, J.B. (1986). Neuropeptide Y, somatostatin and NADPH diaphorase reactive fibers contribute to senile plaque formation in Alzheimer's disease. Neurology 36 (Suppl 1), 224.
72. Armstrong, D.M. and Terry, R.D. (1985). Substance P immunoreactivity within neuritic plaques. Neurosci. Lett. 58, 139–144.
73. Price, D.L., Powers, R.E., Walker, L.C., Struble, R.G., Whitehouse, P.J., Vale, W.W. and DeSouza, E.B. (1986). Corticotropin releasing factor immunoreactivity in senile plaques. Neurosci. Abst. 12, 98.
74. Struble, R.G., Powers, R.E., Casanova, M.F., et al. (1985). Multiple transmitter-specific markers in senile plaques in Alzheimer's disease. Neurosci. Abst. 11, 953.
75. Graveland, G.A., Williams, R.S. and Difiglia, M. (1985). A golgi study of the human striatum: Neurons and afferent fibers. J. Comp. Neurol. 234, 317–333.
76. Graybiel, A.M. and Ragsdale C.W. (1983). Biochemical anatomy of the striatum. In *Chemi-*

cal Neuroanatomy, Emson, P.C., ed., Raven, New York, pp. 427–504.

77. Ribak, C.E., Vaughn, J.E. and Roberts, E. (1979). The GABA neurons and their axon terminals in the rat corpus striatum as demonstrated by GAD immunocytochemistry. J. Comp. Neurol. 187, 261–284.
78. Aronin, N., Difiglia, M., Graveland, G.A., et al. (1984). Localization of immunoreactive enkephalins in GABA synthesizing neurons of the rat neostriatum. Brain Res. 300, 376–380.
79. Difiglia, M., Aronin, N. and Martin, J.B. (1982). Light and electron microscopic localizations of immunoreactive leu-enkephalin in the monkey basal ganglia. J. Neurosci. 2, 203–320.
80. Bolam, J.P., Somogyi, P., Takagi, H., et al. (1983). Localization of substance P-like immunoreactivity in neurons and nerve terminals in the neostriatum of the rat: A correlated light and electron microscopic study. J. Neurocytol. 12, 325–344.
81. Chesselet, M.F. and Graybiel, A.M. (1983). Met-enkephalin-like and dynorphin-like immunoreactivities of the basal ganglia of the cat. Life Sci. 33, 37–40.
82. Zamir, N., Palcovitz, M., Weber, E., et al. (1984). A dynorphinergic pathway of leu-enkephalin production in rat substantia nigra. Nature 307, 643–645.
83. Bolam, J.P., Clarke, D.J., Smith, A.D. and Somogyi, P. (1986). A type of aspiny neuron in the rat neostriatum accumulates [^{3}H]gamma-aminobutyric acid: Peptides derived from prodynorphin are decreased in basal ganglia of Huntington's disease brains. Brain Res. 372, 155–158.
84. Difiglia, M. and Aronin, N. (1984). Quantitative electron microscopic study of immunoreactive somatostatin axons in the rat neostriatum. Neurosci. Lett. 50, 325–331.
85. Kowall, N., Ferrante, R.J., Beal, M.F. and Martin, J.B. (1985). Characteristics, distribution and interrelationships of somatostatin, neuropeptide Y, and NADPH-diaphorase in human caudate nucleus. Neurosci. Abst. 11, 209.
86. Takagi, H., Somogyi, P., Somogyi, J. and Smith, A.D. (1983). Fine structural studies of a type of somatostatin immunoreactive neuron and its synaptic connections in the rat striatum: A correlated light and electron microscopic study. J. Comp. Neurol. 214, 1–16.
87. Vincent, S.R. and Johansson, O. (1983). Striatal neurons containing both somatostatin- and avian pancreatic polypeptide (APP)-like immunoreactivities and NADPH-diaphorase activity. A light and electron microscopic study. J. Comp. Neurol. 217, 264–270.
88. Vincent, S.R., Johansson, O., Hokfelt, T., et al. (1983). NADPH-diaphorase: A selective histochemical marker for striatal neurons containing both somatostatin- and avian pancreatic polypeptide (APP)-like immunoreactivities. J. Comp. Neurol. 217, 252–263.
89. Takagi, H., Mizuta, H., Matsuda, T., et al. (1984). The occurrence of cholecystokinin-like immunoreactive neurons in the rat neostriatum: Light and electron microscopic analysis. Brain Res. 309, 346–369.
90. Theriault, E., Marshall, P.E. and Landis, D.M. (1984). Morphology of neurons containing VIP-like immunoreactivity in the rat striatum. Neurosci. Abst. 10, 701.
91. Vincent, S.R., Staines, W.A. and Fibiger, H.C. (1983). Histochemical demonstration of separate populations of somatostatin and cholinergic neurons in the rat striatum. Neurosci. Lett. 35, 111–114.
92. Zaborszky, L., Alheid, G.F., Beinfield, M.C., et al. (1985). Cholecystokinin innervation of the ventral striatum: A morphological and radioimmunological study. Neuroscience 14, 427–453.
93. Aronin, N., Cooper, P.E., Lorenz, L.J., et al. (1983). Somatostatin is increased in the basal ganglia in Huntington's disease. Ann. Neurol. 13, 519–526.
94. Buck, S.H., Burks, T.F., Brown, M. and Yamamura, H.I. (1981). Reduction in basal ganglia and substantia nigra substance P levels in Huntington's disease. Brain Res. 209, 464–469.
95. Emson, P.C., Arregui, A., Clement-Jones, V., et al. (1980). Regional distribution of methionine-enkephalin and substance P-like immunoreactivity in normal human brain and in Huntington's disease. Brain Res. 199, 147–160.
96. Gale, J.S., Bird, E.D., Spokes, E.G., et al. (1978). Human substance P: Distribution in controls and Huntington's chorea. J. Neurochem. 30, 633–634.
97. Kanazawa, I., Bird, E., O'Connell, R. and Powell, D. (1977). Evidence for a decrease in substance P content of substantia nigra in Huntington's chorea. Brain Res. 120, 387–392.
98. Kanazawa, I., Sasaki, H., Muramoto, O., et al. (1985). Studies on neurotransmitter markers and striatal neuronal cell density in Huntington's disease and dentatorubropallidoluysian

atrophy. J. Neurol. Sci. 70, 151–165.
99. Marshall, P.E., Landis, D.M. and Zalneraitis, E. (1983). Immunocytochemical studies of substance P and leucine-enkephalin in Huntington's disease. Brain Res. 298, 11–26.
100. Dawbarn, D., Zamin, N., Waters, C.M., Hunt, S.P., Emson, P.C. and Brownstein, M.J. (1983). Combination of golgi-staining, autoradigoraphy and electronmicroscopy. J. Comp. Neurol. 213, 121–134.
101. Seizinger, B.R., Leibisch, D.C., Kish, S.J., Arendt, R.M., Hornykiewicz, O. and Herz, A. (1986). Opioid peptides in Huntington's disease: Alterations in prodynorphin and proenkephalin system. Brain Res. 378, 405–408.
102. Nemeroff, C.B., Youngblood, W.W., Manberg, P.J., et al. (1983). Regional brain concentrations of neuropeptides in Huntington's chorea and schizophrenia. Science 221, 972–975.
103. Dawbarn, D., Dequidt, M.E. and Emson, P.C. (1985). Survival of basal ganglia neuropeptide Y/somatostatin neurons in Huntington's disease. Brain Res. 340, 251–260.
104. Beal, M.F., Ellison, D.W., Mazurek, M.F., Malloy, J.R., Bird, E.D. and Martin, J.B. (1986). Neuropeptide Y is increased in Huntington's disease. Ann Neurol.
105. Beal, M.F., Domesick, V.B. and Martin, J.B. (1985). Effects of lesions in the amygdala and periventricular hypothalamus on striatal somatostatin-like immunoreactivity. Brain Res. 330, 309–316.
106. Beal, M.F. and Martin, J.B. (1983). Effect of lesions on somatostatin-like immunoreactivity in the rat striatum. Brain Res. 266, 67–73.
107. Ferrante, R.J., Kowall, N.W., Beal, M.F., et al. (1985). Selective sparing of a class of strial neurons in Huntington's disease. Science 230, 561–563.
108. Ferrante, R.J., Beal, M.F., Kowall, N.W., Richardson, E.P. and Martin, J.B. (1987). Sparing of acetylcholinesterase-containing striatal neurons in Huntington's disease. Brain Res. 411, 162–166.
109. Schwarcz, R., Foster, A.C., French, E.D., et al. (1984). Excitotoxic models for neurodegenerative disorders. Life Sci. 35, 19–32.
110. Beal, M.F., Kowall, N.W., Ellison, D.W., et al. (1986). Replication of the neurochemical characteristics of Huntington's disease with quinolinic acid. Nature 321, 168–171.
111. Schwarcz, R., Whetsell, W.O. and Mangano, R.M. (1983). Quinolinic acid: An endogenous metabolite that produces axon-sparing lesions in rat brain. Science 219, 316–318.

IV. SHORT COMMUNICATIONS

15. DEMONSTRATION OF INDIVIDUAL FIBERS FROM THE SUBSTANTIA INNOMINATA TO THE FRONTAL CORTEX OF THE RAT, USING PHASEOLUS VULGARIS LEUCOAGGLUTININ (PHA-L)*

KENNETH M. CARNES, AND JOSEPH L. PRICE

Kidney bean lectin (PHA-L) was used as an anterograde axonal tracer to label fibers from the magnocellular areas of the basal forebrain (especially the ventral pallidum and other parts of the substantia innominata). Previous studies have reported that cells in these regions provide input to all nonstriatal parts of the telencephalon, including the cerebral cortex, amygdaloid complex, hippocampal formation, and olfactory bulb and cortex [1–5]. Notably, a high proportion of the fibers to the neocortex has been reported to be cholinergic [4].

Iontophoretic or pressure injections of PHA-L were made through glass micropipette syringes; after survival periods of 7–14 days, the animals were killed and their brains reacted immunohistochemically with antibodies against PHA-L [6]. Complete series of sections were taken through the rostral part of the hemisphere in order to allow reconstruction of individual labeled fibers in the frontal cortex; a 1-in-5 series of sections was taken through the remainder of the brain.

Small injections (ca. 500 μm in diameter) in the substantia innominata labeled fibers in many parts of the cerebral cortex, from the frontal cortex to the entorhinal cortex (Figure 15-1). In addition, significant numbers of fibers were labeled in the olfactory bulb, amygdaloid complex, midline and medio-

* Supported by NIH grants NS09518 and AG05681. KMC was also was supported by NIH GM07200, Medical Scientist.

Ferrendelli, J.A., Collins, R.C. and Johnson, E.M. (eds), Neurobiology of Amino Acids, Peptides, and Trophic Factors.

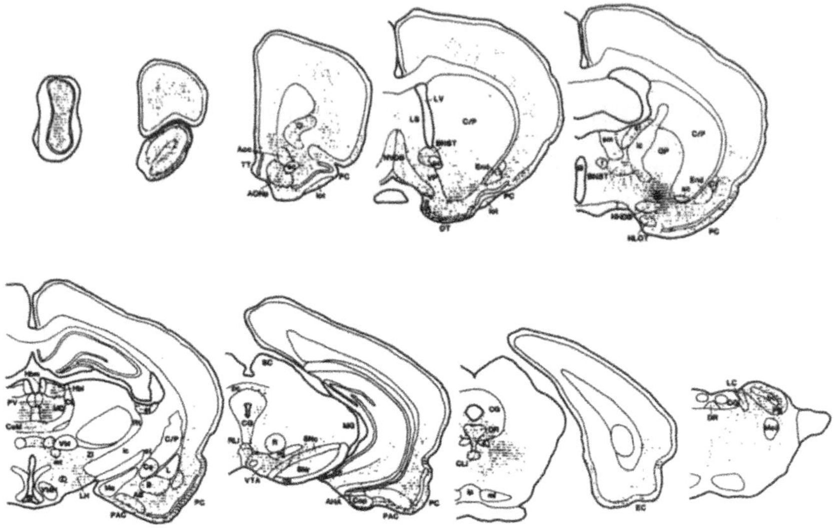

Figure 15-1. The distribution pattern of labeled fiber segements following an iontophoretic injection of PHA-L in the substantia innominata. The sections were scanned in approximately horizontal traverses, 0.1 mm wide. Each dot represents a point where a traverse intersected a labeled fiber segment. 4 = trochlear nucleus; AB = accessory basal nucleus of the amygdala; ac = anterior commissure; Acc = nucleus accumbens; AHA = amygdalo-hippocampal area; AONp = anterior olfactory nucleus, posterior division; B = basal nucleus of the amygdala; bc = brachium conjunctivum; BNST = bed nucleus of the stria terminalis; Ce = central nucleus of the amygdala; CeM = central medial nucleus of the thalamus; CG = central (periaqueductal) grey; CL = central lateral nucleus of the thalamus; Cl = claustrum; CLi = caudal linear nucleus of the raphe; Cop = posterior cortical nucleus of the amygdala; cp = cerebral peduncle; C/P = caudate/putamen; DR-dorsal raphe; EC = entorhinal cortex; End = endopiriform nucleus; f = fornix; GP = globus pallidus; Hbl = lateral habenular nucleus; Hbm = medial habenular nucleus; ic = internal capsule; III = third ventricle; ip = interpeduncular nucleus; L = lateral nucleus of the amygdala; LC = locus coeruleus; LH = lateral hypothalamus; lot = lateral olfactory tract; LS = lateral septum; LV = lateral ventricle; MD = mediodorsal nucleus of the thalamus; Me = medial nucleus of the amygdala; MG = medial geniculate; ml = medial lemniscus; Mo5 = motor trigeminal nucleus; mt = mammillothalamic tract; NHDB = nucleus of the horizontal limb of the diagonal band; NLOT = nucleus of the lateral olfactory tract; NVDB = nucleus of the vertical limb of the diagonal band; OT = olfactory tubercle; PAC = periamygdaloid cortex; PB = parabrachial nuclei; PC = piriform cortex; pc = posterior commissure; PV = paraventricular nucleus of the thalamus; R = red nucleus; RLi = rostral linear nucleus of the raphe; Rt = reticular nucleus of the thalamus; SC = superior colliculus; sm = stria medul-laris; SNc = substantia nigra, pars compacta; SNr = substantia nigra, pars reticularis; st = stria terminalis; TT = taenia tecta; VM = ventromedial nucleus of the thalamus; VMH = ventromedial nucleus of the hypothalamus; VP = ventral pallidum; VTA = ventral tegmental area; ZI = zona incerta.

dorsal thalamic nuclei, lateral habenular nucleus, lateral hypothalamic area, ventral tegmental area and substantia nigra, raphe nucleus, midbrain reticular formation, and the parabrachial nucleus. In the frontal cortex, labeled fiber segments with varicosities were found in all layers, but were concentrated in the superficial (I and II) and deep (V and VI) layers.

Reconstruction of single fibers from serial sections suggests that individual

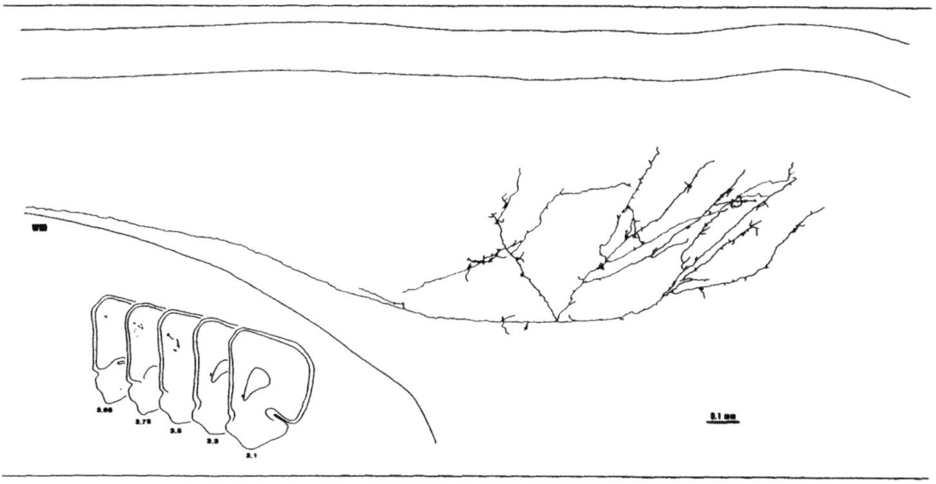

Figure 15-2. Camera lucida reconstruction of an individual fiber from the substantia innominata in the frontal cortex, made from 18 serial 50 μm sections. The small inset drawing of the coronal sections illustrates the location of this fiber in the cortex. The numbers below the sections refer to the position of the sections in mm anterior to bregma.

fibers have different morphologies, with some ramifying in the deeper layers of the cortex, and others concentrated in the superficial layers. The branches of individual fibers appear to be concentrated within an area about 1.0 mm in diameter, although distal fiber segments may extend 0.5 mm beyond this limit. Figure 15-2 illustrates a typical labeled axon in the frontal cortex. In addition, separate fibers labeled from a restricted injection (and therefore arising from nearby cell somata) may be concentrated within the same 1–2 mm area of the cortex. These results are in agreement with previous data from double retrograde tracer experiments, which indicated that individual cells in the substantia innominata project to restricted areas (ca. 1.0–1.5 mm) of the cerebral cortex [7].

REFERENCES

1. Kievit, J. and Kuypers, H.G. (1975). Basal forebrain and hypothalamic connections to frontal and parietal cortex in the rhesus monkey. Science 187, 660–662.
2. Bigl, V., Woolf, N.J. and Butcher, L.L. (1982). Cholinergic projections from the basal forebrain to frontal, parietal, temporal, occipital, and cingulate cortices: A combined fluorescent tracer and acetylcholinesterase analysis. Brain Res. Bull. 8, 727–749.
3. McKinney, M., Coyle, J.T. and Hedreen, J.C. (1983). Topographic analysis of the innervation of the rat neocortex and hippocampus by the basal forebrain cholinergic system. J. Comp. Neurol. 217, 103–121.
4. Mesulam, M.-M., Mufson, E.J., Levey, A.I. and Wainer, B.H. (1983). Cholinergic innervation of cortex by the basal forebrain: Cytochemistry and cortical connections of the septal area, diagonal band nuclei, nucleus basalis (substantia innominata), and hypothalamus in the rhesus monkey. J. Comp. Neurol. 214, 170–197.
5. Saper, C.B. (1984). Organization of cerebral cortical afferent systems in the rat. II. Magnocellular basal nucleus. J. Comp. Neurol. 222, 313–342.

6. Gerfen, C.R. and Sawchenko, P.E. (1984). An anterograde neuroanatomical tracing method that shows the detailed morphology of neurons, their axons and terminals: Immunohistochemical localization of an axonally transported plant lectin, *Phaseolus vulgaris* leucoagglutinin (PHA-L). Brain Res. 290, 219–238.
7. Price, J.L. and Stern, R. (1983). Individual cells in the nucleus basalis — diagonal band complex have restricted axonal projections to the cerebral cortex in the rat. Brain Res. 269, 352–356.

16. DETERMINATION OF THE PHARMACOKINETICS OF 2-AMINO-7-PHOSPHONOHEPTANOATE IN PLASMA AND CEREBROSPINAL FLUID

R.P. COMPTON, P.A. KREITER, R.G. SMITH, R.D. HARKEN, AND J.B. MONAHAN

The N-methyl-D-aspartate (NMDA) receptor subclass of excitatory amino acid receptors has been implicated in pathological conditions such as epilepsy, ischemia, and hypoglycemia. Antagonists of the NMDA receptor have been shown to block these conditions when induced in experimental animals. One of the most specific and potent NMDA antagonists is 2-amino-7-phosphonoheptanoate (APH), with the majority of the activity residing in the D-isomer. The racemic mixture of APH, injected intraperitoneally into mice at doses of 0.33–1.0 mmol/kg, is effective against either sound or chemically induced seizures [1]. APH has also been shown to protect against ischemia induced by bilateral carotid occlusion [2] and neuronal damage due to hypoglycemia [3]. Although these studies have demonstrated the effectiveness of APH in these pathological conditions, only limited information on the pharmacokinetics of APH is available, and it is not clear whether D,L-APH and D-APH would demonstrate different pharmacokinetic properties in blood and appearance in cerebrospinal fluid. The present study describes an analytical method for the quantification of APH in plasma and cerebrospinal fluid. Additionally, the pharmacokinetics of D-APH and D,L-APH in the rat are reported.

Male Sprague-Dawley rats were prepared by cannulation of the femoral vein and artery with polyethylene tubing. These cannulations allowed ease of drug injection and frequent sampling of blood. Two days after surgery, APH was administered via the venous cannula in a 500 μl bolus, followed by 100–150 μl of heparinized saline. At specified times, 300 μl of blood was with-

Ferrendelli, J.A., Collins, R.C. and Johnson, E.M. (eds), Neurobiology of Amino Acids, Peptides, and Trophic Factors.

drawn from the arterial cannula and replaced by an equal volume of saline. For the collection of cerebrospinal fluid, rats were anesthetized with sodium pentobarbital (i.v.) and placed in a stereotaxic apparatus to allow easy access to the cisterna magna at the base of the skull. A 22-gauge needle attached to a micrometer syringe was used to remove approximately 250 μl of blood-free cerebrospinal fluid. Each rat was sampled several times for plasma but only once, at the end of the experiment, for cerebrospinal fluid.

The analysis of APH in the plasma and cerebrospinal fluid was performed by fluorescence derivatization followed by reverse phase HPLC. Samples were deproteinated by precipitation with sulfosalicylic acid containing 2-amino-4-phosphonobutanoate as an internal standard, with greater than 95% recovery of the APH. The deproteinated supernatants were derivatized with 9-fluorenylmethyl-chloroformate, and the fluorescent derivatives were separated and analyzed by reverse phase HPLC on a 5 micron, C18 column using a modification of published procedures [4]. Under these conditions, APH could be measured over a concentration range of 1.5–250 pmoles/μl.

In plasma, the clearance rate of D-APH and D,L-APH are 16 and 43 ml/min/kg, respectively. At a 1 mmol/kg dose of either compound, the maximal plasma concentration occurred at the earliest time point taken and subsequently decreased to less than 5% of the initial value after 4 hours. The plasma half-life of D-APH and D,L-APH were 37 and 20 minutes, respectively. A linear relationship between the APH concentration in plasma and the dose administered exists over the range tested (0.188–2.5 mmol/kg).

Both D-APH and D,L-APH were maximal in the cerebrospinal fluid 10–15 minutes post injection, with a peak concentration of 12–15 μM following a 1 mmol/kg dose (i.v.). This represents less than 2% of the APH present in the plasma at that time. Two hours following a 1 mmol/kg dose, significant quantities (3 μM) of APH were present in the cerebrospinal fluid, but no APH was detectable after 4 hours. A linear relationship between the APH concentration in cerebrospinal fluid (2–53 μM) and the amount administered (0.188–2.5 mmol/kg i.v.) was observed. The concentrations of APH found in the cerebrospinal fluid are in the range of the Ki's of D-APH and D,L-APH for the NMDA receptor, which are 4.0 and 5.4 μM, respectively [5].

The method described here represents a sensitive analytical procedure that can be used to quantify APH in physiological fluids. This will allow studies of the relationship between the effectiveness of APH in animal models of neurodegenerative disorders and its concentration in the CNS.

REFERENCES

1. Croucher, M.J., Collins, J.F., and Meldrum, B.S. (1982). Anticonvulsant actions of excitatory amino acid antagonists. Science 216, 899–901.
2. Simon, R.P., Swan, J.H., Griffiths, T., and Meldrum, B.S. (1984). Blockade of N-methyl-D-aspartate receptors may protect against ischemic damage in the brain. Science 226, 850–852.
3. Wieloch, T. (1985). Hypoglycemic-induced neuronal damage prevented by an N-methyl-D-aspartate antagonist. Science 230, 681–683.

4. Cunico, R.L., Dimson, P., Mayer, A., and Wehr, C.T. (1985). Automated amino acid analysis using precolumn derivatization with FMOC. In *Proceedings of The Fifth International Symposium on HPLC of Proteins, Peptides and Polynucleotides*, in press.
5. Monahan, J.B., and Michel, J. (1987). Identification and characterization of an N-methyl-D-aspartate specific L-[^{3}H]Glutamate recognition site in synaptic plasma membranes. J. Neurochem. 48, 1699–1708.

17. AFFERENTS TO THE HORIZONTAL DIAGONAL BAND OF THE RAT*

TERRY A. FULLER, KENNETH M. CARNES, AND JOSEPH L. PRICE

The magnocellular nuclei of the basal forebrain (MNBF) contain cholinergic and other neurons that innervate most of the forebrain [1]. Previous studies have identified the sources of afferents, including presumptive glutamergic/aspartergic projections, to the ventral striatopallidal region [2]. The present studies were undertaken to identify the inputs to another part of the MNBF, the horizontal limb of the diagonal band (NHDB).

Following injections of the nonspecific tracer wheat germ agglutinin conjugated to horseradish peroxidase (WGA-HRP), retrogradely labeled cells were found in the orbital, insular, and piriform cortices; the olfactory tubercle; and the ventrally and medially placed amygdaloid nuclei (Figure 17-1). In addition, significant numbers of cells were labeled in the lateral and caudal hypothalamus, the ventral tegmental area, the pedunculopontine and dorsolateral tegmental nuclei, and other brainstem structures.

In the contralateral hemisphere, the densest collection of WGA-HRP labeled cells were found in the NHDB and in the magnocellular area, caudal and medial to it. In order to further characterize the extent of this contralateral projection, the anterograde axonal tracer *Phaseolus vulgaris* leucoagglutinin (PHA-L) was injected in the caudal NHDB. This indicated that the fibers travel through the stria medullaris and habenular commissure and terminate in a dense plexus of labeled axons, with numerous boutons in the contralateral

* Supported by RSDA MH00330; ADRC AG05681; NIH GM07200, Medical Scientist; and NIH NS09518.

Ferrendelli, J.A., Collins, R.C. and Johnson, E.M. (eds), Neurobiology of Amino Acids, Peptides, and Trophic Factors.

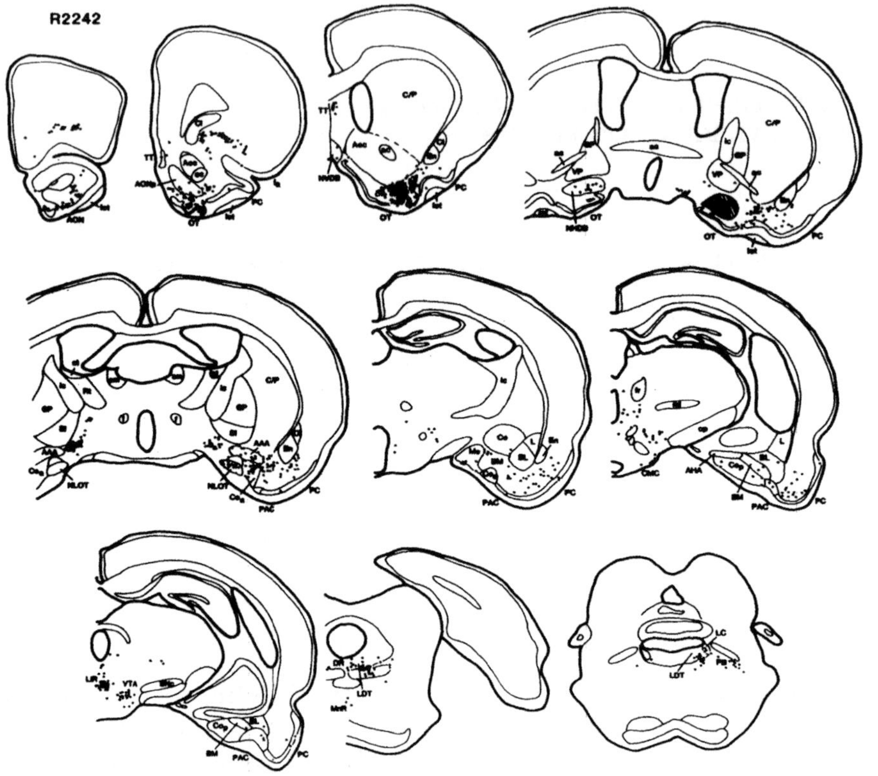

Figure 17-1. The distribution of retrogradely labeled cells following an injection of the non-specific tracer WGA-HRP into the horizontal diagonal band. Each dot represents one labeled cell.

NHDB and the area caudal and medial to it. Attempts to double label the contralaterally projecting cells in the homologous area of the basal forebrain with the retrograde fluorescent tracer True Blue and choline acetyltransferase immunohistochemistry suggested that the vast majority of commissural cells are not cholinergic.

To determine which of the afferents to the NHDB may use one of the excitatory amino acids (glutamate or aspartate) as a neurotransmitter, injections of 3H-D-aspartate were made into the NHDB and surrounding area. This retrograde tracer is apparently specific for cells that possess a high affinity uptake mechanism for glutamate and/or aspartate and are therefore presumed to be glutamergic or aspartergic [3]. In these experiments, cells were labeled in the orbital, insular, and olfactory cortices; in the nucleus of the lateral olfactory tract and other amygdaloid nuclei; and in the midline thalamic nuclei and the hypothalamus (Figure 17-2). However, many of the areas that contained cells labeled by WGA-HRP were not labeled with 3H-D-aspartate. These included

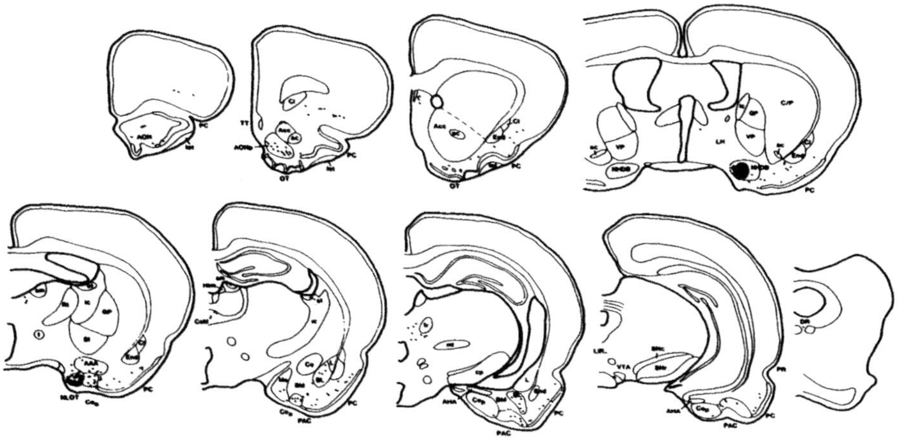

Figure 17-2. The distribution of retrogradely labeled cells following an injection of the "transmitter specific" tracer ^{3}H-D-aspartate into the horizontal diagonal band. Each dot represents one labeled cell.

the contralateral NHDB, the caudal magnocellular nuclei of the hypothalamus, the ventral tegmental area, and, with rare exception, other parts of the brainstem.

REFERENCES

1. Mesulam, M.-M., Mufson, E.J., Wainer, B.H. and Levey, A.I. (1983). Central cholinergic pathways in the rat: An overview based on an alternative nomenclature (Ch1–Ch6). Neuroscience 10, 1185–1201.
2. Fuller, T.A., Russchen, F.T. and Price, J.L. (1987). Sources of presumptive glutamergic/aspartergic afferents to the rat ventral striatopallidal region. J. Comp. Neurol. 258, 317–338.
3. Streit, P. (1980). Selective retrograde labeling indicating the transmitter of neuronal pathways. J. Comp. Neurol. 191, 429–463.

18. MALE INFERTILITY: PRELIMINARY EVIDENCE FOR TWO NEUROENDOCRINE MEDIATORS OF STRESS ON GONADAL FUNCTION

D.H. HELLHAMMER AND I. GUTBERLET

In West Germany, approximately 15% of all couples are involuntarily barren, and psychological factors seem to be relevant in about one-third of them [1]. Thus, a series of studies were conducted to investigate the role of stress in male sterility. So far, both an adrenergic activation of the nervous system and enhanced levels of corticosteroids are considered possible mechanisms involved in the transfer of stress to gonadal function.

1. POSSIBLE ADRENERGIC EFFECTS ON GONADAL FUNCTION

Relationships among personality attitudes, sex steroids, gonadotropins, and seminal parameters were investigated in 218 husbands of barren couples [2, 3]. Interestingly, we observed significant correlations between low sperm count, low serum testosterone levels, and the profile of an active, competitive personality. Depressed patients, on the other hand, showed no impaired fertility. An analysis of psychological data suggest that infertile men show similarities to patients with coronary prone behavior.

On the basis of these findings, rats were exposed to two different stress paradigms, "learned helplessness" [4] and "activity-wheel-stress" [5, 6], respectively. Behavioral, neurochemical, endocrinological, and histological analyses were performed to study stress effects on the nervous, endocrine, and gonadal systems.

Helpless rats, which behaved passively after being exposed to uncontrollable

Ferrendelli, J.A., Collins, R.C. and Johnson, E.M. (eds), Neurobiology of Amino Acids, Peptides, and Trophic Factors.

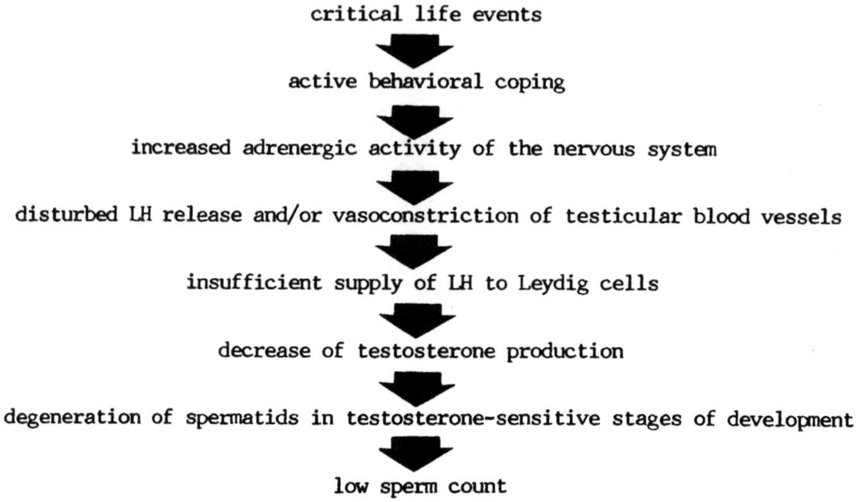

Figure 18-1. A possible adrenergic mechanism in male infertility.

shock, showed no abnormalities with respect to levels of testosterone, luteinizing hormone (LH), or testicular histology. Neurochemical data suggested an enhanced turnover of serotonin in the cortex and brain stem, while levels of catecholamines and their metabolites remained normal [4]. These findings agree with the above findings in infertile men and support the view that behavioral depression is associated with a functional increase of serotonin in the central nervous system and a trophotropic status of the organism [7].

Activity-stress, on the other hand, resulted in a decrease of blood supply to the gonads and a drop of testosterone levels in both serum and testes. In the brain, a strong increase of norepinephrine turnover was observed in the hypothalamus, thalamus, striatum, hippocampus, neocortex, midbrain, pons-medulla, and cerebellum [5, 6]. Histologically, a degeneration of spermatids in testosterone sensitive stages of spermiogenesis was demonstrated [8]. Again, the animal data agreed with the human findings, suggesting that active behavioral coping under stress is associated with impaired sperm count (Figure 18-1).

Active behavioral coping associated with high adrenergic arousal may either disturb a regular pulsatile release of LH or a vasoconstriction of testicular blood vessels, resulting in an insufficient supply of LH to Leydig cells. A study of monoamine turnover in discrete hypothalamic nuclei and LH in animals exposed to activity stress, however, did not support the view that the pituitary-gonadal axis is primarily involved in the observed disturbance of testicular function [9]. In any case, there is strong evidence that Leydig cells can not provide appropriate amounts of testosterone, and this may explain

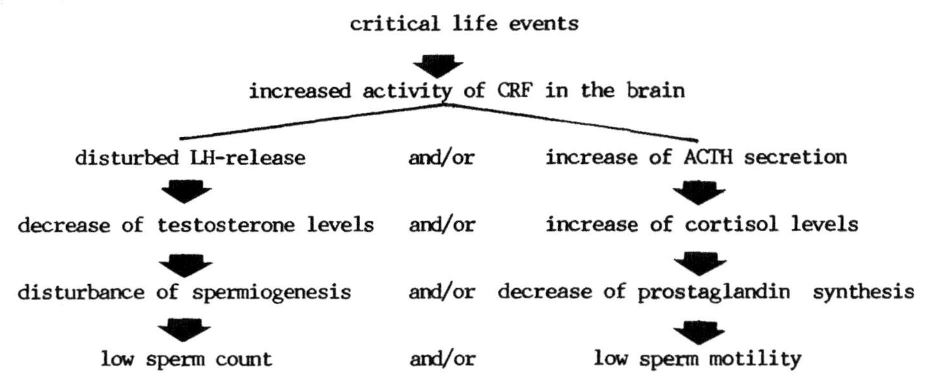

Figure 18-2. A hypothetical peptidergic mechanism in male infertility.

the observed degeneration of spermatids in testosterone sensitive stages of development.

To investigate a proposed causal relationship between active behavioral coping and low sperm count, we designed a study employing behavioral therapy to improve sperm count in 16 patients who showed both the relevant behavior and oligozoospermia without pathological findings [10]. After therapy, we observed reduced distress accompanied by a significant increase in sperm count. Additionally, six pregnancies occurred within a period of 4 months after therapy.

Taken together, there is preliminary evidence now that adrenergic arousal can impair spermiogenesis. From a phylogenetic viewpoint, this may not simply reflect a negative effect of stress, but rather a significant biological mechanism preventing reproduction under disadvantageous enviromental conditions.

2. POSSIBLE PEPTIDERGIC EFFECTS ON GONADAL FUNCTION

Recently, a negative correlation between cortisol levels and both testosterone ($r = -.56$) and sperm motility ($r = -.32$) was observed in 88 infertile men (Bents et al., unpublished data). In addition, an increase of cortisol, accompanied by a decrease of testosterone, was found in saliva of normal volunteers under experimental stress [11, 12]. Thus, it is not unlikely that an increase of cortisol may also affect gonadal function in patients with oligoasthenozoospermia (Figure 18-2).

A study from Rivier and associates [13] suggests that a stress-induced activation of corticotropin-releasing factor (CRF) disturbs the regular release of gonadotropins. Thus, a release of CRF under stress may indirectly result in both an increase of cortisol and a drop of testosterone. Since cortisol is known to inhibit prostaglandin synthesis, one may expect an indirect impairment of sperm motility [14].

REFERENCES

1. Bents, H. (1985). Int. J. Andrology 8, 325–336.
2. Hellhammer, D.H. et al. (1985). Psychosomatic Medicine 47, 58–66.
3. Hubert, W. et al. (1985). J. Psychosom. Res. 29, 161–165.
4. Hellhammer, D.H. et al. (1984). Pharmacol. Biochem. Behav. 21, 481–485.
5. Hellhammer, D.H. et al. (1984). Neuropsychobiology 11, 251–254.
6. Rea, M. and Hellhammer, D.H. (1984). Psychoth. Psychosom. 42, 218–223.
7. Hellhammer, D.H. (1983). In *The Origins of Depression*, Angst, J. ed., Springer, New York, pp. 147–161.
8. Hellhammer et al. (1982). XIV Europ. Conf. Psychosom. Res., Nordwijkerhout.
9. Hellhammer et al. (1984). XXIV Ann. Meet. Soc. Neuroscience, Anaheim.
10. Bents, H. (1985). XV Ann Meet. Europ. Assoc. Beh. Therapy, Munich.
11. Hellhammer, D.H. et al. (1985). Psychoneuroendocrinology 10, 77–81.
12. Hellhammer, D.H. et al. (1987). In Verhaltens medizin, W.D. Gerber et al. Eds; VCH, Weinheim, 7–18.
13. Rivier, C. et al. (1986). Science 231, 607–609.
14. Schlegel, W. and Meyer, J. (1986). Prostaglandines, 31, 735–744.

19. SPECIFIC (D, L)-[^{3}H]2-AMINO-4-PHOSPHONOBUTYRIC ACID BINDING TO FROZEN SYNAPTIC PLASMA MEMBRANES

W.F. HOOD, L.M. PULLAN, J.B. MONAHAN, AND J. MICHEL

In pathways where acidic amino acids, such as glutamate, are thought to be the endogenous neurotransmitter, electrophysiological studies have demonstrated that L-2-amino-4-phosphonobutyrate (L-APB) is a potent antagonist of the excitatory responses [1–3]. The binding of (D, L)-[^{3}H]APB to its putative receptor can be readily differentiated from the binding to other subclasses of glutamate receptors by its dependence upon chloride. Furthermore, binding of APB to its recognition site has been reported to be sensitive to freezing. [4].

We report here conditions whereby freezing of synaptic plasma membranes (SPM) does not eliminate the APB sensitive chloride-dependent glutamate subclass of binding sites. Using a buffer comprised of 5mM Tris/sulfate (pH 7.4), 1 mM $MgSO_4$, 0.32 M sucrose, and 0.5 mM EDTA [5] to freeze synaptic plasma membranes, a binding site kinetically and pharmacologically indistinguishable to that reported for fresh SPM has been demonstrated.

The method involved the preparation of SPM from rat forebrains, which were either resuspended in 50 mM Tris/acetate and stored at 4°C overnight (fresh SPM) or resuspended in a buffer of 0.32 M sucrose, 0.5 mM EDTA, 1 mM $MgSO_4$, and 5 mM Tris/sulfate (pH 7.4), at a protein concentration of 10–15 mg/ml, and stored under liquid nitrogen (frozen SPM), as previously described [5].

Prior to use in the ligand binding assay, fresh or frozen SPM (thawed at room temperature) were diluted with 50 mM Tris/acetate (pH 7.4), incubated at 37°C for 30 minutes and centrifuged. This washing procedure was repeated

Ferrendelli, J.A., Collins, R.C. and Johnson, E.M. (eds), Neurobiology of Amino Acids, Peptides, and Trophic Factors.

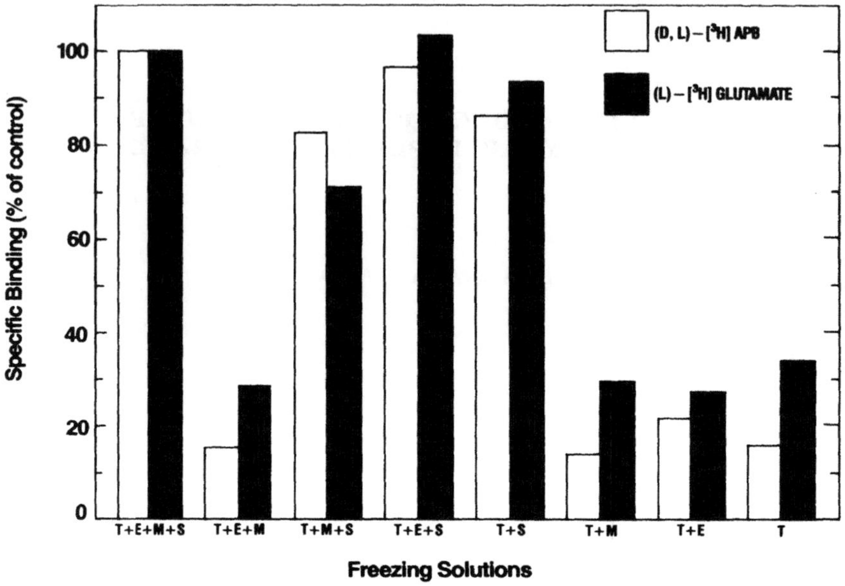

Figure 19-1. (D,L)-[^{3}H]APB and (L)-[^{3}H]glutamate binding to frozen SPM. SPM were frozen in solutions comprised of 5mM Tris/SO_4 (T), 1.0mM $MgSO_4$ (M), 0.5mM EDTA (E), or 0.32M sucrose (S) and assayed 6 days later for chloride-dependent binding. Results are expressed as a percentage of the specific binding determined in SPM frozen in the complete freezing solution.

three times. For the binding assay, incubations contained 10 nM (D, L)-[^{3}H]APB, 3.0 mM $CaCl_2$, and 0.2–0.4 mg of SPM in 50 mM Tris/acetate (pH 7.4). After an incubation period of 30 minutes at 37°C, the samples were centrifuged for 15 minutes at 12,000 xg, the supernatant aspirated, and the tube tip cut off and agitated in tissue solubilizer prior to liquid scintillation counting. Nonspecific binding was defined as the residual binding in the presence of 0.4 mM glutamate or 0.4 mM APB and usually was 25%–35% of the total binding. The binding was analyzed using Scatchard and Hill transformations, and the inhibition constants (Ki) for the compounds were determined using logit-log analysis. Calculations and regression analysis were done using templates developed for Lotus 1-2-3, as previously described [6].

In order to ascertain the conditions necessary to maintain the APB site in frozen SPM, the SPM fraction was isolated and frozen under various conditions. Synaptic plasma membranes frozen in the presence of 5 mM Tris, 0.5 mM EDTA, or 1 mM $MgSO_4$ retained minimal APB-sensitive binding, whereas SPM frozen in solutions containing 0.32 M sucrose displayed maximal APB chloride-dependent binding (Figure 19-1).

Initial experiments utilizing frozen SPM at 37°C revealed a L-[^{3}H]glutamate binding site that was dependent on $CaCl_2$. This site appeared to be of the APB subclass since 20 μM APB inhibited more than 70% of the specific binding. When competition experiments were performed with L-APB on the frozen SPM, we obtained a similar Kd (3.3 ± 0.2 μM) but a higher Bmax (92 ± 13 pmol/mg) than that observed in fresh SPM (2.2 ± 0.2 μM and 53 ± 9 pmol/mg). The time dependency of the binding of (D, L)-[^{3}H]APB to frozen SPM was similar to that of fresh SPM. The association rate constant (k_{+1}) was 3.37×10^4 M^{-1} min^{-1}. The dissociation rate constant (k_{-1}), measured in the presence of 0.4 mM APB was determined to be 14×10^{-3} min^{-1}. Using these two constants, a dissociation constant (Kd = k_{-1}/k_{+1}) of 0.41 μM can be calculated.

Compounds that are specific for other acidic amino acid subclasses (N-methyl-D-aspartate, α-amino-3-hydroxy-5-methylisoxazole-4-propionate (AMPA), and kainate caused only minimal displacement of (D, L)-[^{3}H] APB binding to frozen SPM (Ki's > 300 μM). The binding of (D, L)-[^{3}H] APB was stereoselective and displaced by L-APB (Ki = 3.3 μM) and L-glutamate (Ki = 0.99 μM), with their D-isomers being somewhat weaker, Ki = 43 μM and 13 μM, respectively. The Ki's of a series of ω-phosphono derivatives of glutamate are similar for fresh and frozen SPM (L-2-amino-5-phosphonovalerate in fresh Ki = 18 μM and frozen Ki = 15 μM; D-2-amino-5-phosphonovalerate 22 μM and 20 μM; D,L-2-amino-6-phosphonohexanoate 3.8 μM and 3.3 μM; and D, L-2-amino-7-phosphonoheptanoate 6.8 μM and 6.9 μM).

The pharmacological specificity and the kinetics of APB binding to frozen SPM correlate well with that observed in fresh SPM. Thus when SPM fractions are frozen in solutions containing 0.32 M sucrose, they retain a APB-sensitive chloride-dependent glutamate recognition site similar to that observed in fresh SPM.

REFERENCES

1. Fagg, G.E. and Lanthorn, T.L. (1985). Cl^-/Ca^{+2}-dependent L-glutamate binding sites in synaptic membranes do not correspond to 2-amino-4-phosphonobutanoate-sensitive receptors. Br. J. Pharmacol. 86, 743–751.
2. Hori, N., Auker, C.R., Braitman, D.J., and Carpenter, D.O. (1982). Pharmacologic sensitivity of amino acid responses and synaptic activation of in vitro prepyriform neurons. J. Neurophysiol. 48, 1289–1301.
3. Davies, J. and Watkins, J.C. (1982). Actions of the D- and L-forms of 2-amino-5-phosphonovalerate and 2-amino-4-phosphonobutyrate in the cat spinal cord. Brain Res. 235, 378–386.
4. Monaghan, D.T., McMills, M.C., Chamberlin, A.R., and Cotman, C.W. (1983). Synthesis of [^{3}H]2-amino-4-phosphonobutyric acid and characterization of its binding to rat brain membranes: A selective ligand for the chloride/calcium-dependent class of L-glutamate binding sites. Brain Res. 278, 137–144.
5. Michaelis, E.K., Magruder, C.D., Lampe, R.A., Galton, N., Ghang, H.H., and Michaelis, M.L. (1984). Effects of amphipathic drugs on L-[^{3}H]glutamate binding to synaptic membranes and the purified binding protein. Neurochem. Res. 9, 29–44.
6. Pullan, L.M., Monahan, J.B., Hood, W.F., and Michel, J. (1986). Automated receptor ligand binding analysis with data from an NMDA specific assay. Transactions of the Am. Soc. Neurochem. 17, 169.

20. L-[^{3}H]GLUTAMATE BINDING TO AN N-METHYL-D-ASPARTATE RECOGNITION SITE IN SYNAPTIC PLASMA MEMBRANES

J.B. MONAHAN, J. MICHEL, W.F. HOOD, L.M. PULLAN, AND R.P. COMPTON

The N-methyl-D-aspartate (NMDA) receptor is the best defined subclass of excitatory amino acid receptors with regard to both its electrophysiological properties and the functional consequences of its stimulation and inhibition. However, straightforward radioligand binding assays that specifically label the NMDA receptor are lacking. Specific binding of the NMDA selective antagonist D,L-[^{3}H]-2-amino-7-phosphonoheptanoate has been demonstrated, but the pharmacological profile of this site does not correspond to the NMDA receptor [1]. The NMDA specific antagonist D-[^{3}H]-2-amino-5-phosphonopentanoate does label a recognition site that shows the pharmacological characteristic expected of the NMDA receptor [2]. However, the high ratio of nonspecific to specific binding with this ligand makes it less than ideal for receptor binding studies. The nonselective ligand L-[^{3}H]glutamate has been used to label NMDA receptors. A study using postsynaptic densities demonstrated that 58% of the specific L-[^{3}H]glutamate binding was displaceable by NMDA [3]. Recently, a report has appeared that compared the pharmacological profile of L-[^{3}H]glutamate binding to an NMDA site in brain slices using autoradiography and in homogenates where the majority of the binding was displaceable by NMDA [4]. The present study describes conditions for an L-[^{3}H]glutamate binding assay in which 85%–95% of the specific binding is to a site that corresponds to the NMDA subclass of excitatory amino acid receptors.

Binding studies were carried out on frozen synaptic plasma membranes

Ferrendelli, J.A., Collins, R.C. and Johnson, E.M. (eds), Neurobiology of Amino Acids, Peptides, and Trophic Factors.

prepared from rat forebrain that were thawed and washed sufficiently to remove endogenous glutamate and aspartate. These membrane were then incubated with L-[^{3}H]glutamate in 50 mM Tris/acetate at pH 7.4 and centrifuged for 15 minutes at 12,000 g to separate bound from free radioligand.

The fraction (0.85–0.95) of specific L-[^{3}H]glutamate binding that was displaced by 0.5 mM NMDA was maximal at 2°C. A decreased contribution of NMDA specific binding relative to total specific binding was observed as the time and temperature increased. Less than 30% of the specific L-[^{3}H] glutamate binding was displaced by NMDA following an 80-minute incubation at 37°C. The NMDA specific, L-[^{3}H]glutamate binding reached equilibrium rapidly (maximal binding was observed after 2 minutes) and was readily reversible. The L-[^{3}H]glutamate binding increases linearly with increasing protein concentration over the concentration range of 0.15–0.95 mg/ml. The pH optimum for this binding is near the physiological pH of 7.0–7.4, with only 30% of the maximal binding observed at the pH extremes tested (pH = 5 and 10). The subcellular localization studies showed that this NMDA specific binding is localized in the synaptic plasma membranes, with the myelin and mitochondrial fractions exhibiting less than 20% of the total binding present in the synaptic membranes. From these results, optimal conditions for specific L-[^{3}H]glutamate labeling of the NMDA recognition site were obtained (incubation time 2–20 minutes, 2°C in 50 mM Tris/acetate, pH 7.4). Under these conditions, the equilibrium constants for L-[^{3}H]glutamate at this site, calculated from Scatchard and Hill analysis, are Kd = 0.62 μM, Bmax = 8.9 pmole/mg protein, and Hill coefficient = 1.03.

The pharmacological characteristics of this binding site correspond to the electrophysiologically defined NMDA receptor. Analysis of the log-dissociation curve for NMDA gave a Ki = 7.4 μM, while the other electrophysiologically defined, acidic amino acid subclass specific ligands, L-2-amino-4-phosphonobutanoate, kainate, and alpha-amino-3-hydroxy-7-methylisoxazole-4-propionate (AMPA) show a lower affinity for this site (Ki's > 300 μM). Stereoselectivity of this NMDA specific site was observed, with the D-isomers of both aspartate (Ki = 0.9 μM) and N-methylaspartate (Ki = 7.4 μM) having a higher affinity than the corresponding L-isomers (Ki = 2.6 μM and 66 μM, respectively), whereas the L-isomer of glutamate (Ki = 0.62 μM) has a higher affinity than the D-isomer (Ki = 14.5 μM). The omega-phosphono amino acids tested have affinities that correspond with their physiological potencies as NMDA specific antagonists [5]. Thus the D-isomers of the C-5 (Ki = 1.2 μM) and C-7 (Ki = 4.0 μM) analogues have the highest affinities for this binding site, while the corresponding L-isomers (Ki = 20 μM and 21 μM, respectively), along with the C-4 (Ki > 300 μM) and C-6 (Ki = 74 μM) compounds, have significantly lower affinities.

Several sulfer-containing amino acids have been shown to be excitants in the mammalian CNS, and it has been suggested that the L-isomers may be endogenous neuro-transmitters [2]. Some of the sulfur-containing acidic amino acids tested in the present study exhibited high affinity for the NMDA binding site, with the D- and L-isomers of homocysteinesulfinic acid (Ki = 1.8 μM and 3.4 μM, respectively) and the D- and L-isomers of homocysteic acid (Ki = 3.3 μM and 1.2 μM, respectively) being the most active.

An ionic effect on L-[^{3}H]glutamate binding has frequently been observed, most notably with the ions calcium, chloride, and sodium [7]. An analysis of the NMDA specific L-[^{3}H]glutamate binding indicates a differential effect of cations and anions. At a concentration of 1 mM, the anions Cl^-, Br^-, SCN^-, CH_3COO^-, NO_3^-, SO_4^{2-}, and HPO_4^{2-} have no effect on NMDA-specific binding. The monovalent cations K^+ and NH_4^+ also have no effect, while 1 mM Na^+ inhibited the binding by 27%. Several of the divalent cations tested at 1 mM also inhibited L-[^{3}H]glutamate binding, with copper, cadmium, and zinc the most effective, reducing the binding to 54%, 58%, and 76% of the control, respectively. Magnesium and calcium at a concentration of 1 mM had no effect on the binding.

In summary, this study describes an accurate, reproducible method to analyze a recognition site for L-[^{3}H]glutamate that has the pharmacological and biochemical characteristics of the NMDA receptor.

REFERENCES

1. Ferkany, J.W. and Coyle, J.T. (1983). Specific binding of [^{3}H]±2-amino-7-phosphonoheptanoic acid to rat brain membranes in vitro. Life Sci. 33, 1295–1306.
2. Olverman, H.J., Jones, A.W. and Watkins, J.C. (1984). L-glutamate has a higher affinity than other amino acids for [^{3}H]-D-AP5 binding sites in rat brain membranes. Nature 307, 460–462.
3. Fagg, G.E. and Matus, A. (1984). Selective association of N-methylaspartate and quisqualate types of glutamate receptors with brain postsynaptic densities. Proc. Natl. Acad. Sci. USA 81, 6876–6880.
4. Monaghan, D.T., Yao, D., Nguyen, L. and Cotman, C.W. (1985). Excitatory amino acid binding sites: Correspondence between autoradiographic and membrane fraction preparations. Soc. Neurosci. Abst. 11, 110.
5. Evans, R.H., Francis, A.A., Jones, A.W., Smith, D.A. and Watkins, J.C. (1982). The effects of a series of ω-phosphonic α-carboxylic amino acids on electrically evoked and excitant amino acid-induced responses in isolated spinal cord preparations. Br. J. Pharmacol. 75, 65–75.
6. Do, K.Q., Mattenberger, M., Streit, P. and Cuenod, M. (1986). In vitro release of endogenous excitatory sulfur-containing amino acids from various rat brain regions. J. Neurochem. 46, 779–786.
7. Mena, E.E., Wittemore, S.R., Monaghan, D.T. and Cotman, C.W. (1984). Ionic regulation of glutamate binding sites. Life Science 35, 2427–2433.

21. ANTAGONIST EFFECTS OF Y-GLUTAMYL-AMINOMETHYLSULFONATE IN THE IN VITRO HIPPOCAMPAL SLICE

RANDY K. RADER, AND TOM H. LANTHORN

Two types of nonselective acidic amino acid antagonists have been reported to block non-NMDA receptors more potently than NMDA receptors in the spinal cord. These are y-glutamyl-aminomethylsulfonate (GAMS) [1] and the N-(p-chlorobenzoyl) and N-(p-bromobenzoyl) derivatives of piperazine-2,3-dicarboxylate (pCB-PzDA and pBB-PzDA, respectively) [2]. Recently, the effects of the piperazine dicarboxylate derivatives have been evaluated in the hippocampal slice. In contrast to the spinal cord, these compounds were shown to more effectively block NMDA responses than responses induced by kainate or quisqualate [3].

This difference in the antagonist spectrum of the piperazine dicarboxylate derivative antagonists could be due to a number of factors, one of which is the possible existence of subtypes of NMDA receptors [4]. In order to assess whether these anomalies in antagonist activity are specific to the piperazine dicarboxylate antagonists or are more general, we have tested the antagonist activity of GAMS in the in vitro hippocampal slice.

Hippocampal slices were prepared from male, Sprague-Dawley albino rats and maintained as described previously [5]. Slices were maintained in experimental medium (124 mM NaCl, 2.5 mM KCl, 1.0 mM KH_2PO_4, 26.4 mM $NaHCO_3$, 2 mM $CaCl_2$, 1.5 mM $MgSO_4$, and 10 mM D-glucose) at 35–36°C. As needed, slices were transferred from a static bath to a small perfusion chamber. During testing of GAMS, slices were secured with an upper net and completely submerged in continuously flowing (2 ml/min) medium. The

Ferrendelli, J.A., Collins, R.C. and Johnson, E.M. (eds), Neurobiology of Amino Acids, Peptides, and Trophic Factors.

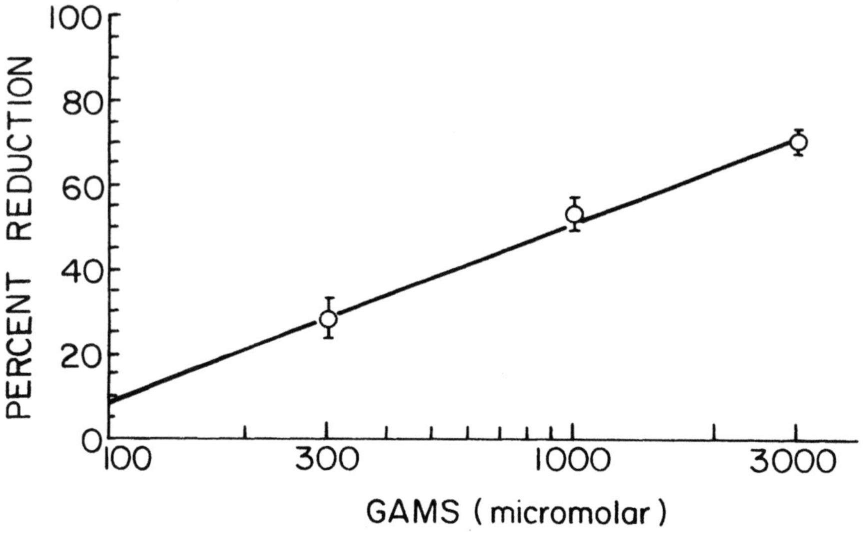

Figure 21-1. Reduction of Schaffer collateral/commissural CA1 field EPSP by bath application of GAMS.

Schaffer collateral/commissural-CA1 (S/C-CA1) synaptic response was stimulated (0.05 Hz; 0.05 msec duration single shock) from stratum radiatum at the CA2–CA3 border and recorded in stratum radiatum in the middle portion of CA1. Focal potentials were induced and recorded in stratum radiatum of CA1. GAMS was obtained from Tocris neuramin.

GAMS was able to block the S/C-CA1 synaptic response in the hippocampus. The concentration of GAMS needed to antagonize the synaptic response by 50% (IC_{50}) was between 1 and 3 mM (Figure 21-1). GAMS was also able to block focal potentials induced by NMDA, kainate, and AMPA. The IC_{50} for the blockade of all these focal potentials was between 1 and 3 mM (Figure 21-2). None of the agonist-induced responses exhibited selective vulnerability.

Although GAMS and the piperazine dicarboxylate derivatives preferentially block non-NMDA receptors in the spinal cord, this is clearly not the case in the hippocampus. Data from site-selective radioligand binding indicate that GAMS has a higher affinity for NMDA binding sites than for kainate or AMPA sites (K_i's of 90 μM, > 300 μM and > 300 μM, respectively) [Monahan, Michel, and Hood, unpublished observations]. In addition, GAMS is a more effective blocker of retinal neurotoxicity induced by NMDA than by kainate or quisqualate [Olney and Price, unpublished observations]. These data indicate that the usefulness of GAMS for functional and behavioral studies of non-NMDA receptors is limited, and its actions must be determined in each test system.

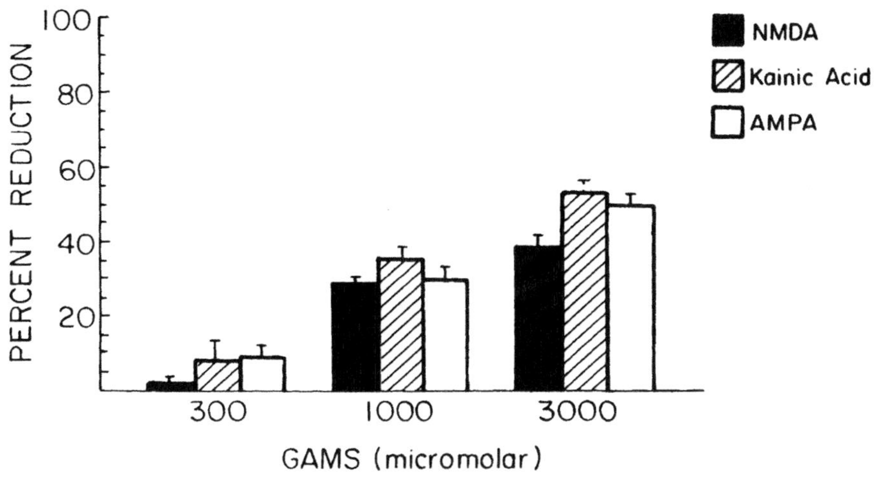

Figure 21-2. Reduction of focal potentials induced by pressure ejection of NMDA, kainate, and AMPA (all at 100 μM) in the hippocampal slice by bath application of GAMS.

From the present data, there is no way to determine whether this difference in antagonist selectivity between the hippocampus and spinal cord is due to differences in techniques or due to differences in the receptors present. However, GAMS is reported to be about equipotent to gamma-D-glutamylglycine (yDGG) in blocking kainate and quisqualate in the spinal cord, and yDGG has an IC_{50} of 0.5–2 mM against these responses in the spinal cord. This value is similar to the potency of GAMS in the hippocampal slice. GAMS is further reported to be about ten times less potent against NMDA responses in the spinal cord than non-NMDA responses. Since GAMS is about equipotent in its ability to block NMDA and non-NMDA responses in the hippocampus, this suggests that the NMDA antagonist activity of GAMS is increased in the hippocampus. It is interesting to note that the activity of NMDA agonists is also increased 10–20 times relative to non-NMDA agonists in the hippocampal slice versus what has been reported in the spinal cord [6].

REFERENCES

1. Jones, A.W., Smith, D.A. and Watkins, J.C. (1984). Structure-activity relations of dipeptide antagonists of excitatory amino acids. Neuroscience 13, 573–581.
2. Davies, J., Jones, A.W., Sheardown, M.J., Smith, D.A. and Watkins, J.C. (1984). Phosphono dipeptides and piperazine derivatives as antagonists of amino acid-induced and synaptic excitation in mammalian and amphibian spinal cord. Neuroscience Letts. 52, 79–84.
3. Ganong, A.H., Cotman, C.W., Jones, A.W. and Watkins, J.C. (1984). Analogues of piperazine-2-3-dicarboxylic acid inhibit excitatory synaptic transmission in rat hippocampal slices. Abs. Neurosci. Soc. 10, 228.
4. Perkins, M.N. and Stone, T.W. (1983). Quinolinic acid: Regional variations in neuronal sensitivity. Brain Res. 259, 172–176.

5. Ganong, A.H., Lanthorn, T.H. and Cotman, C.W. (1983). Kynurenic acid inhibits synaptic and acidic amino acid-induced responses in rat hippocampus and spinal cord. Brain Res. 273, 170–174.
6. Lanthorn, T.H. and Cotman, C.W. (1983). Relative potency of analogues of excitatory amino acids on hippocampal CA1 neurons. Neuropharmacology 22, 1343–1348.

22. "TRANSMITTER SPECIFIC" INPUTS TO THE MEDIODORSAL THALAMIC NUCLEUS IN THE RAT*

J.P. RAY, F.T. RUSSCHEN, T.A. FULLER, AND J.L. PRICE

[^{3}H]D-aspartate ([^{3}H]D-Asp) and [^{3}H]gamma-aminobutyric acid ([^{3}H]GABA) have been used as "transmitter specific" retrograde tracers to identify projections to the mediodorsal thalamic nucleus (MD) that may use glutamate and/or aspartate, or GABA as their neurotransmitter. Following injections of the "nonspecific" tracer WGA-HRP into MD, retrogradely labeled cells are found in a wide variety of forebrain and brainstem areas, including layer VI of the frontal and agranular insular cortex, the thalamic reticular nucleus, the ventral pallidum (including the polymorphic zone of the olfactory tubercle), the deepest layers of the piriform cortex, periamygdaloid cortex and entorhinal cortex, the amygdaloid complex, the superior colliculus, substantia nigra, and dorsal raphe nucleus. Following injections of [^{3}H]D-Asp or [^{3}H] GABA, different subsets of these cells are labeled.

Injections of [^{3}H]D-Asp into MD result in substantial numbers of labeled cells in layer VI of the frontal and agranular insular cortex. With injections in the medial part of MD, cells are also labeled in the piriform and entorhinal cortices and in the amygdaloid complex, while injections in the more lateral part of MD produce labeled cells in the superior colliculus. Labeled cells are also found in the nucleus triangularis of the septum, possibly due to involvement of the medial habenular nucleus in the injections [1].

In contrast, the only projection to MD that was definitely labeled by in-

* Supported by NIH grants NS09518 and AG05681. TAF is also supported by RSDA MH00330.

Ferrendelli, J.A., Collins, R.C. and Johnson, E.M. (eds), Neurobiology of Amino Acids, Peptides, and Trophic Factors.

jections of [^{3}H]GABA arises from the reticular thalamic nucleus. Injections that involve the habenular nuclei also produce some labeled cells in the nucleus triangularis of the septum, and in the endopeduncular nucleus and adjacent parts of the hypothalamus. Although a few, scattered cells are also labeled in the ventral pallidum in some cases, such cells are much more numerous following injections in which the habenular nuclei are heavily involved and are not found after injections restricted to MD. Therefore, these cells appear to be related to the endopeduncular nucleus and to project to the habenular nuclei instead of MD.

A few cells in the posterior hypothalamus are also labeled following injections of either [^{3}H]D-Asp and [^{3}H]GABA.

REFERENCE

1. Swanson, L.W. and Cowan, W.M. (1979). The connections of the septal region in the rat. J. Comp. Neur. 186, 621–656.

23. CHARACTERIZATION OF NERVE GROWTH FACTOR RECEPTOR-BEARING CELLS IN CULTURES OF BRAIN TISSUE

DIKLA ROUFA, STEVE RAPP, AND WAYNE ENGLEMAN

Recent studies have demonstrated the presence of NGF, NGF specific mRNA [1], and NGF receptors (NGFR) [2, 3] in the central nervous system (CNS). Cholinergic nerve terminals within the hippocampus and cortex have been shown to internalize iodinated NGF and retrogradely transport it to their cell bodies in the septum and magnocellular basal forebrain [4, 5]. In addition, NGF has been shown to selectively increase choline acetyltransferase (ChAT) activity of basal forebrain both in vivo [6] and in vitro [7]. However, survival or fiber outgrowth of cultured fetal septal cholinergic neurons was not affected by exogenous NGF [7]. The present study utilized cell cultures of septal, hippocampal, and cortical tissue to identify and characterize the NGFR bearing cells and to determine the effect of exogenously added NGF on NGFR positive cells.

Primary cultures of dissociated septal, hippocampal, and cortical tissue obtained from embryonic (E15–E20) or postnatal (P2–P12) rat brain were grown in either serum-containing or chemically-defined N2 medium [8] and maintained in culture for several weeks. A monoclonal antibody (192–IgG), which binds specifically to rat NGFR (a gift from Dr. Eugene Johnson), was used in combination with immunocytochemical visualization with ABC-alkaline phosphatase to localize NGFR-containing cells. To characterize the cells present in the cultures, immunocytochemical localization of neurofilaments (NF), glial fibrillary acidic protein (GFAP), and ChAT, and cytochemical visualization of acetylcholinesterase (AChE) activity was utilized.

Ferrendelli, J.A., Collins, R.C. and Johnson, E.M. (eds), Neurobiology of Amino Acids, Peptides, and Trophic Factors.

A subpopulation of neuronal cells in both embryonic and postnatal septal area cultures were found to contain NGFR positive cells. The antibody intensely labeled the cell body, as well as what appears to be the entire neuritic arbor. Only a few neuronal-like cells in cortical cultures were labeled with the anti-NGFR antibody, and labeled neurons were rarely found in hippocampal cultures. To further characterize the NGFR positive cells, the immunocytochemical staining of the cultures with 192-IgG was followed by staining with anti-ChAT antibodies and by cytochemical visualization of AChE. The majority of NGFR positive cells in septal area cultures were also labeled with ChAT or AChE. Similarly, most, but not all, of the AChE positive cells were NGFR positive. Some cells that labeled with both NGFR antibodies and AChE were found in cortical cultures.

Septal area neurons obtained from embryonic (E17) or postnatal (P2) rats and grown on polylysine coated 96-well plates in serum-containing medium in the presence of 100 ng/ml 2.5S NGF for 32 days had significantly larger mean number of NGFR positive neurons per well as compared to cultures grown in the absence of NGF. The number of NGFR positive neurons per well for embryonic cultures was 212 ± 15 (mean ± SD, n = 7) with NGF and 145 ± 10 in the absence of NGF. Likewise, the number of ChAT positive cells was significantly greater when the septal area neurons were grown in the presence of NGF. In addition to the increase in the number of ChAT positive cells, the mean staining intensity (quantified with a computer-assisted image analysis system) of the ChAT positive neurons was significantly greater for cells grown in the presence of 100 ng/ml NGF, suggesting that NGF induces the synthesis of ChAT and may in addition increase its activity. One of the NGF effects on responsive cells within the peripheral nervous system is cellular hypertrophy [9]. A similar response was found with NGF responsive CNS neurons. The mean detected area of NGFR positive neuronal cell soma (measured using a computer-assisted image analysis system) was significantly larger in cultures of both embryonic (37%) and postnatal (48%) septal area neurons grown in the presence of NGF than in its absence.

In addition to neuronal cells, antibody (192-IgG) identified a subpopulation of non-neuronal cells. These cells ranged in morphology from very large "flat" cells to both large and small neuronal-like cells. The stained non-neuronal cells constituted only a small percent of the non-neuronal cells present and were found at higher frequency in septal area cultures as compared to cortical or hippocampal cultures. Exogenous NGF appeared to also have an effect on the non-neuronal cells. A larger number of a subpopulation of darkly staining GFAP positive cells were found in septal area cultures grown in the presence of NGF.

In summary, the presence of NGFR has been demonstrated on the surface of a subpopulation of cultured central neuronal and non-neuronal cells. The majority of the NGFR positive neurons were also ChAT or AChE positive. Both the neuronal and non-neuronal NGFR positive cells in septal area cultures are NGF responsive.

REFERENCES

1. Korsching, S., Auburger, G., Heumann, R., Scott, J. and Thoenen, H. (1985). Levels of nerve growth factor and its mRNA in the central nervous system of the rat correlate with cholinergic innervation. EMBO J. 4, 1389–1393.
2. Richardson, P.M., Verge Issa, V.M. and Riopelle, R.J. (1986). Distribution of neuronal receptors for nerve growth factor in the rat. J. Neurosci. 6, 2312–2321.
3. Taniuchi, M., Schweitzer, J.B. and Johnson E.M., Jr. (1986). Nerve growth factor receptor molecules in rat brain. Proc. Natl. Acad. Sci. USA 83, 1950–1954.
4. Schwab M.E., Otten, U., Agid, Y. and Thoenen, H. (1979). Nerve growth factor (NGF) in the rat CNS: Absence of specific retrograde axonal transport and tyrosine hydroxylase induction in locus coeruleus and substantia nigra. Brain Res. 168, 473–483.
5. Seiler M. and Schwab, M.E. (1984). Specific retrograde transport of nerve growth factor (NGF) from neocortex to nucleus basalis in the rat. Brain Res. 300, 33–39.
6. Mobley, W.C., Ruthowski, J.L., Tennekoan, G.I., Buchanan, K. and Johnston, M.V. (1985). Choline acetyltransferase activity in striatum of neonatal rats increased by nerve growth factor. Science 229, 284–287.
7. Hefti, F., Hartikka, J., Eckenstein, F., Gnahn, H., Heumann, R. and Schwab, M. (1985). Nerve growth factor increases choline acetyltransferase but not survival or fiber outgrowth of cultured fetal septal cholinergic neurons. Neuroscience 14, 55–68.
8. Bottenstein, J.E. and Sato, G.E. (1979). Growth of a rat neuroblastoma cell line in serum-free supplemented medium. Proc. Natl. Acad. Sci. USA 76, 514–517.
9. Angeletti, P.U., Levi-Montalcini, R. and Caramia, F. (1971). Ultranstructural changes in sympathetic neurons of newborn and adult mice treated with nerve growth factor. J. Ultrastruct. Res. 36, 24–36.

24. ROLE OF HYPOTHALAMIC GABA IN AVERSIVELY MOTIVATED BEHAVIORS*

A. SHEKHAR, J.N. HINGTGEN, AND J.A. DIMICCO

Recent studies have shown that blockade of GABA in the posterior hypothalamic nucleus of rats elicits increases in heart rate, respiratory rate, and, to a lesser extent, arterial pressure [1, 2]. These autonomic changes are similar to those seen in emotional defense reactions in conscious rats [3]. The present study was aimed at testing the hypothesis that GABA blockade in this cardiostimulatory area of the posterior hypothalamus in conscious animals would elicit aversively motivated behaviors.

Experiments were conducted on male Sprague-Dawley or Wistar rats. Two stainless steel microinjection cannulae were stereotaxically implanted in the posterior hypothalamic nucleus, where microinjection of the GABA antagonist, bicuculline methiodide (BMI) 25 ng, caused an increase in heart rate under anesthesia (pentobarbital 50 mg/kg i.p.). At least 2 days later, each of these animals was placed in a rectangular container (18″ × 10″ × 8″) that was divided by a line on the floor into two equal parts. After an initial period of acclimatization, a saline control and one of the drugs randomly selected were bilaterally injected, and the behavior of the animal was observed for the following 30 minutes. The drugs used were two postsynaptic GABA antagonists, BMI (1, 5, and 25 ng) and picrotoxin (PIC, 4, 20, and 100 ng); a GABA synthesis inhibitor, isoniazid (INH 35 and 70 μg); and a non-GABAergic CNS stimulant, strychnine sulphate (38 ng, a dose equimolar to BMI 25 ng). Similar experiments were conducted with BMI alone with the microinjection cannulae im-

* Supported by grants USPHS NS 19883 and PHS MH 17107, NIMH.

Ferrendelli, J.A., Collins, R.C. and Johnson, E.M. (eds), Neurobiology of Amino Acids, Peptides, and Trophic Factors.

Table 24-1. Number of crossings and rearings (mean ± SEM) by rats during the 30-minute period following administration of saline, BMI, PIC, or INH.

	Saline (n = 8)	BMI 25 ng (n = 4)	PIC 100 ng (n = 4)	INH 70 ug (n = 4)
Crossings/30 min	5 ± 1	135 ± 19*	150 ± 30*	145 ± 11*
Rearings/30 min	1 ± 1	122 ± 17*	234 ± 35*#	231 ± 19*#

* Significantly different from saline $p < 0.001$
# Significantly different from BMI $p < 0.025$

planted in the lateral hypothalamic area. All microinjection sites were later verified by histology.

Microinjection of either of the GABA antagonists BMI or PIC as well as INH, but not of saline, into the posterior hypothalamus caused dose-related locomotor arousal, which included jumping from the observation chamber at the highest doses (Table 24-1). This effect was quantified as the number of crossings (i.e., of a line bisecting the floor) and rearings. The effects of BMI and PIC appeared immediately after injection, attaining peak effects between 6 to 12 minutes, while the effects of INH appeared much more slowly, attaining peak effects 24 ± 1 minutes after injection. The time course of the behavioral effects of BMI in conscious rats was correlated significantly with the heart rate responses in the same rats under anesthesia (heart rate and crossings, $r = 0.9128$, $p < 0.001$; heart rate and rearings, $r = 0.9473$, $p < 0.001$).

Microinjection of either strychnine (38 ng) into the posterior hypothalamus or BMI (25 ng) into the lateral hypothalamic area failed to increase locomotor behavior.

Although the well coordinated "escape" oriented locomotor stimulation suggested that this behavior was aversively motivated, it is not possible to determine, by observing gross locomotor behavior alone, whether it is actually motivated by a specific drive (in this case, aversive) or represents nonspecific arousal. In order to clarify the motivation behind the locomotor stimulation, rats were trained in two schedules, where the same motor response (lever pressing) was motivated by an aversive drive in the first schedule and by an appetitive drive in the second schedule. Rats were trained in a Sidman avoidance schedule (measuring aversive drive) in which they pressed a lever in order to avoid a foot shock presented at a constant interval (RS 20:SS10) and an approach schedule (measuring appetitive drive) in which they obtained sweetened milk by pressing a lever [4, 5]. The performance of these rats in both behavioral schedules was assessed after microinjection of drugs that either block (BMI 25 ng) or stimulate (muscimol 25 ng) GABA receptors into the cardiostimulatory area of the posterior hypothalamic nucleus.

Microinjection of BMI significantly increased avoidance responding without affecting the approach responding, while muscimol decreased responding in both schedules (Table 24-2). Again, the time course of the effects of BMI

Table 24-2. Total approach and avoidance responses (mean ± SEM) of rats during the 20-minute period following microinjection of saline, BMI, or muscimol.

	No injection (n = 4)	Saline (n = 4)	BMI 25 ng (n = 4)	Muscimol 25 ng (n = 4)
Avoidance	131 ± 6	153 ± 16	301 ± 27*	77 ± 15#
Approach	364 ± 54	428 ± 92	425 ± 103	48 ± 28#

* Significantly different from saline $p < 0.001$
# Significantly different from saline $p < 0.025$

on responding in the avoidance schedule and on heart rate were significantly correlated ($r = 0.9273$, $p < 0.05$).

Microinjection of strychnine (38 ng) into the posterior hypothalamus did not significantly affect the avoidance behavior. Microinjection of BMI into the lateral hypothalamic area had no effect on either approach or avoidance responding, while microinjection of muscimol into the lateral hypothalamus reduced approach responses without significantly affecting avoidance behavior. Even though BMI appeared to selectively enhance avoidance responding, it is possible that the higher baseline responding in the approach schedule as compared to avoidance responses (Table 24-2) may have precluded our ability to detect a stimulatory effect in this schedule. However, treatment with amphetamine sulphate (0.1 mg/kg), a nonspecific behavioral stimulant, significantly increased responding in both schedules in spite of the higher baseline in the approach schedule.

These results suggest that blockade of GABA in the posterior hypothalamic nucleus that elicits cardiorespiratory changes typical of an emotional defense reaction also elicits behavioral arousal that is characterized by an aversive motivational state.

REFERENCES

1. DiMicco, J.A., Abshire, V.M., Hankins, K.D., Sample, R.H. and Wible, J.H. Jr. (1986). Neuropharmacol. 25, 1063–1066.
2. DiMicco, J.A. and Abshire, V.M., (1987). Brain Res. 402, 1–10.
3. Hilton, S.M., (1982). J. Exp. Biol. 100, 159–174.
4. Hingtgen, J.N. and Aprison, M.H., (1970). Neuropharmacol. 9, 419–425.
5. Hingtgen, J.N., Hendrie, H.C., and Aprison, M.H. (1984). Pharmacol. Biochem. Behav. 20, 425–428.

25. CHOLECYSTOKININ RELEASE FROM RAT CAUDATOPUTAMEN SLICES INCUBATED IN VITRO IS INHIBITED BY EXCITATORY AMINO ACIDS*

JUDITH M. STONE, LLOYD R. ALLARD,
SONG PING HAN, AND MARGERY C. BEINFELD

Cholecystokinin (CCK) was originally isolated from the intestine and was later discovered to be widely distributed in gut endocrine tissue and the central and peripheral nervous systems. Numerous studies have concluded that CCK displays many properties of a neurotransmitter or neuromodulator [1]. CCK is very abundant in the caudato-putamen (cp) of the rat, where it appears to be mainly extrinsic. In the rat, some dopamine neurons in the substantia nigra also contain CCK [2]. These neurons are known to be, at best, a minor source of CCK for the cp [3, 4]. The precise CCK cell groups projecting to the cp have not been conclusively identified, but it appears that the claustrum-piriform cortex area or the amygdala are likely sites for these CCK perikarya [3, 4].

Previous studies on CCK release from cp have focused on the role of dopamine agonists [5–7], vasoactive intestinal polypeptide, VIP [8], and GABA [9]. Dopamine D-2 agonists and GABA increased the release of CCK, while dopamine D-1 agonists and VIP inhibited release of CCK. Recent studies in our laboratory [10] have focused on other factors regulating CCK release. Based on several lines of evidence, it was apparent that the release of CCK from cp is under strong inhibitory control by a substance or substances released from cp or cerebral cortex by potassium in a Ca^{2+}-dependent manner. Further studies on the chemical nature of the unknown inhibitory substance,

* This work was supported in part by NIH grants NS 18667 and RS 05388 to St. Louis University.

Ferrendelli, J.A., Collins, R.C. and Johnson, E.M. (eds), Neurobiology of Amino Acids, Peptides, and Trophic Factors.

Table 25-1. Effect of excitatory amino acids on CCK release from rat caudatoputamen.

	Inhibition of CCK release (control = 0%)		
	Glutamate	NAAG	Aspartate
10^{-5}	22%**	16%**	0%
10^{-4}	41%*	47%*	30%*

* $p < .001$; ** $p < .02$

which we call *X*, have indicated that it is likely to be a small, polar substance that is not degraded by trypsin, possibly an amino acid or small peptide.

The cp is known to contain high levels of both excitatory and inhibitory amino acids [11] as well as the excitatory dipeptide N-acetyl-aspartyl-glutamate [NAAG, Ref. 12]. The possibility that *X* is an amino acid was examined. Slices from rat cp of 200 microns were incubated in a Krebs Ringer phosphate buffer. Release was elicited by 40 mM potassium. In all experiments, CCK release from drug-treated and control slices from the same rat were compared. The methodology of the release experiments has been published [10]. CCK release was quantitated by a CCK RIA [13]. The inhibitory amino acids glycine (10^{-4} and 10^{-5} M) and GABA (10^{-4} and 10^{-5} M) and the GABA agonist muscimol (10^{-6} M) did not alter CCK release; neither did the GABA antagonist picrotoxin (10^{-4} M).

The ability of the excitatory amino acids glutamate, aspartate, and the excitatory dipeptide, NAAG, to alter CCK release was tested. The results are summarized in Table 25-1. Percentage inhibition was calculated as: (control-drug) control × 100. All these agents produced a significant inhibition at 10^{-4} M, and only glutamate and NAAG produced an inhibition at 10^{-5} M.

The observation that NAAG is equipotent with glutamate may perhaps be explained by its rapid conversion to glutamate during the incubation [14], although this was not examined in this study. Glutamate, but none of the other excitatory amino acids studied, produced a significant elevation (doubling) of the basal CCK release at 10^{-4} M.

Further studies will be required to establish a connection between these compounds and *X* and to define the receptor type and possible mediator of this inhibition. These results suggest a possible mechanism whereby one corticostriatal excitatory neurotransmitter (glutamate or aspartate) [15, 16] can regulate the activity of another excitatory neurotransmitter (CCK) by modulating its release.

REFERENCES

1. Beinfeld, M.C. (1983). Cholecystokinin in the central nervous system: A minireview. Neuropeptides 3, 411–427.
2. Hokfelt, T., Rehfeld, J.F., Skirboll, L., Ivemark, B., Goldstein, M. and Markey, K. (1980). Evidence for coexistence of dopamine and CCK in meso-limbic neurons. Nature 285, 476–478.

3. Meyer, D.K., Beinfeld, M.C., Oertel, W.H. and Brownstein, M.J. (1982). Origin of the cholecystokinin-containing fibers in the rat caudato-putamen. Science 215, 187–188.
4. Zaborsky, L., Alheid, G.F., Beinfeld, M.C., Eiden, L.E., Heimer, L.R., Palkovits, M. (1985). Cholecystokinin innervation of the ventral striatum: A morphological and radioimmunological study. Neurosci. 14, 110–116.
5. Meyer, D.K. and Krauss, J. (1983). Dopamine modulates cholecystokinin release in neostriatum. Nature 301, 338–340.
6. Meyer, D.K., Holland, A. and Conzelmann, U. (1984). Dopamine D_1-receptor stimulation reduces neostriatal cholecystokinin release. Eur. J. Pharmacol. 104, 387–388.
7. Conzelmann, U., Holland, A., and Meyer, D.K. (1984). Effects of selective dopamine D_2-receptor agonists on the release of cholecystokinin-like immunoreactivity from rat neostriatum. Eur. J. Pharmacol. 101, 119–125.
8. Allard, L.R. and Beinfeld, M.C. (1986). Vasoactive intestinal polypeptide (VIP) inhibits potassium-induced release of cholecystokinin (CCK) from rat caudato-putamen (cp) but not from cerebral cortex. Neuropeptides 8, 287–293.
9. Conzelmann, U., Meyer, D.K. and Sperk, G. (1986). Stimulation of receptors of gamma-aminobutyric acid modulates the release of cholecystokinin-like immunoreactivity from slices in rat neostriatum. Br. J. Pharmac. 89, 845–852.
10. Gysling, K. and Beinfeld, M.C. (1987). The regulation of cholecystokinin release from rat caudato-putamen in vitro. Brain Res. 407, 110–116.
11. Graybiel, A.M. and Ragsdale, C.W. Jr. (1983). Biochemical anatomy of the striatum. In *Chemical Neuroanatomy*, Emson, P.C., ed., Raven Press, New York, pp. 427–504.
12. Koller, K.J., Zacek, R. and Coyle, J.T. (1984). N-acetyl-aspartyl-glutamate: Regional levels in rat brain and the effects of brain lesions as determined by a new HPLC method. J. Neurochem. 43, 1136–1142.
13. Beinfeld, M.C., Meyer, D.K., Eskay, R.L., Jensen, R.T. and Brownstein, M.J. (1981). The distribution of cholecystokinin in the central nervous system of the rat as determined by radioimmunoassay. Brain Res. 212, 51–57.
14. Baud, J. and Fagg, G.E. (1986). Glutamate-containing dipeptides do not modulate ligand binding at excitatory amino acid receptors. Neuroscience Letts. 70, 228–233.
15. Spencer, J.J. (1976). Antagonism of cortical excitation of striatal neurons by glutamic acid diethyl-ester: Evidence for glutamic acid as an excitatory transmitter in the rat striatum. Brain Res. 102, 91–101.
16. Druce, D., Peterson, D., DeBelleroche, J. and Bradford, H.F. (1982). Differential amino acid neurotransmitter release in rat neostriatum following lesioning of the cortico-striatal pathway. Brain Res. 247, 303–307.

26. LUMINESCENT IMMUNOASSAY FOR SALIVARY CORTISOL MEASUREMENT IN PSYCHOENDOCRINE STUDIES

C.J. STRASBURGER, C. KIRSCHBAUM, C. BECKER-CARUS,
W.G. WOOD, AND D.H. HELLHAMMER

Salivary cortisol levels reflect the biologically active, "free" portion of total plasma cortisol [1]. The determination of salivary cortisol levels is of growing interest in psychology due to the noninvasive, stress-free, and simple sampling method. The chemiluminescence immunoassay described here overcomes the disadvantages of radioimmunoassay such as restricted places of application, limited stability of the assay kits due to isotope half-life, and the problem of radioactive waste deposal. The method only requires 10 μl of salivary sample per tube and thus allows frequent sampling where this is needed.

1. MATERIALS AND METHODS

The assay follows the Solid Phase Antigen Luminescence Technique (SPALT) principle [2], using a suspension of paramagnetic particles as solid support for the solid phase antigen. This competes with the sample-antigen for the antigen-specific antibody (rabbit anti-cortisol-3CMO-BSA). After a wash step, the amount of antigen-specific antibodies bound by the solid phase antigen is inversely proportional to the amount of sample antigen. In a second incubation, an excess of luminescent labeled species-specific antibody [donkey anti-rabbit-IgG labeled with an active ester of N-(4-aminobutyl-N-ethyl) isoluminol hemisuccinamide (DARS-ABEI-H)] is added [3]. After a further wash step, the chemiluminescence reaction is initiated by addition of a catalyst such as hemin or catalase and injection of alkaline hydrogen peroxide [4] in the light protected measuring chamber of the luminometer (Berthold 9500).

Ferrendelli, J.A., Collins, R.C. and Johnson, E.M. (eds), Neurobiology of Amino Acids, Peptides, and Trophic Factors.

Table 26-1.

Salivary cortisol SPALT assay flow sheet
10 µl standard or sample
+100 µl rabbit anti cortisol serum 1:20,000 in assay buffer
+100 µl cortisol coated MAIA particles 1:200 in assay buffer—incubate 25 ± 5 minutes, wash with 0.8 ml wash solution, put on magnetic rack for 3 minutes, repeat with 1 ml wash solution
+200 µl labeled donkey anti-rabbit IgG 1:1000 in assay buffer—incubate >40 minutes and wash as above, add acidic catalyst solution, and measure in luminometer by injection of alkaline H_2O_2

To autoreactive paramagnetic particles consisting of iron oxide coated with polyacrolein (Serono), an ovalbumin-cortisol conjugate is coupled and remaining aldehyde functions of the solid phase are subsequently saturated with 1% BSA and 50 mmol/L ethanolamin in 0.1 mol/L carbonate buffer pH 9.0. The second antiserum (RD17) was purchased from Wellcome, ABEI-H is from LKB-Wallac.

The wash steps and bound-free separation are carried out by putting the assay tubes on a magnetic separator (Ciba-Corning) for 3 minutes and decanting the supernatant. Thus, throughout the assay no centrifugation step is required. A flow sheet of the assay procedure is given in Table 26-1.

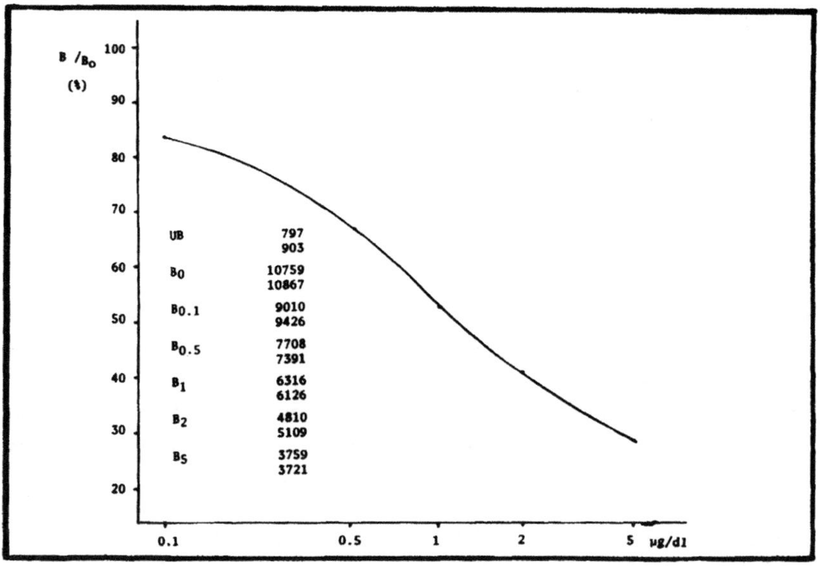

Figure 26-1. A representative standard curve and the related data of the salivary cortisol SPALT assay.

Table 26-2.

Mean Cortisol concentrations (nmol/l)

Time	n	concentration	sd	t-value
Baseline	41	17.39		
5 min after task	41	20.38	6.5	2.94**
25 min after task	41	16.77	9.8	0.29$^{n.s.}$
45 min after task	41	13.99	8.8	2.33*

* $p = 0.025$; ** $p = 0.005$; $^{n.s.}$ not significant

Mean heart rate (beats/min)

Time	n	heart rate	sd	t-value
5 min before task	43	79.63		
1. trial	43	95.91	14.1	8.88***
2. trial	43	92.05	14.8	6.87***
3. trial	43	92.67	16.1	5.86***
4. trial	43	91.42	14.2	5.89***

*** $p = 0.001$

Pearsons correlation table

	Diff. Cortisol	Diff. HR	State-anxiety^{+}	Trait-anxiety^{+}
Diff. Cortisol (sample 2–sample 1)	—	−0.04	−0.07	−0.34*
Diff. Heart rate (HR) (mean trial 1–4 before task)	−0.04	—	−0.11	−0.12

* $p = 0.02$; $^{+}$ following STAI quetionnaire

2. RESULTS AND DISCUSSION

Under optimized assay conditions, the total assay time was 2 hours. Sensitivity defined as mean minus 2s of a tenfold determination of the zero-standard was < 1 nmol/L using 10 μl of sample, which corresponds to < 4 pg/tube. A good correlation was found with the RIA previously used for salivary cortisol determination (Mallinckrodt SPAC RIA using 100 μl salivary samples): $r = 0.96$; for $y(LIA) = a + bx(RIA)$: $a = 0.08$ ug/dl, $b = 1.13$, $n = 68$. In a study, students were submitted to psychomotor stress, having to answer a high frequency series of optical and acoustical signals by pushing related bottoms. A significant increase of the heart rate ($p < 0.001$) during, and salivary cortisol ($p < 0.005$) immediately after, the task were observed. After peaking the average cortisol level declined continuously and fell below baseline level ($p < 0.03$). As the experiments were carried out during the afternoon, this reflects the overall decay of cortisol concentration analogous to the circadian rhythm of the hormone. In Table 26-2 the physiological and the STAI-questionnaire related data found in this experiment are presented. Figure 26-2 schematically illustrates the test procedure and the related salivary cortisol levels.

In a control group just playing with the bottoms without receiving signals, but also being connected to a Dynograph recorder, no increase in heart rate, but a similar cortisol pattern could be observed. As a possible explanation for this phenomenon, the anticipation of a potentially stressful event may have provoked a cortisol elevation [5].

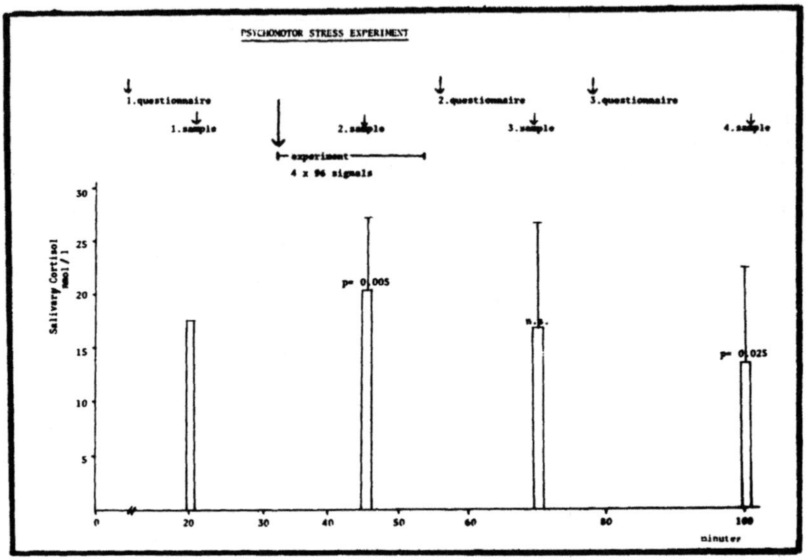

Figure 26-2. Scheme of the psychomotor test and related salivary cortisol levels.

There was no direct correlation of heart rate and cortisol patterns, which might refer to the fact that cortisol was measured before and after the task, while the heart rate was recorded during the task.

We conclude that the chemiluminescence immunoassay for salivary cortisol measurement is a useful tool for stress-related behavioral studies in humans, while fundamental work still has to be done on the standardization of stressors and on the correlation of individual stress-response with salivary cortisol level alterations.

REFERENCES

1. Riad-Fahmy, D., Read, G.F., Walker, R.F. and Griffiths, K. (1982). Endocrine Reviews 3, 367.
2. Wood, W.G., Fricke, H., Haritz, J., Gadow, A., Krausz, H.S., Tode, B., Strasburger, C.J. and Scriba, P.C. (1984). J. Clin. Chem. Clin Bochem. 22, 349.
3. Wood, W.G. and Gadow, A. (1983). J. Clin. Chem. Clin. Biochem. 21, 789.
4. Wood, W.G., Hantke, U. and Gross, A.J. (1985). J. Clin. Chem. Clin. Biochem. 23, 47.
5. Mason, J.W. (1973). Psychosom. Med. 35 (5), 406.

27. A QUANTITIVE STUDY OF THE DEVELOPMENTAL EXPRESSION OF NERVE GROWTH FACTOR RECEPTORS IN RATS

QIAO YAN AND EUGENE M. JOHNSON

A quantitative immunoprecipitation assay was conducted to study the developmental expression of nerve growth factor (NGF) receptor by using a monoclonal antibody (192-IgG) against rat NGF receptor. Either homogenates or plasma membrane enriched preparations from isolated tissues or whole rat embryos were bound with ^{125}I-NGF and crosslinked by 1-ethyl-3-(3-dimethylaminopropyl)carbodiimide. The receptor was then solubilized by 2% octylglucoside, bound with 192-IgG, and precipitated by secondary antibodies against mouse IgG prebound to Pansorbin. The complex, ^{125}I-NGF/receptor/antibodies/Pansorbin, was separated from free ligand by rapid centrifugation through a 0.15 M sucrose cushion. The tube was frozen, and the tip containing the radioactivity was cut and counted. In some cases, the pellet was resuspended in SDS-PAGE sample buffer and subjected to a SDS-PAGE autoradiographic analysis.

The NGF receptor was found in whole embryo homogenates as early as embryonic day 10 (E10) (earliest age examined). The NGF receptor content in whole embryos increased about six-fold from E10 to E18 (35 fmole/mg protein). SDS-PAGE autoradiography showed that the molecular weights of ^{125}I-NGF-bound receptor from different ages were the same as that of adult (a major band at 92 kD and a minor band at 220 kD). The NGF receptor content in sciatic nerve homogenates decreased 23-fold from newborn rats (276 fmole/mg protein) to adult rats. The change of NGF receptor level in hindleg muscle had a similar profile as that seen in sciatic nerve. The NGF receptor contents in

Ferrendelli, J.A., Collins, R.C. and Johnson, E.M. (eds), Neurobiology of Amino Acids, Peptides, and Trophic Factors.

superior cervical ganglion (SCG) or dorsal root ganglion (DRG) homogenates were expressed in two ways: 1) On a per mg protein basis, in DRG, the receptor density was relatively constant from E15 through postnatal day zero (PND-0) (average of 100 fmole/mg protein) and then dropped 6.7-fold in adults; in SCG, it decreased slightly from E20 (80 fmole/mg protein) to adulthood. 2) On a per ganglion basis, in DRG, it increased nine-fold from E15 to PND-0 (1.7 fmole/mg protein) and then stayed constant through adulthood; in SCG, it increased 4.4-fold from E20 to adult (7.9 fmole/SCG). The NGF receptor was also found in the central nervous system. In brain membrane preparations, the NGF receptor level decreased 11-fold from E15 (68.9 fmole/mg protein) to adulthood. In spinal cord membrane preparations, it dropped seven-fold from E18 (174.5 fmole/mg protein) to adulthood.

The present study shows that: 1) The NGF receptor appeared very early in development, and the apparent molecular weights of the receptor did not change. 2) Prenatally, the temporal changes of NGF receptor content varied with different tissues; it increased slightly in whole embryo, stayed relative constant in DRG, SCG, and spinal cord, and decreased in brain and muscle. 3) The NGF receptor density dramatically decreased postnatally in all the tissues examined except SCG. These data suggest that alterations in the NGF receptor density may play a role in changes in tissue responsiveness to NGF during development.

INDEX

GPSR Compliance

The European Union's (EU) General Product Safety Regulation (GPSR) is a set of rules that requires consumer products to be safe and our obligations to ensure this.

If you have any concerns about our products, you can contact us on ProductSafety@springernature.com

In case Publisher is established outside the EU, the EU authorized representative is:

Springer Nature Customer Service Center GmbH
Europaplatz 3
69115 Heidelberg, Germany

Batch number: 10755284

Printed by Printforce, the Netherlands